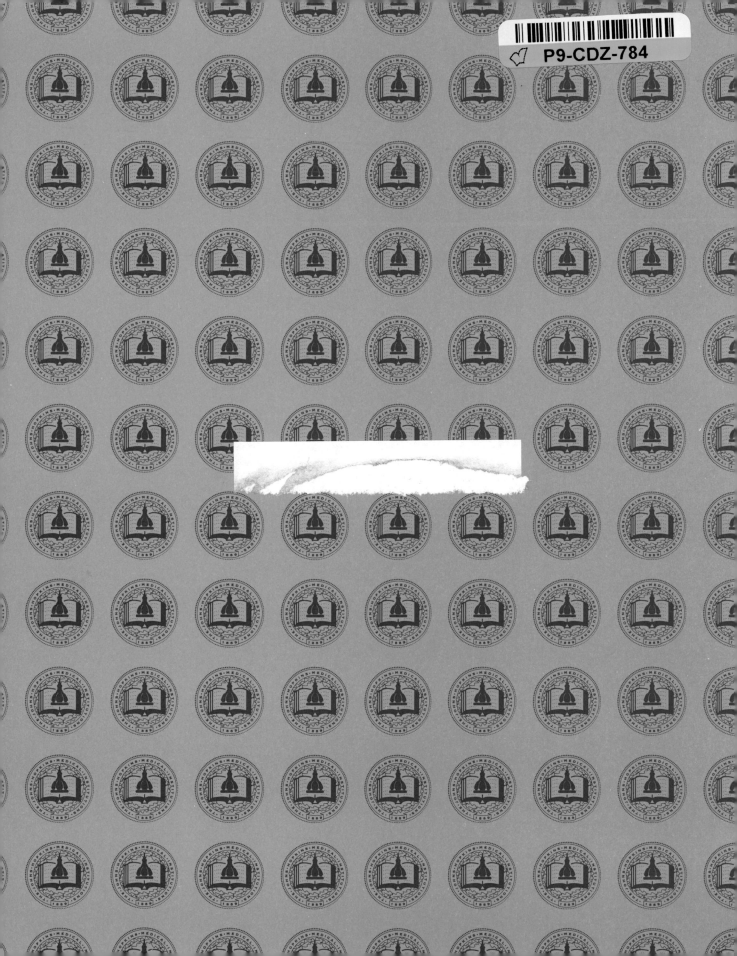

P9-CDZ-784

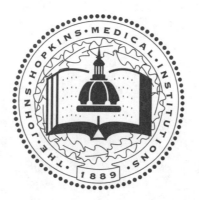

THE JOHNS HOPKINS
CONSUMER GUIDE TO MEDICAL TESTS

RC
71.3
.J64
2001

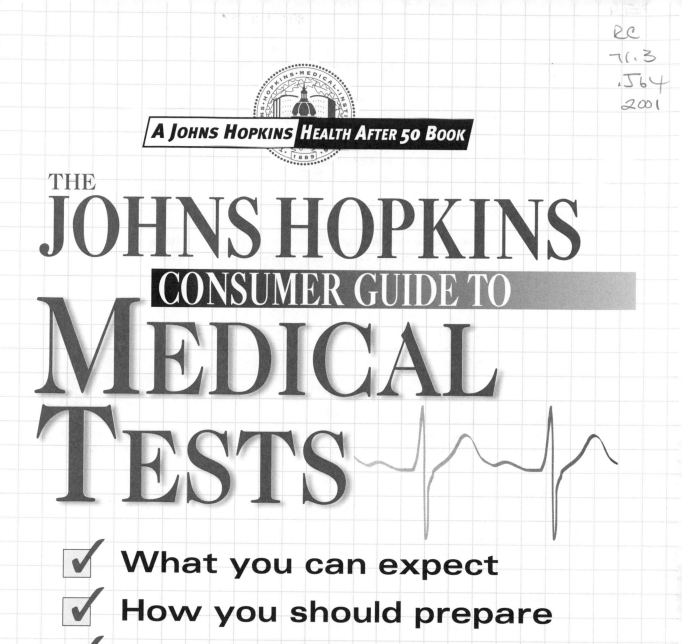

A JOHNS HOPKINS HEALTH AFTER 50 BOOK

THE JOHNS HOPKINS
CONSUMER GUIDE TO
MEDICAL TESTS

✓ What you can expect

✓ How you should prepare

✓ What your results mean

Simeon Margolis, M.D., Ph.D., *Medical Editor*

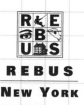

REBUS

NEW YORK

WITHDRAWN LEHIGH VALLEY COMMUNITY COLLEGE LIBRARY

NOV 1 3 2001

THE JOHNS HOPKINS MEDICAL LETTER
HEALTH AFTER 50

THE JOHNS HOPKINS CONSUMER GUIDE TO MEDICAL TESTS *is published in association with* THE JOHNS HOPKINS MEDICAL LETTER HEALTH AFTER 50. *This monthly eight-page newsletter provides practical, timely information for anyone concerned with taking control of his or her own health care. The newsletter is written in clear, nontechnical, easy-to-understand language and comes from the century-old tradition of Johns Hopkins excellence. For information on how to subscribe to this newsletter, please write to Medletter Associates, Inc., Department 1106, 632 Broadway, New York, New York 10012.*

Get subscription information online—along with the latest perspectives from our experts—at our Web site:

www.hopkinsafter50.com

This book is not intended as a substitute for the advice of a physician. Readers who suspect they may have specific medical problems should consult a physician about any suggestions made in this book.

Copyright © 2001 Medletter Associates, Inc.

All rights reserved.
No part of this book may be reproduced or transmitted in any form or by any means, electronic, mechanical, photocopying, recording, or otherwise, without the prior written permission of the publisher.

For information about permission to reproduce selections from this book, write to Permissions, Medletter Associates, Inc., 632 Broadway, New York, New York 10012.

Johns Hopkins was ranked America's best overall medical center in a survey conducted by *U.S. News & World Report*, published July 17, 2000.

Library of Congress Cataloging-in-Publication Data

The Johns Hopkins consumer guide to medical tests : what you can expect, how you
should prepare. what your results mean / Simeon Margolis, medical editor.
    p. cm.
"A Johns Hopkins health after 50 book."
Includes index.
ISBN 0-929661-63-X
  1. Diagnosis--Popular works. I. Margolis, Simeon, 1931- II. Johns Hopkins medical
health letter health after 50.

RC71.3 .J64 2001
616.07'5--dc21

                                     2001019980

Printed in the United States of America
10 9 8 7 6 5 4 3 2 1

WITHDRAWN

**Johns Hopkins Medical Books
are published under the auspices of**
The Johns Hopkins Medical Letter
HEALTH AFTER 50.

RODNEY FRIEDMAN
Editor and Publisher

EVAN HANSEN
Editorial Director

PATRICE BENNEWARD
Executive Editor

DEVON SCHUYLER
Senior Editor

SUZANNE R. UNDY
Senior Writer

JEREMY D. BIRCH
Production Assistant

TOM R. DAMRAUER, M.L.S.
Chief of Information Resources

LESLIE MALTESE-MCGILL
Copy Editor

_____

HELEN MULLEN
Circulation Director

BARBARA MAXWELL O'NEILL
Associate Publisher

DAVID ALEXANDER
Circulation Manager

JERRY LOO
Product Manager

ALLISON HORDOS
Promotions Coordinator

**The Johns Hopkins Consumer
Guide to Medical Tests**

RODNEY FRIEDMAN
Publisher

EVAN HANSEN
Editorial Director

ANDREA MORGAN
Executive Editor

JEREMY D. BIRCH
Managing Editor

MAUREEN O'SULLIVAN
Senior Writer

TIMOTHY JEFFS
Art Director

BREE ROCK
Production Associate

CARNEY W. MIMMS III
Production Database Designer

JOHN VASILIADIS
Production Database Programmer

ROBERT DUCKWALL
Medical Illustrator

DONALD HOMOLKA
Copy Editor

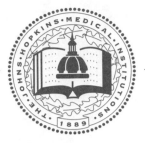

The Johns Hopkins Medical Institutions
Baltimore, Maryland 21205

MEDICAL EDITOR

SIMEON MARGOLIS, M.D., PH.D.
Professor, Medicine &
Biological Chemistry

EDITORIAL BOARD OF ADVISORS

MARTIN D. ABELOFF, M.D.
Professor, Oncology
Director, Oncology Center

MICHELE F. BELLANTONI, M.D.
Associate Professor, Medicine
Medical Director, Long Term Care,
Johns Hopkins Geriatrics Center

BARBARA DE LATEUR, M.D.
Professor & Director
Physical Medicine & Rehabilitation

JOHN A. FLYNN, M.D.
Associate Professor, Medicine
Clinical Director, Division of General
Internal Medicine

H. FRANKLIN HERLONG, M.D.
Associate Dean, School of Medicine
Associate Professor, Medicine

KEITH D. LILLEMOE, M.D.
Professor & Vice-Chairman, Surgery

PETER RABINS, M.D.
Professor, Psychiatry
Director, Division of Geriatric &
Neuropsychiatry

ANDREW P. SCHACHAT, M.D.
Professor, Ophthalmology
Director, Retinal Vascular Center

EDWARD E. WALLACH, M.D.
Professor, Gynecology & Obstetrics

PATRICK C. WALSH, M.D.
Professor & Chairman, Urology

JAMES WEISS, M.D.
Associate Dean
Professor, Medicine, Cardiology Division

OFFICE OF COMMUNICATIONS &
PUBLIC AFFAIRS

ELAINE FREEMAN
Executive Director

JOANN RODGERS
Deputy Director

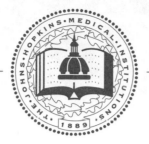

Consultants for The Johns Hopkins Consumer Guide to Medical Tests

CHIEF OF MEDICAL ADVISORY BOARD

SIMEON MARGOLIS, M.D., PH.D.
*Professor of Medicine &
Biological Chemistry
Johns Hopkins School of Medicine*

N. FRANKLIN ADKINSON, M.D.
Asthma & Allergy Medicine

IVAN M. BORRELLO, M.D.
Oncology

LAWRENCE J. CHESKIN, M.D.
Gastroenterology & Nutrition

MICHAEL J. CHOI, M.D.
Nephrology

CHRISTOPHER J. EARLEY, M.D., PH.D.
Neurology

JOHN ENG, M.D.
Diagnostic Imaging

JOHN A. FLYNN, M.D.
Internal Medicine & Rheumatology

DANIEL E. FORD, M.D., M.P.H.
Internal Medicine

H. FRANKLIN HERLONG, M.D.
Hepatology

SUZANNE JAN DE BEUR, M.D.
Endocrinology

KHALED M. KEBAISH, M.D.
Orthopedics

LANDON S. KING, M.D.
Pulmonary Medicine

DAVID L. KNOX, M.D.
Ophthalmology

LAWRENCE R. LUSTIG, M.D.
Otolaryngology

ROBERT E. MILLER, M.D.
Pathology

WENDY S. POST, M.D., M.S.
Cardiovascular Medicine

GEORGE H. SACK JR., M.D., PH.D.
Genetics

JERRY L. SPIVAK, M.D.
Hematology

TIMOTHY R. STERLING, M.D.
Infectious Disease

PETER B. TERRY, M.D.
Pulmonary Medicine

EDWARD E. WALLACH, M.D.
Obstetrics & Gynecology

S. ELIZABETH WHITMORE, M.D.
Dermatology

G. MELVILLE WILLIAMS, M.D.
Vascular Medicine

E. JAMES WRIGHT, M.D.
Urology

Contents

INTRODUCTION

Each year, technological advances and scientific discoveries lead to the development of new and ever-more-sophisticated medical tests, as well as refinements to existing ones. These developments come at a time when many people are seeking to take a more active role in their own health care. *The Johns Hopkins Consumer Guide to Medical Tests* was created to help you understand the essentials of modern diagnostic testing, particularly the tests that are commonly done in adults over the age of 50. Inside, you'll find concise and authoritative information on more than 170 medical tests, including how they work, why they're used, and the implications of the results. Armed with this knowledge, you'll be well prepared to ask informed questions of your doctors, raise any concerns with your managed care plan or insurance company, and generally make more educated decisions about your health and medical care.

The information contained in this book was compiled by a board of Johns Hopkins physicians drawn from multiple fields of medicine. Based on the clinical experience of these experts, only the most relevant tests are included. For example, we do not cover extremely rare tests and outmoded procedures that have been replaced with safer or more accurate techniques.

Medical tests serve a variety of purposes. Used as part of a regular check-up, they can help to screen for possible risks to your health before any symptoms occur. They may also play an essential role in pinpointing the correct diagnosis when symptoms of an illness do develop. Or, they may help to select the proper treatment, assess the success of therapy, or monitor the course of an illness over time.

It is important to remember, however, that no matter how state-of-the-art the technology may be, all medical tests have limitations. The accuracy of any given test depends on how well it is performed and interpreted, as well as the nature of the test itself. And, although modern medical tests are less invasive than ever before, many tests still pose real and serious risks. Before undergoing any invasive procedure, it is essential that the procedure be fully explained to you, in person, by a doctor or other medical professional—including why it's necessary, what new information will be learned, what risks are entailed, and what the potential benefits are. In some cases, you must also sign a consent form verifying that you understand this information and give your permission for the test to be performed.

Typically, a physician will only recommend a particular specialized test (or tests) after conducting a thorough physical exam and obtaining the details of your medical history. In many situations, test results alone can determine abnormal function of a particular organ and are sufficient to make a diagnosis. At other times, your doctor must evaluate the test results in the context of your history and physical exam, and possibly additional tests, in order to arrive at an accurate diagnosis.

How to use this book

The information in this book is arranged to make it useful in a variety of circumstances. For example, if your doctor orders a particular medical test, you may want to read about it in advance to learn what to expect and how to prepare yourself. If you are reluctant to undergo a certain test for some reason, you may want to check and see if there are any alternatives. Or, if you are told that you have a specific disease, you may want reassurance that all the appropriate and relevant tests have been recommended.

The book is organized into four main sections, beginning with a detailed body atlas to use as a reference when reading about the different testing procedures. Secondly, you will find five introductory chapters that cover some of the major aspects of medical testing: laboratory testing, diagnostic imaging, screening for disease, home testing, and genetic testing and screening. Chapters 1 and 2 provide broad overviews of the specific techniques that are used for laboratory analysis and imaging procedures such as x-rays and CT scans. Chapter 3 discusses the current controversies over screening for disease in individuals without symptoms, describes the most common screening tests recommended for use in the general population, and lists specific screening guidelines issued by various organizations. Chapter 4 reviews the tests that you may perform yourself at home and provides tips on when they're appropriate and how to use them accurately. Chapter 5 reviews the concepts behind genetic tests and their growing role in diagnosis and screening for disease.

The third section, the Index of Tests by Subject, lists all of the diagnostic tests included in this book, organized in groups according to the organ systems or specific medical fields they are commonly used to evaluate—for example, the digestive system or cancer.

The fourth section of the book contains detailed descriptions of more than 170 relevant diagnostic tests that are arranged alphabetically. Each entry is organized in a concise, easy-to-follow format:

• *Description* provides a brief and basic summary of the test.

• *Purpose of the Test* describes the most common reasons why the test is ordered and what diseases and conditions it may detect.

• *Who Performs the Test* indicates which types of health-care professionals normally carry out the procedure.

• *Special Concerns* includes any special information that may be relevant to the test, including reasons why it may not be safe or appropriate for certain individuals (contraindications), situations where another test might be preferred, and factors that can interfere with the accuracy of results.

• *Before the Test* addresses any specific steps you need to take to prepare for the test, such as dietary restrictions or discontinuing certain drugs.

• *What You Experience* offers a step-by-step description of the testing procedure, including what you will feel, what equipment is used, and how long it takes (which refers only to how long you are involved).

• *Risks and Potential Complications* lists both common and rare risks and complications that are associated with the test.

• *After the Test* describes immediate post-procedure care, any steps you should take to speed your recovery, as well as warning signs of possible complications.

• *Results* describes how the test results are evaluated, whether the findings are definitive, whether follow-up tests may be needed, and what the next step may be. Specific values are not usually given for laboratory tests because "normal" ranges can vary widely from laboratory to laboratory, and because there may be considerable need for interpretation based on your doctor's analysis of your complete health profile. In addition, we do not estimate how long it takes to receive test results, since this factor may differ a great deal based on how and where the results are analyzed.

• *Estimated Cost* gives an approximation of the average cost for the test, given as a range:

Estimated Cost Legend
$ = Less than $100
$$ = $100 to $500
$$$ = $500 to $1,000
$$$$ = More than $1,000

These ranges refer to the costs for the tests themselves and do not include any fees that may be charged by the medical professionals who perform and interpret them. In addition, keep in mind that costs for particular tests vary dramatically across different geographic regions and between different testing facilities.

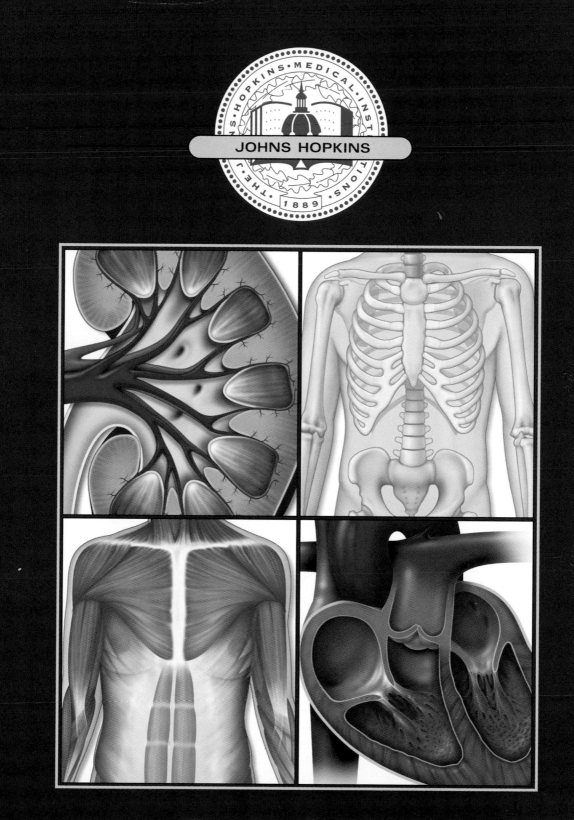

Body Atlas

Body Atlas

The integumentary system is made up of the skin and its associated structures—hair, nails, and the sweat and sebaceous (oil) glands. Composed of two layers (the inner dermis and outer epidermis), the skin forms an external body covering that serves as a barrier to injury and infectious microbes, regulates body temperature and water balance, receives sensory stimuli such as pressure and pain, and synthesizes vitamin D when exposed to sunlight.

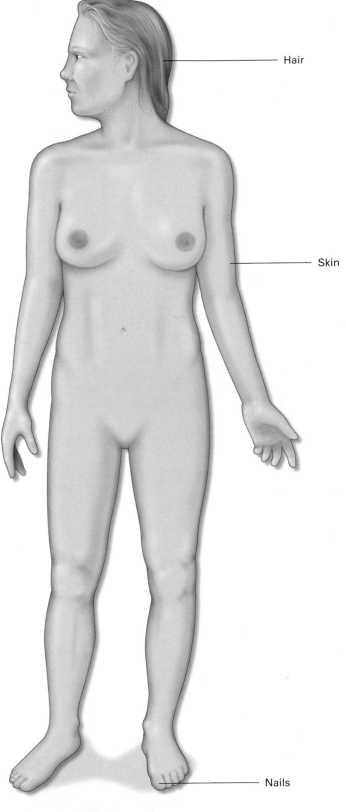

Hair

Skin

Nails

The human skeleton contains 206 bones, forming a rigid framework that provides shape and form for the body, protects and supports the internal organs, and works with the muscles to allow bodily movement. The bones are largely composed of living tissue that is constantly being remodeled. They also store important minerals, such as calcium and phosphorus, and house the bone marrow, which manufactures new blood cells. Bones are attached to each other by fibrous bands of connective tissue called ligaments. The junctions where two or more bones meet, or joints, are lined with cartilage, a tough, elastic connective tissue that is also found in various other parts of the body, such as the outer ear.

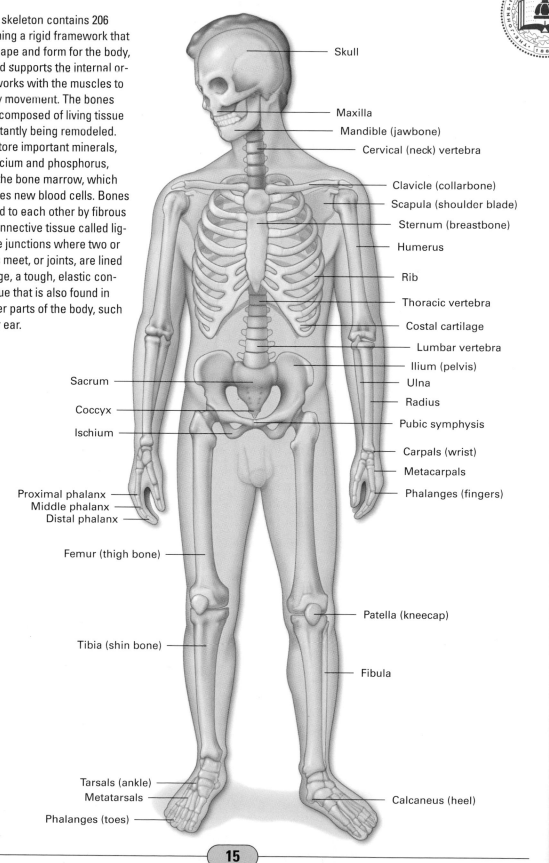

- Skull
- Maxilla
- Mandible (jawbone)
- Cervical (neck) vertebra
- Clavicle (collarbone)
- Scapula (shoulder blade)
- Sternum (breastbone)
- Humerus
- Rib
- Thoracic vertebra
- Costal cartilage
- Lumbar vertebra
- Ilium (pelvis)
- Ulna
- Radius
- Pubic symphysis
- Carpals (wrist)
- Metacarpals
- Phalanges (fingers)
- Patella (kneecap)
- Fibula
- Calcaneus (heel)

- Sacrum
- Coccyx
- Ischium
- Proximal phalanx
- Middle phalanx
- Distal phalanx
- Femur (thigh bone)
- Tibia (shin bone)
- Tarsals (ankle)
- Metatarsals
- Phalanges (toes)

Body Atlas

Body Atlas

The central nervous system consists of the brain, the body's primary control center, and the spinal cord, the main conduction pathway for nerve signals to and from the brain. The peripheral nervous system refers to the complex network of nerves that branch out from the brain and spinal cord; it includes the sensory nerves, the nerves that carry the signals for muscle contraction, and the autonomic nerves that control involuntary functions such as breathing, heartbeat, and digestion. In addition, the sense organs (such as the eyes and ears) are considered part of the nervous system. Together, this system receives and processes information from external and internal sources, and transmits messages to the body's organs, glands, and muscles so that they respond appropriately.

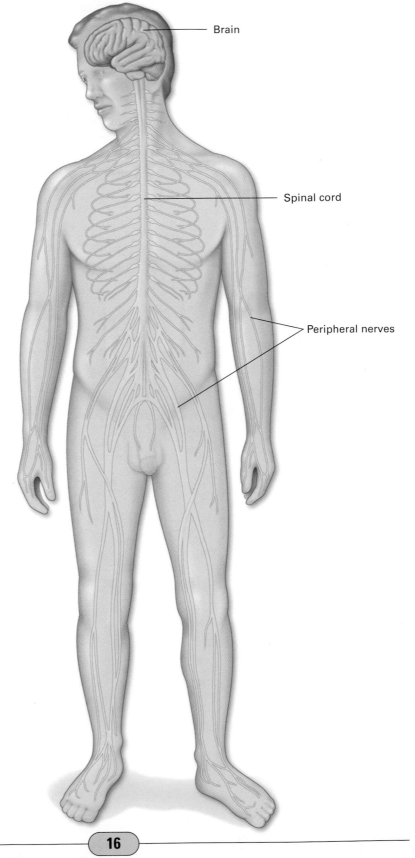

Brain

Spinal cord

Peripheral nerves

More than 600 muscles cover the skeleton, giving the human body its characteristic shape. The muscular system consists of the large skeletal muscles that provide support and enable us to move; the cardiac muscles of the heart; and the smooth muscles found in our internal organs. Only skeletal muscles, which are attached to bone by strong bands of fibrous tissue called tendons, are under our voluntary control. Responding to signals from the nervous system, they contract and relax to allow movement, locomotion, and facial expression. The involuntary contractions of the cardiac and smooth muscles are stimulated by signals from the nervous system and hormones from the endocrine system.

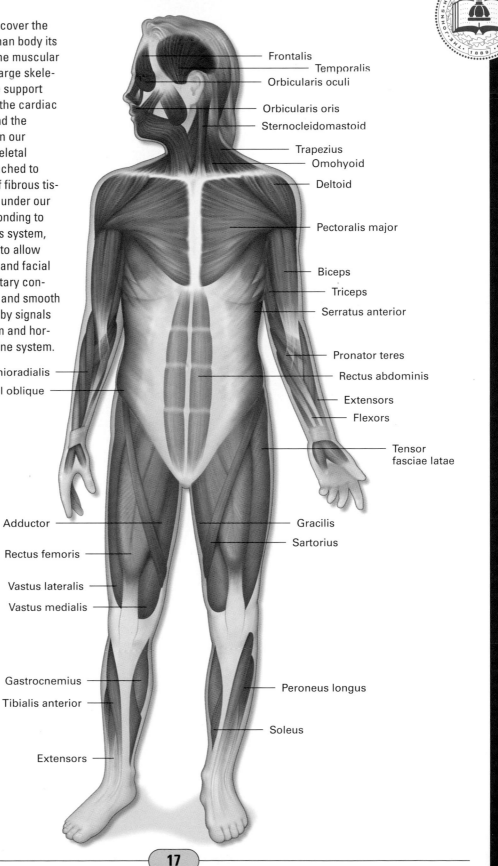

Frontalis
Temporalis
Orbicularis oculi
Orbicularis oris
Sternocleidomastoid
Trapezius
Omohyoid
Deltoid
Pectoralis major
Biceps
Triceps
Serratus anterior
Pronator teres
Rectus abdominis
Extensors
Flexors
Tensor fasciae latae

Brachioradialis
External oblique

Adductor
Rectus femoris
Vastus lateralis
Vastus medialis

Gracilis
Sartorius

Gastrocnemius
Tibialis anterior

Peroneus longus

Soleus

Extensors

Body Atlas

Body Atlas

The endocrine system—which, along with the nervous system, oversees the body's internal communications—consists of glands that produce hormones and secrete them into the bloodstream. Hormones act as chemical messengers that travel to their target organs or tissues and trigger specific reactions. Together with nerve signals, hormones help to regulate various body functions and rhythms, including growth and repair of tissues, metabolism, blood pressure, sexual development and reproduction, and the body's response to stress. In addition to the glands and organs pictured here, specialized cells in other organs, such as the kidneys, heart, and lungs, also secrete hormones.

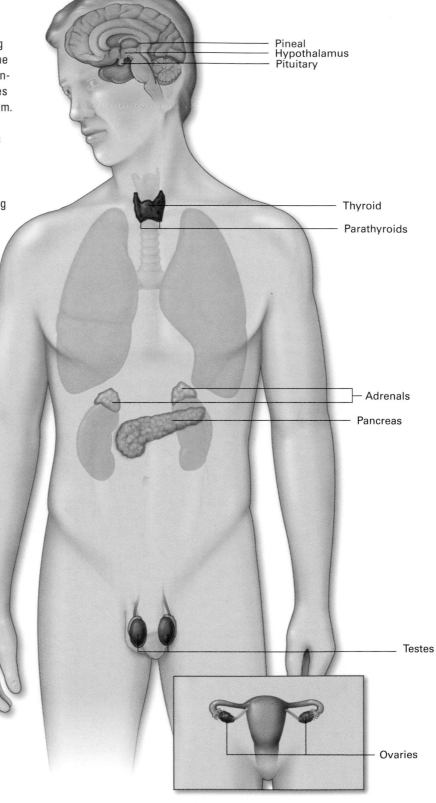

Pineal
Hypothalamus
Pituitary

Thyroid
Parathyroids

Adrenals
Pancreas

Testes

Ovaries

The lymphatic system is a secondary circulatory system made up of a complex network of vessels, nodes, and ducts, as well as certain organs. This system performs various filtering and transporting functions, including the return of excess tissue fluid, or lymph, and proteins to the bloodstream. (Most lymphatic drainage, as well as fat absorbed from the intestine, passes into the thoracic duct—the main lymphatic channel—which drains into veins in the chest.) In addition, the lymphatic system plays an important role in immunity: Blood and lymph carry white blood cells called lymphocytes that help to defend the body against disease-causing agents, such as bacteria and viruses. (Lymphocytes are produced by the bone marrow and concentrated in the spleen, thymus, and lymph nodes.) Contraction of skeletal muscles moves lymph through the lymphatic vessels, while valves within the vessels help to prevent any backflow.

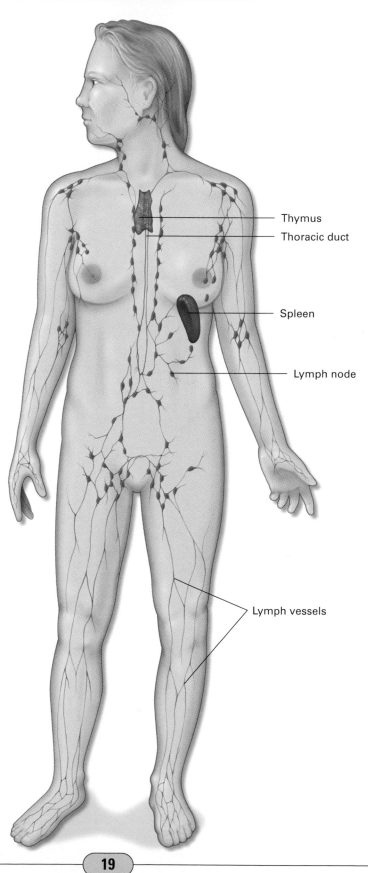

Thymus

Thoracic duct

Spleen

Lymph node

Lymph vessels

Body Atlas

The cardiovascular system, which includes the heart and blood vessels, is the main transportation system in the body, responsible for supplying oxygen and nutrients to all cells in the body. With its perpetual contractions, the heart is a tireless pump that maintains a continuous flow of oxygen-rich blood to tissues and organs throughout the body while simultaneously sending blood to the lungs to pick up oxygen and be recycled. The blood vessels that transport blood from the heart are called arteries, while those that return blood to the heart are called veins. Each day, the heart pumps the equivalent of 2,000 gallons of blood through about 60,000 miles of blood vessels.

Body Atlas

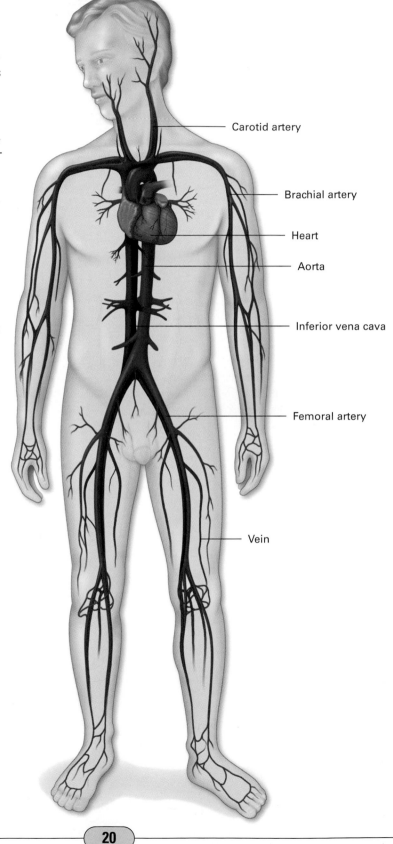

Carotid artery

Brachial artery

Heart

Aorta

Inferior vena cava

Femoral artery

Vein

The heart, which beats 60 to 80 times a minute, is a muscular organ with four chambers: the left and right atria and the left and right ventricles. With each contraction, the left side of the heart pumps oxygen-rich blood through the aorta, the body's largest artery, to smaller arteries throughout the body. These arteries, in turn, branch into even smaller vessels, called arterioles, and eventually into the microscopic capillaries that deliver oxygen and nutrients to every cell and pick up carbon dioxide and other waste products. Blood returns to the right side of the heart via the veins and is then sent through the pulmonary arteries to the lungs. Inside the lungs, carbon dioxide is removed, fresh oxygen is added, and the blood returns to the left chambers of the heart. The heart muscle itself is fed a continuous supply of oxygenated blood via the coronary arteries, which branch off at the root of the aorta.

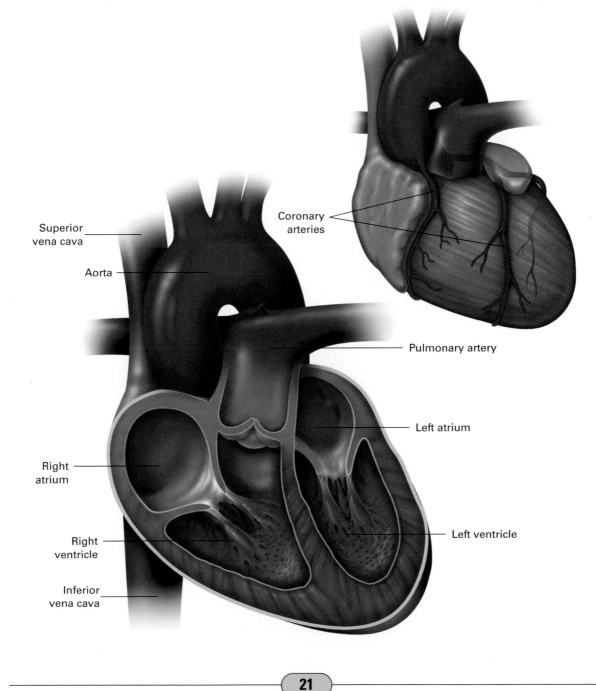

Coronary arteries

Superior vena cava

Aorta

Pulmonary artery

Left atrium

Right atrium

Right ventricle

Left ventricle

Inferior vena cava

Body Atlas

Body Atlas

The respiratory system, made up of the lungs and air passages, provides the body with a continuous supply of oxygen and an efficient means of removing the cellular waste gas carbon dioxide. The oxygen we breathe in with air passes from the lungs to the bloodstream, which carries it to cells throughout the body. At the same time, the blood picks up carbon dioxide and returns it to the lungs to be exhaled. The diaphragm and chest muscles help to control the breathing process, or respiration.

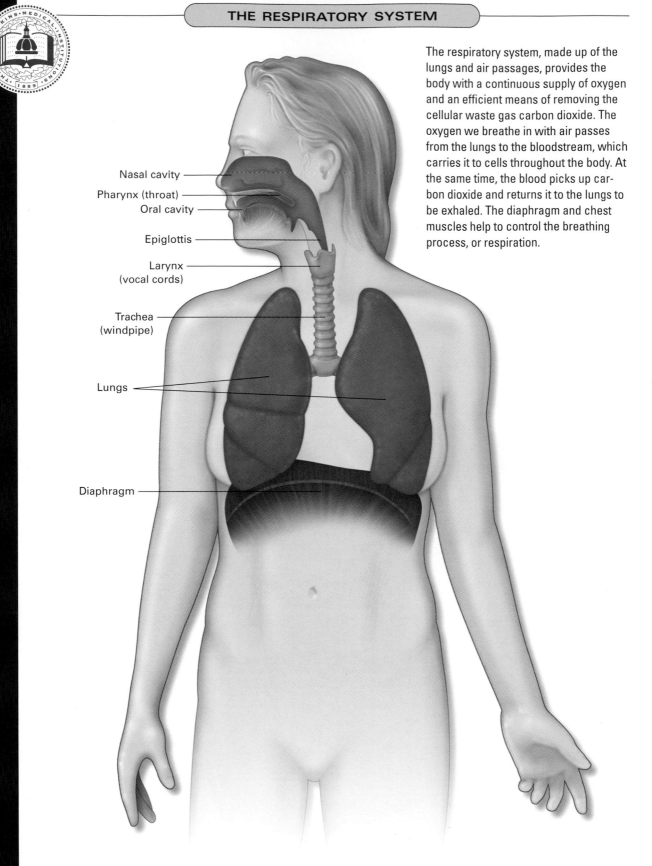

Nasal cavity

Pharynx (throat)

Oral cavity

Epiglottis

Larynx
(vocal cords)

Trachea
(windpipe)

Lungs

Diaphragm

The trachea, or windpipe, branches into two primary tubes, or bronchi, one leading into each lung. Each of these bronchi divides into progressively smaller bronchi, which branch into thousands of bronchioles, and finally culminate in some 300 million tiny air sacs, or alveoli. The grapelike clusters of alveoli are covered with a dense network of tiny blood vessels, or capillaries; it is here that the exchange of oxygen and carbon dioxide occurs. The lung on the right side of the body has three lobes, while the left lung has only two. Both lungs are covered with a layer of moist membranes, called the pleura, which allows them to inflate and deflate smoothly.

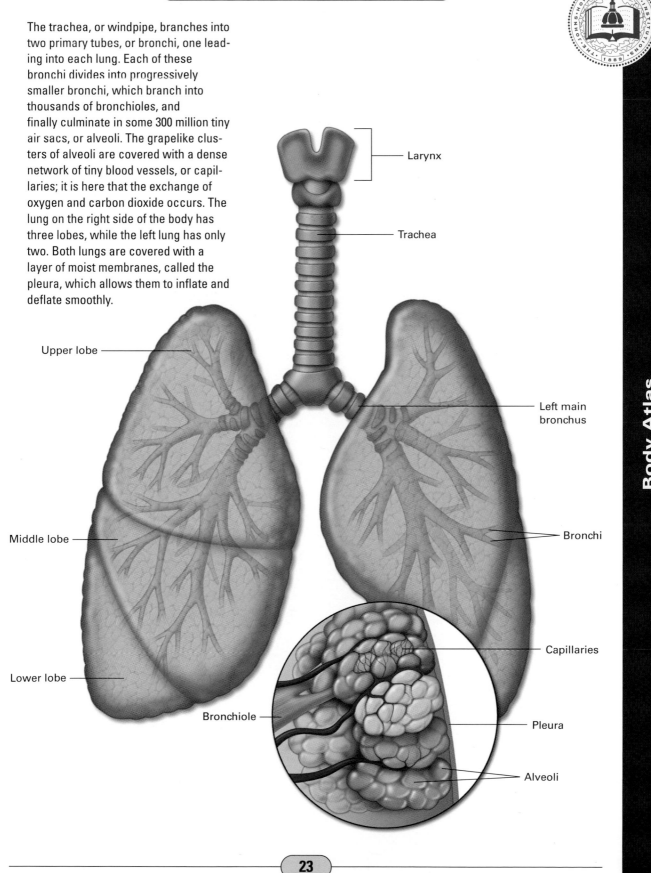

Larynx

Trachea

Upper lobe

Left main bronchus

Middle lobe

Bronchi

Lower lobe

Capillaries

Bronchiole

Pleura

Alveoli

Body Atlas

Body Atlas

The digestive (or gastrointestinal) system consists of a series of connected hollow organs and the organs and glands that secrete digestive juices into this tract. This system breaks food down into absorbable units that enter the bloodstream to nourish cells and provide energy. Food is crushed, mixed, and pushed forward with the wave-like muscular contractions, or peristalsis, of the esophagus, stomach, and intestine. In addition, it is broken up by digestive enzymes secreted by the salivary glands, stomach lining, and intestine. Digested nutrients are absorbed through the walls of the small intestine; the waste products that remain (primarily plant fiber) are propelled into the large intestine and eliminated as feces.

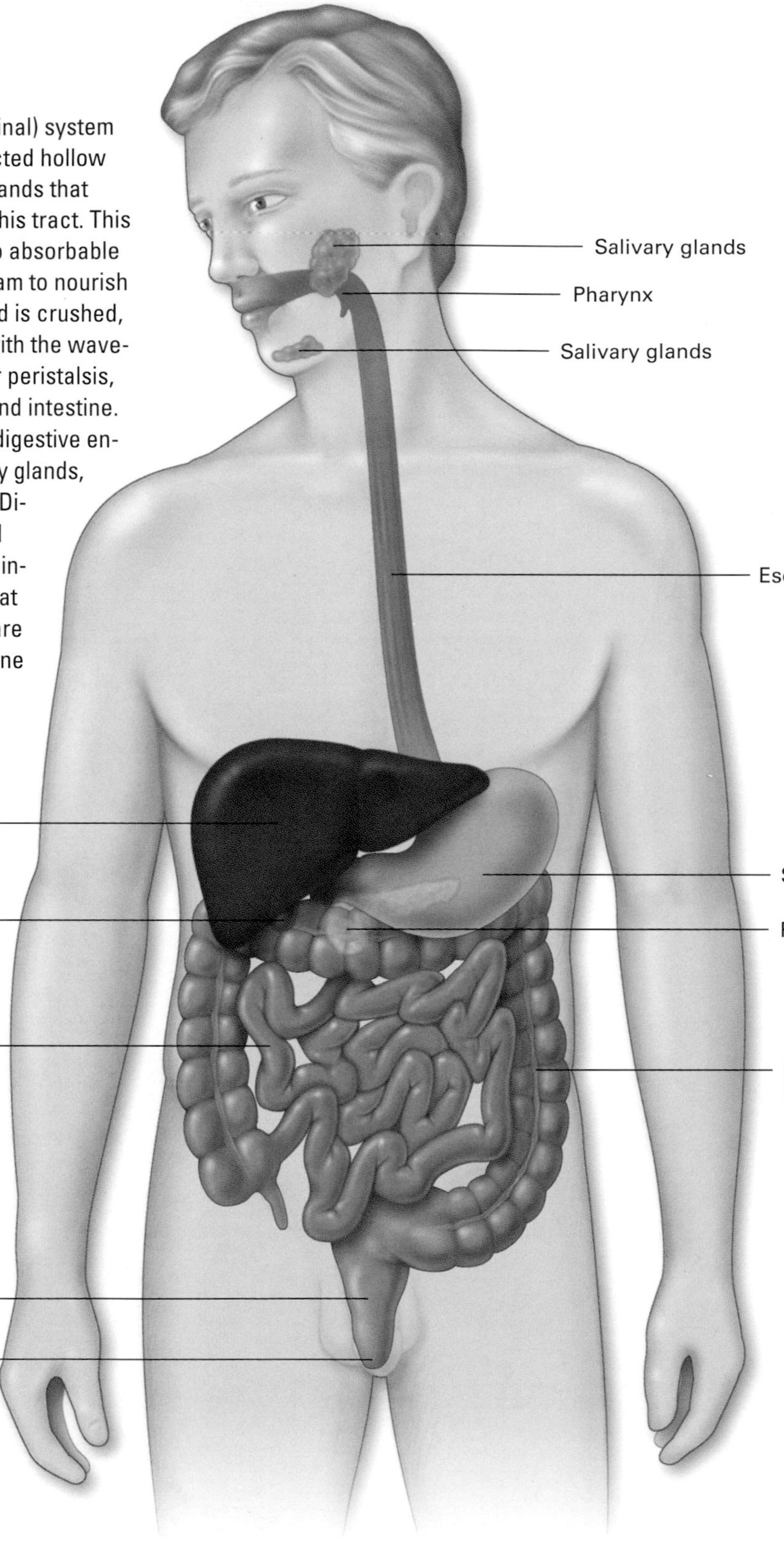

Salivary glands

Pharynx

Salivary glands

Esophagus

Liver

Stomach

Gallbladder

Pancreas

Small intestine

Large intestine

Rectum

Anus

More than 99% of digestion takes place in the small intestine (or small bowel), a coiled muscular tube ranging from 12 to 22 feet in length. This organ consists of three segments: the duodenum, jejunum, and ileum. In the duodenum, pancreatic enzymes and bile from the liver and gallbladder break food down into simple, absorbable components. Almost all the nutrients present in food are then absorbed into the bloodstream through the walls of the jejunum and ileum; the residue passes into the large intestine, a 5-foot tube also known as the colon or large bowel. Here, excess water and electrolytes are absorbed from the waste material, which is broken down further by intestinal bacteria and stored until it is excreted from the body. The large intestine is divided into the cecum, colon, rectum, and anal canal.

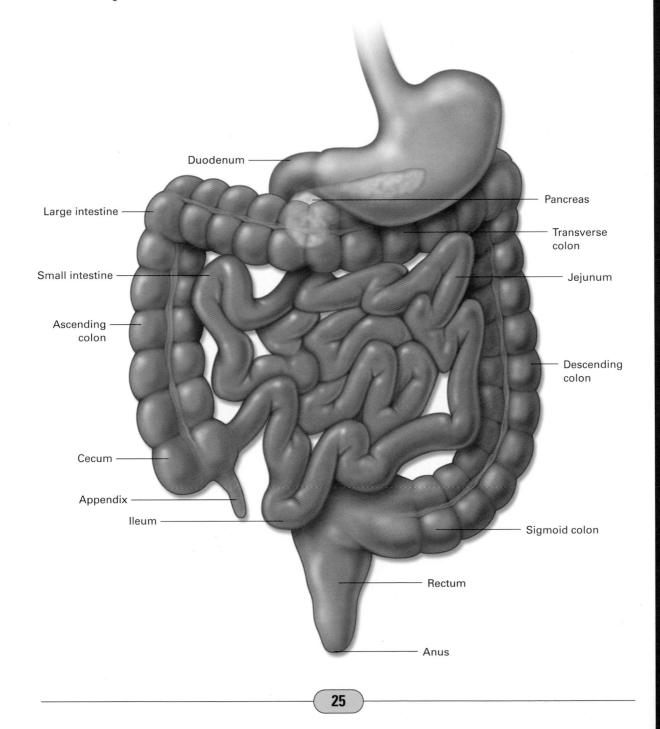

Duodenum

Large intestine

Small intestine

Ascending colon

Cecum

Appendix

Ileum

Pancreas

Transverse colon

Jejunum

Descending colon

Sigmoid colon

Rectum

Anus

Body Atlas

Body Atlas

The urinary system removes wastes from the body and helps to regulate body chemistry and fluid balance. The kidneys filter excess fluid, waste products, and drugs from the bloodstream and form urine for excretion from the body. Urine passes from the kidneys to the bladder through slender, muscular tubes called ureters. When the bladder is about half full, nerves in the bladder signal the urge to urinate and muscles at the bladder outlet relax, allowing urine to be expelled through the urethra.

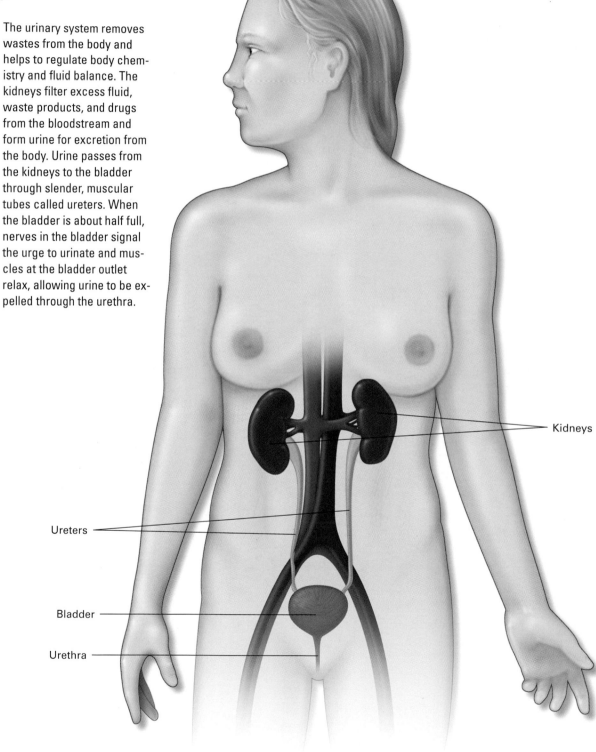

Kidneys

Ureters

Bladder

Urethra

Nearly one quarter of the volume of blood pumped with each heartbeat passes through the kidneys, where it is cleansed of waste products such as urea, uric acid, and excess salts. The outer part of the kidney is known as the cortex, and the inner part is the medulla. The renal artery brings blood into the kidney, where it passes through a series of complex filtering units, called nephrons. Inside the 1 million nephrons in either kidney, blood is filtered through tiny capillary blood vessels, called glomeruli, into small collecting tubes (renal tubules). As the filtrate passes through the renal tubules, urine is formed from wastes and excess water and eventually collects in a reservoir called the renal pelvis; from there, it is channeled through the ureter to the bladder. Filtered blood re-enters the circulation via the renal vein.

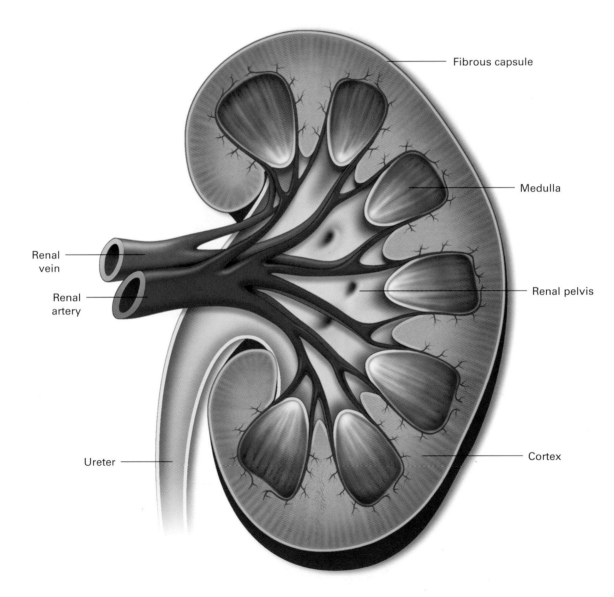

Fibrous capsule

Medulla

Renal vein

Renal artery

Renal pelvis

Ureter

Cortex

Body Atlas

Male Reproductive System

The testes produce male sex hormones and sperm, the male reproductive cell. Sperm cells mature for two to four weeks in the epididymis, a tightly coiled tube on top of each testis. A thin, muscular tube called the vas deferens transports sperm from the testis to the ejaculatory duct (which empties into the urethra just inside of the prostate gland). Semen that is ejaculated through the urethra during sexual activity is made up of sperm cells mixed with fluids from the prostate and seminal vesicles.

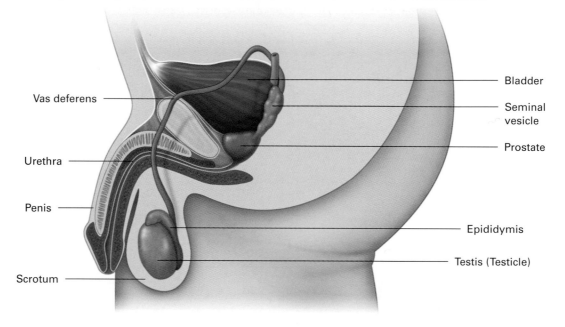

Vas deferens

Urethra

Penis

Scrotum

Bladder

Seminal vesicle

Prostate

Epididymis

Testis (Testicle)

Female Reproductive System

The ovaries, which produce female sex hormones and the eggs needed for reproduction, are small oval organs located on either side of the uterus, a hollow organ with muscular walls. Eggs released during each menstrual cycle travel down the fallopian tubes to the uterus. If an egg is fertilized, it is implanted in the uterine lining, or endometrium. If fertilization does not occur, the endometrium is shed through the vaginal canal during menstruation.

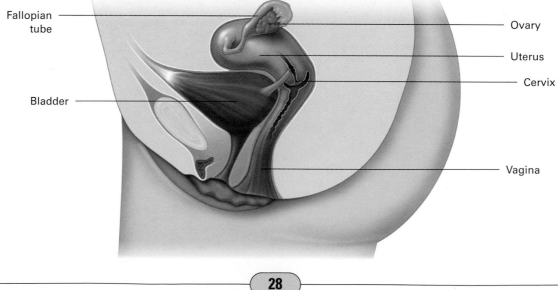

Fallopian tube

Bladder

Ovary

Uterus

Cervix

Vagina

Body Atlas

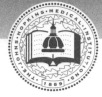

LABORATORY TESTING

An integral part of modern medicine, laboratory testing involves the analysis of blood, urine, other body fluids, and tissue samples. With the help of sophisticated, computerized equipment, laboratory technologists and physician-experts called pathologists—who specialize in analyzing changes in the body produced by disease—examine these specimens to answer questions about your body and your health. Such laboratory investigations provide valuable information that may help pinpoint the cause of an illness, as well as determine optimal treatments. This chapter will explain how body fluid and tissue samples are collected and analyzed in diagnostic laboratories.

THE ROLE OF LABORATORY TESTING IN MEDICINE

Physicians today rely heavily on the results of laboratory tests as a source of objective, reliable information to help them make medical decisions. These findings can be of the first importance for a variety of purposes, such as to screen patients for potential health problems (see page 48); to establish or confirm a diagnosis; to rule out a particular illness; to select a treatment; to monitor the course of a disease; or to assess the effects of therapy. Even so, laboratory data alone are not typically sufficient to make a definitive diagnosis because of the nonspecific nature of some tests. Instead, test results must be combined with the doctor's careful and expert assessment of a patient's symptoms, physical exam, and medical history to reach an accurate diagnosis and prescribe appropriate treatment.

When a patient is first seen for an undiagnosed problem, laboratory tests are rarely ordered singly—instead, the doctor usually requests a group, or battery, of general tests. These initial tests tend to be ones that can be performed quickly and reliably, and which may show abnormalities resulting from a broad range of diseases. If an abnormality is found, additional, more specific tests may then be done to identify the cause of the particular health problem. For example, if a patient experiences a nonspecific symptom such as fatigue, the physician often sends a blood sample to the laboratory for a battery of general tests. These test results may reveal an abnormality, such as altered kidney function, that suggests underlying kidney disease. Once this potential problem is identified, more specific tests are then performed to determine whether kidney disease is present, and if so, its nature and severity.

Pathology laboratories may be part of a hospital or may be independent entities. They include two separate, but overlapping, fields: clinical pathology and anatomical pathology.

CLINICAL PATHOLOGY

Clinical pathologists evaluate the body's biochemical and physiological processes by measuring levels of various substances—such as electrolytes, enzymes, hormones, and antibodies—in the blood, urine, and other body fluids. These substances may be produced as part of normal body functions, arise as metabolic waste products, or come from organs or tissues affected by injury or disease. Using diverse technologies, clinical pathologists most often look for abnormally high or low levels of substances in the bloodstream, the body's main transportation system for delivering

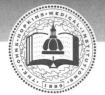

nutrients and other materials to and from tissues and cells. These test results can help identify specific disorders, determine whether further diagnostic procedures are needed, and assist in monitoring the course of an illness.

THE BRANCHES OF CLINICAL PATHOLOGY

The field of clinical pathology encompasses a number of subspecialties. Blood samples and other specimens are sent to specific laboratories, depending on the types of tests desired.

Hematology laboratories study the cellular components of blood, such as red blood cells (which carry oxygen to tissues and organs), white blood cells (which fight infection), platelets (cells involved in blood clotting), hemoglobin (the oxygen-carrying pigment in red blood cells), and coagulation factors (that cause blood to clot). These laboratories specialize in diagnosing and following the course of blood disorders such as anemia, leukemia, and hemophilia, as well as monitoring patients who take anticlotting drugs. In addition, physical and chemical analysis of urine samples (urinalysis) is usually performed in these laboratories.

Clinical chemistry laboratories use a wide range of procedures to measure levels of various chemical substances in the blood or urine. The following are the most commonly performed clinical chemistry tests.

• **Electrolytes,** including sodium, potassium, chloride, calcium, phosphorus, and bicarbonate (carbon dioxide), are measured to identify and monitor certain metabolic, endocrine, heart, liver, and kidney disorders.

• **Enzymes** may be released into the blood when organs or tissues are diseased or damaged. Elevated levels of particular enzymes may indicate problems with a specific organ or tissue. The enzyme creatine kinase, for example, may signal a heart attack and can help to determine the extent of heart damage.

• **Glucose,** the major sugar in the blood, is measured to diagnose hypoglycemia (low blood sugar) and to diagnose and follow the treatment of diabetes mellitus.

• **Hormones** are substances produced by the endocrine glands, such as the pituitary, thyroid, and adrenals (see page 18 of the body atlas). An abnormally high or low level may indicate an endocrine disorder, such as an overactive or underactive gland.

• **Lipids** are fatty substances in the blood, including cholesterol and triglycerides. Elevated blood lipid levels indicate an increased risk of coronary artery disease and may result from kidney or liver disease, diabetes, and other disorders.

• **Proteins** are measured to identify or evaluate metabolic and nutritional disorders. Low levels of albumin, for example, may indicate liver disease, kidney disease, or malnutrition. High globulin levels can point to chronic infection or inflammation, or to some blood cancers.

• **Other metabolic substances** are measured to assess the function of various organs. High blood urea nitrogen (BUN) and creatinine levels indicate kidney dysfunction, while elevated uric acid levels may signal gout or kidney disease.

Immunology and serology laboratories focus on identifying antibodies (protective proteins usually made in response to foreign invaders such as bacteria and other microorganisms); diagnosing autoimmune disorders, such as rheumatoid arthritis, that occur when the body's immune system attacks healthy tissues; and diagnosing immunodeficiency disorders, such as HIV infection.

Microbiology laboratories perform tests to identify disease-causing microorganisms— bacteria, viruses, parasites, and fungi—in the blood, urine, other body fluids, stool, and tissues. Bacteria and fungi are identified by placing specimens in culture dishes containing

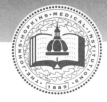

special media, under conditions that encourage microorganisms to multiply. Chemical tests and microscopic examination can then identify the disease-causing agent. Small amounts of antibiotics or other medications may be added to the culture to determine which is most effective in killing that particular microorganism.

Blood banking laboratories ensure the safety of donated blood, prepare special blood products such as platelets, and match the blood type of a donor with that of a patient receiving a transfusion.

TESTING TECHNOLOGIES

Because of extensive automation, modern clinical pathology laboratories can generate vast quantities of information both rapidly and with a high degree of accuracy. Large, computerized machines (called multichannel analyzers) can produce up to 20 different test results from a single specimen of blood or other fluid in seconds to minutes. These sophisticated instruments, run by expert laboratory technicians, have greatly increased the efficiency of clinical pathology laboratories and reduced the opportunity for human error. (More complicated, technically demanding tests, however, are still performed manually.) In addition, computerization has allowed electronic linkages between different laboratories to combine test results into comprehensive reports that can be sent directly to physicians by computer.

Clinical pathology laboratories employ a wide variety of methods to identify and quantitate substances in blood and other body fluids. The following are some of the more important analytic technologies used.

Spectrophotometry determines the concentration of a substance based on the intensity of color that occurs when specific reagents are added to blood or other samples. Special instruments use spectrophotometry to measure the color produced as the two substances react. This process provides the results for many of the automated tests performed on multichannel analyzers.

Immunoassays are used principally to diagnose infectious diseases and to measure substances that are present in extremely low amounts in the body. These highly sensitive tests can identify antigens (proteins found on the surface of foreign invaders such as bacteria, viruses, or allergens) and antibodies (proteins formed by the immune system in response to particular antigens), as well as determine the concentrations of hormones or drugs for which specific antibody-reagents have been developed.

These assays rely on the fact that there is a specific antibody for each antigen; thus, each one can be used to detect the presence of the other. In a typical immunoassay test system, the surface of a plate or test tube is covered with a particular antigen (or antibody), and a patient's specimen is added. If the corresponding antibody (or antigen) is present in the specimen, the two proteins will bind together. This interaction can be identified and quantitated by using various markers—for example, a radioisotope, enzyme, or fluorescent chemical.

Electrophoresis utilizes the characteristic movement of proteins when they are placed in an electrical field to identify and measure the amounts of particular proteins in blood and urine. Electrophoresis can assist in the diagnosis and management of multiple myeloma (a type of bone marrow cancer) and chronic inflammatory disorders of the liver and kidney.

Chromatography separates substances—such as drugs, proteins, and hormones—from the blood and quantitates them by virtue of their molecular size, physical structure, and chemical properties. Chromatography is performed by adding blood specimens to a glass chromatography column packed with specific

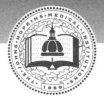

materials. Substances in the blood, which absorb or adhere to the column more or less tightly, are identified and measured by how quickly they travel through the chromatography medium when various liquids or gases are added.

Mass spectroscopy, used together with chromatography, can identify a substance by the mass and charge of its fragments. This technique, which is sometimes referred to as "molecular fingerprinting," is commonly used to test for illicit drugs, usually to confirm the results of a positive immunoassay screening test for a particular drug.

Ion-selective electrodes are devices that provide accurate and precise measurements of certain electrically charged blood components—including the electrolytes sodium, potassium, bicarbonate, and calcium. When blood specimens are exposed to special electrodes, the strength of the generated current depends on the concentration of the substance being measured.

Automated blood cell counters are computerized instruments used by hematology laboratories to measure the number and type of blood cells and their physical characteristics. Automated blood cell counters assist in identifying conditions such as anemia, infection, leukemia, and bleeding disorders, and in monitoring the progress of chemotherapy for cancer.

Flow cytometry is a newer technology used both in clinical and anatomical pathology laboratories (see page 38).

COLLECTING A BLOOD SAMPLE

Blood—made up of blood cells and the liquid that carries them—is the most common body fluid used to assess normal function and to detect the presence of disease. While there are hundreds of different blood tests, they fall into two general categories: those that look for changes in the normal constituents of the

blood (such as electrolytes, lipids, and hormones) and those that detect abnormal blood constituents, such as antibodies characteristic of a particular disease or tumor markers like prostate specific antigen (PSA).

The type of blood sample required depends on the nature of the test. Many studies use whole blood, which contains all the blood elements (these samples are collected in tubes that contain an anticoagulant to prevent clotting). Some tests require only plasma, the liquid part of whole blood that contains hundreds of dissolved substances, including glucose, electrolytes, proteins, and hormones. Others use serum, the clear liquid that remains after whole blood clots and the cells are removed. (Both plasma and serum are obtained by spinning the blood in a centrifuge to separate the blood components.) Whatever the type of sample needed, blood is drawn by three general methods: venipuncture, skin puncture, and arterial puncture.

Venipuncture, the drawing of blood from a vein, is most common because veins are closer to the surface of the skin and more easily accessible than arteries. A vein on the front of the arm near the elbow is used most often; alternatives include veins on the back of the hands and, rarely, the ankles and feet. Venipuncture can be performed by a doctor, nurse, or technician. Usually, no special preparation is required, though some tests, such as a lipid profile, require overnight fasting beforehand.

During venipuncture, you sit in a chair with your arm supported on an armrest or table. A soft, rubber tourniquet is tied around your upper arm, causing a temporary stoppage of blood flow so that the veins below it bulge. You may then be asked to make a fist, distending the veins even further so they will be easier to puncture. After the site is cleansed with an antiseptic and dried with gauze, a sterile needle is inserted into the vein. (While the needle

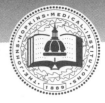

stick may cause mild, brief discomfort, most people feel no pain once the needle is in place.) When blood begins to flow adequately, the tourniquet is released.

In most cases, the needle is attached to a glass collection tube. (Less often, a needle and syringe are used.) A vacuum within the tube draws blood into the tube; when it is full, the tube may be removed and replaced with an empty one (depending on how much blood is needed) while the needle is still in place. The quantity of blood required depends on the type and number of tests to be done.

Once the sample is collected, a gauze pad or cotton ball is placed over the puncture site and the needle is withdrawn. You will be asked to maintain gentle pressure on the site for a few minutes to help stop the bleeding, and then a small bandage is applied. In general, venipuncture takes only 5 minutes or less to perform.

Drawing blood is easier in some people than in others. Be sure to inform the person collecting the sample if you've had problems before, or if you've ever felt faint during a blood test (if so, blood will be drawn while you are lying down). Serious complications are rare. A small mass of blood (hematoma) may collect under the skin at the puncture site and cause transient bruising or swelling. (Applying pressure after the needle is withdrawn helps to prevent this problem.) If a hematoma does develop, ice may be applied at first to stop any active bleeding. Then, warm, moist compresses may be applied to enhance blood reabsorption.

Skin puncture is performed if only a small amount of blood is needed—for example, to measure glucose or test for anemia—or for a special coagulation test called bleeding time (see page 157). First, a warm, moist compress may be applied to the puncture site—usually the tip of a finger or an earlobe—for a few minutes to improve blood flow. After being cleansed, the skin is punctured with a tiny sterile lancet and a few drops of blood are collected. At the end of the blood collection, brief pressure is applied to the puncture site, and then you will be asked to hold a sterile gauze pad over the site until bleeding has stopped. A small bandage may then be applied.

Arterial puncture causes more discomfort and carries more risk of hemorrhage than venipuncture because the blood is under higher pressure in the arteries. Therefore, arterial puncture is rarely performed for routine studies, and then only by a doctor or specially trained technician or nurse. Its primary use is to obtain a specimen for arterial blood gases (see page 93), since arterial blood has been freshly reoxygenated by the lungs. Arterial specimens are usually drawn from an artery inside the wrist.

For this procedure, you sit with your arm extended on a table and your wrist on a small pillow or rolled towel. The person taking blood feels the pulse in your wrist to determine if there is adequate blood flow, cleanses the area with an antiseptic, and may inject a small amount of local anesthetic to numb the puncture site. A needle is inserted into the artery and the blood sample is drawn into a syringe. The needle stick may cause brief, sharp pain (this procedure causes more discomfort than venipuncture because arteries are deeper and have more nerve fibers than veins).

After the needle is removed, the person drawing blood will apply firm pressure on the puncture site for 5 minutes or longer in order to prevent a hematoma, which is a significant risk with arterial blood collection. (Pressure should be maintained for at least 15 minutes in patients who tend to bleed excessively, such as those who take anticoagulants or have a bleeding disorder.) A bandage is then firmly taped to the area. Inform your doctor if you feel any pain, numbness, or tingling in your hand after this procedure.

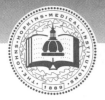

COLLECTING A URINE SAMPLE

Urine—produced by the filtration of blood through the kidneys (see page 27)—carries waste products, excess chemicals, and water out of the body. Simple and relatively inexpensive, urine tests—which include both chemical analysis and microscopic examination of the urine—can help to detect infections and other disorders of the kidneys and urinary tract, as well as some metabolic diseases unrelated to the kidneys (for example, glucose levels in the urine can help in the diagnosis of diabetes). Depending on what tests must be done, different methods may be used to collect urine. Be sure to follow your doctor's instructions carefully, since the accuracy of test results relies on proper collection of the specimen.

Random urine specimens are used for many common tests—for example, to look for glucose, blood, or white blood cells (which are a sign of infection). Random testing is quick and convenient: You are simply asked to collect a few ounces of urine in a clean, dry container. However, random urine samples may not be as reliable as timed collections (see below) for measuring substances that are excreted by the kidneys at varying rates throughout the day.

Midstream, clean-catch specimens are preferred when a kidney or bladder infection is suspected because this technique reduces the numbers of bacteria that could contaminate the sample and cause misleading results. (This method is increasingly common for random urine samples as well.) To obtain the specimen, you must first thoroughly cleanse and dry the opening of the urethra and adjacent genital area, using special antiseptic swabs or tissues. You begin urinating into the toilet, and then collect 3 or 4 ounces of urine into a sterile container from the middle point of the urine flow—called the "midstream." You

may then finish urinating into the toilet. Care should be taken not to touch the inside of the specimen container or lid.

First morning specimens are collected immediately after awakening. Because first morning urine reflects the urine produced overnight, it is typically more concentrated than samples taken later in the day and may be preferred for certain tests of kidney function.

Double-voided specimens, which obtain freshly produced urine, are typically used to measure levels of glucose (sugar) or ketones in people with diabetes (since fresh urine most accurately reflects blood levels of these substances at a particular point in time). After emptying the bladder completely, you consume a glass or two of liquid and wait 30 minutes. A second urine specimen is then collected for testing.

Timed collections are preferred over random specimens for measuring the overall kidney excretion of substances such as hormones, proteins, and electrolytes, since the concentrations of most urine constituents vary throughout the day. In this technique, urine is collected over a designated period, usually 24 hours. You begin by urinating into the toilet and noting the "start time" for the collection. From that point on, all urine is collected into a special container, which may contain a preservative and may need to be refrigerated throughout the testing period. In some instances, certain foods or drugs must be avoided during this test.

Catheter specimens may be necessary in people who are unable to urinate voluntarily—for example, due to a urethral obstruction. While you are lying down, a thin, flexible tube is inserted through the urethra and into the bladder, and urine is drained into a sterile container. This procedure may cause some discomfort, especially in men, but it only lasts a few minutes. There is a small chance that the

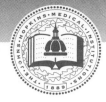

catheter will introduce bacteria into the bladder, risking a urinary tract infection that could require treatment with antibiotics.

COLLECTING A STOOL SAMPLE

Stool tests are valuable for diagnosing gastrointestinal disorders, such as intestinal bleeding, infections, and parasites. Stool may be collected once or several times over a designated period, depending on which tests are to be performed. Specimens are typically collected by the patient into a sterile container and sent promptly to the laboratory, since fresh specimens yield the most accurate results.

OTHER BODY FLUIDS

A variety of other body fluids may be examined for information about your health or to detect the presence of infection or disease. Sputum, or phlegm, is obtained by coughing into a special container. Sputum specimens typically are cultured (see page 166) to identify the cause of a respiratory infection, or they may be examined under a microscope in a microbiology or cytopathology laboratory. Other fluid samples—including cerebrospinal, pleural (from around the lungs), abdominal, and joint fluids—are obtained by needle aspiration (see page 38). These fluids may also be cultured for infectious agents, as well as examined under a microscope.

TEST RESULTS AND IMPLICATIONS

Test results from a clinical pathology laboratory are typically expressed as a number—usually, the amount of a substance found in a certain volume of body fluid (for example, a blood glucose level would be expressed as 140 milligrams of glucose per deciliter of blood, or 140 mg/dL). Occasionally, a test may be labeled either "positive" or "negative," as when screening for a particular infection. The implications of any abnormal finding depend on a variety of factors, including the accuracy of the test and the existence of other symptoms or conditions.

Reference ranges. Test results are compared to a range of "normal" or average values, known as a reference range. Because laboratory techniques, instruments, and other factors can result in significant variations in test results, each laboratory publishes its own set of reference ranges that have been specifically established for its own analytical procedures.

Many factors—including age, sex, body weight, race, and general health—can influence your results. With computers, laboratories can adjust reference ranges according to some of these parameters. However, it is important to remember that reference ranges are only guidelines—not strict separations between normal and abnormal or healthy and diseased. A "normal" value for one person may not be normal for another. In practice, reference ranges represent values for the middle 95% of a test population—which, by definition, means that 5% of healthy patients will have values that are arbitrarily categorized as abnormal.

False-positives and false-negatives. Virtually no tests can detect abnormalities with certainty, but the most reliable ones have a high degree of both sensitivity and specificity. Diagnostic *sensitivity* refers to a test's ability to detect a disease or disorder when it is in fact present. In other words, a test with a 90% sensitivity will correctly identify 90 out of 100 people with a disease; however, the other 10 people with the disease will have normal test values that are known as false-negative results. The diagnostic *specificity* of a test is its ability to appropriately exclude people who do not have a disease. If a test has a 90% specificity, it will produce normal test results in 90 out of 100 healthy people. However, the remaining 10% will have a false-positive result—that is, they will have abnormal test

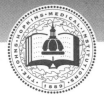

values even though no disease is present.

The diagnostic sensitivity and specificity are inherent characteristics of the test methodology, which is why research continues to develop new testing techniques that have fewer false-positive and false-negative errors. Even with the most sensitive and specific tests, a variety of other factors may cause misleading results for a particular patient. Test results may be influenced by certain foods, drugs, the time of day, stress, climate, and even your posture while the test is performed. Finally, although laboratory quality control procedures are employed to minimize avoidable errors, equipment may occasionally malfunction, and patients' specimens may sometimes be mislabeled or misidentified.

The role of your doctor. The limitations of laboratory testing make it clear that test results require the skilled interpretation of your doctor, who will view them in the context of your medical history, symptoms, overall health, and the results of other tests. For example, if you have a single abnormal test result, but all other findings are normal, your doctor will assess the likelihood that this finding reflects an underlying health problem. If he or she suspects a false-positive, the test may be repeated or an alternative test may be ordered to determine if the initial result is due to a previously unrecognized condition. By the same token, if your test results are normal, but the doctor nonetheless suspects a particular disorder, he or she may order additional tests to rule out the suspected condition.

Laboratory tests cannot always provide a definitive answer. While some tests serve as precise indicators of specific diseases, others give only general information and clues to potential underlying health problems. In many cases, combinations of several tests are required, and in other instances, comparing your current test results to previous ones—to determine any significant change over time—can be far more telling than relying on a single test value.

ANATOMICAL PATHOLOGY

Anatomical pathology involves the examination of tissue samples or cells to identify structural changes that indicate disease. Specimens are most often obtained with a biopsy, a procedure that removes a representative portion of tissue or cells from an area that appears altered due to injury or disease, or from an identifiable lesion, such as a tumor or cyst. (The term "biopsy" refers to both the procedure and the specimen itself.) Depending on the site and other factors, biopsy samples may be obtained through a needle or may require surgical removal.

Anatomic pathologists use a variety of techniques to inspect biopsy specimens, both with the naked eye and with powerful microscopes. Microscopic analysis is essential to establish a diagnosis of cancer, since malignant (cancerous) tumors exhibit microscopic features that distinguish them from benign (noncancerous) conditions. If cancer is detected, biopsies from the surrounding tissue and lymph nodes are generally done to determine whether the disease has spread. A biopsy may also be needed to determine the cause of an unexplained infection, inflammation, or other disorder.

THE BRANCHES OF ANATOMICAL PATHOLOGY

Anatomical pathology includes three major divisions: surgical pathology, cytopathology, and autopsy service.

Surgical pathology is the investigation of biopsies and other tissues that have been surgically removed. After specimens are examined with the naked eye (gross inspection), they are processed for microscopic evaluation. In some cases, surgical pathologists work with the surgeon during an operation using a technique called frozen sectioning (see page 39), which permits rapid microscopic examination of tissue. The results can be used to guide the subsequent course of the surgery.

Cytopathology is the microscopic inspection of specimens containing individual cells for changes that indicate cancer, a precancerous condition, or infection. Specimens are obtained by scraping the surface of tissues, from body fluids, or by fine needle aspiration (see page 38). Examples of cytopathology specimens include those obtained from the neck of the uterus (cervix) with a Pap smear (see page 39) and sputum samples (which are examined for the presence of cancer cells or features indicating infection).

Autopsy service is the branch of anatomical pathology involved in the examination of organs and tissues after death to establish the cause and mechanism of death, to evaluate the accuracy of diagnosis, and to assess the efficacy of therapy. A significant benefit of the autopsy examination is the potential identification of unrecognized infections and other diseases, including hereditary or familial disorders that may be pertinent to living relatives of the deceased.

TESTING TECHNOLOGIES

Anatomical pathologists use various techniques to prepare and inspect tissue and cellular specimens. Some of the primary methods are described here.

Histology is the microscopic study of tissue. After a biopsy specimen is weighed, measured, and inspected, the pathologist selects representative portions to examine under a microscope. These portions of the specimen are placed into an automatic processor where they are preserved and embedded in blocks of paraffin wax. Extremely thin slices are then cut from the block and affixed to glass microscope slides. The tissues on the slides are then stained with chemical dyes; various stains reveal different components of the tissues when examined under a microscope. Histopathologists are skilled in recognizing specific structural alterations caused by inflammation, infection, or cancer. If needed, additional portions of tissue (recuts) may be sliced from the paraffin blocks and stained with a variety of special stains for further microscopic evaluation.

Immunohistochemistry also involves processing tissue and making slides for microscopic examination, but the slides are treated with antibodies in order to detect the presence of specific antigens in the tissue specimen. (Antigens are proteins found on the surface of foreign invaders such as bacteria, viruses, or allergens, while antibodies are proteins formed by the immune system in response to particular antigens.) By observing the presence and patterns of antigen-antibody reactions in tissue specimens, the pathologist can better assess the nature and prognosis of some types of kidney disease and autoimmune disorders (which occur when the body's immune system attacks healthy tissues), or can identify a specific type of infectious agent or tumor.

Electron microscopy involves examining tissue samples under a very powerful microscope that uses a stream of electrons to produce highly magnified images on a fluorescent screen or photographic film. Because the electron microscope provides far greater magnification than standard microscopes (which use ordinary light to allow viewing of objects), pathologists can see characteristic features of some tumors, abnormal aggregations of cells and proteins in kidney disease, or evidence of viral or other infections.

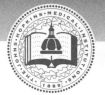

Cytology or cytopathology, the study of individual cells, is distinct from histology, which looks at collections of cells that make up tissues. Cytopathology specimens are smeared onto glass slides (fluid samples are first spun in a centrifuge to separate out the cells), and are then stained and inspected under a microscope. The cytopathologist looks for cellular and other abnormalities, paying particular attention to the size, shape, and structure of the cell nuclei, which show characteristic alterations in precancerous conditions and cancers. Cytopathology can also aid in the diagnosis of some types of infections and other disorders.

Flow cytometry is an emerging technology that uses laser light to scan cells in a flowing stream. Cells from a patient's blood or other body fluid are suspended in liquid, mixed with fluorescent-tagged antibodies that bind to specific components on the cell surfaces, and then pumped through a laser detector system for counting and measurement. Some flow technologies use multiple antibody tags and/or dyes; still others sort cells based on their size and staining characteristics, so that further analyses can be performed. The principal advantage of flow cytometry is the rapid examination of large numbers of cells to reveal detailed information about cell size and structure—even the amount and arrangement of genetic material (deoxyribonucleic acid, or DNA) within cells. Flow cytometry has broad applicability in both clinical and anatomical pathology. Assessment of immune status by flow analysis is often performed on patients with HIV infection. Flow studies can also assist in characterizing some types of malignancies and their prognoses, and can help to monitor the effectiveness of antiviral or anticancer drug therapy.

HOW BIOPSIES ARE PERFORMED

Thanks to modern surgical techniques, including minimally invasive procedures such as nee-dle biopsy, biopsy specimens can be obtained from nearly any part of the body. The most common sites are the bone marrow, breast, gastrointestinal tract, kidney, liver, lung, lymph nodes, skin, thyroid, and brain. Usually only a small sample of tissue is required. In some cases, however, a biopsy may involve total removal of a lesion; excision of a lump in the breast, for example, not only aids in diagnosis but also serves as the primary treatment.

Which of the many different techniques for performing biopsies is selected depends on the type of specimen needed and the overall health of the patient. In many cases, only a local anesthetic is required. The following are the most common biopsy procedures.

Excisional biopsy is the surgical removal of an entire lesion, such as a skin growth or breast lump. This procedure has the advantage of combining both diagnosis and treatment; however, it may require major surgery and general anesthesia. Thus, excisional biopsy is typically performed only on smaller lesions that can be easily and completely removed.

Incisional biopsy removes part of a lesion surgically or with a needle (the two types of needle biopsy are covered in more detail below). This technique is typically used when there are large, multiple, or hidden lesions. The outcome of microscopic examination determines whether subsequent, more invasive surgery is needed to remove the entire lesion.

Fine needle aspiration uses a needle and syringe to extract a small amount of cells or fluid. Frequently used in the diagnosis of breast and thyroid disease, this procedure causes less discomfort and carries fewer risks than more invasive biopsy techniques.

Needle biopsy, or core needle biopsy, is similar to fine needle aspiration, but uses a thicker needle fitted with a cutting tip to remove a larger sample of tissue for microscopic examination. An imaging technique such as ultra-

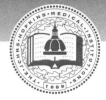

sound or CT scanning (see Chapter 2) may be used to help guide needle placement for both types of needle biopsies.

Endoscopic biopsy is performed with a thin, flexible tube called an endoscope that is inserted into a body cavity (such as the esophagus or colon) or through a small surgical incision. The endoscope is equipped with a fiberoptic system that permits the physician to see the tissue being biopsied. In addition, a forceps or other instrument can be inserted through the endoscope to remove a tissue sample for microscopic examination. This procedure typically requires sedation or local, but not general, anesthesia.

Frozen section examination allows rapid diagnosis of suspicious lesions during surgery. A specimen removed in the operating room is sent immediately to the pathology laboratory, where it is quickly frozen, cut into thin slices, and examined under a microscope. The procedure generally takes less than 10 or 15 minutes, and the results can be used to determine the subsequent course of the surgical procedure. For example, during surgery for prostate cancer, tissues surrounding the prostate are typically analyzed by a pathologist for evidence of cancer. If the cancer is still confined within the gland, the entire prostate is removed (a procedure called total prostatectomy); if, on the other hand, the disease has spread beyond the gland, alternative treatments are initiated.

Pap smear is a test named after Dr. George Papanicolaou, who devised the technique as a screening test for cancer of the uterine cervix (see page 28 of the body atlas). This test involves wiping a tiny brush and small wooden spatula over the cervix to collect cells. The cells are smeared onto a glass slide, which is sent to a laboratory for microscopic analysis. Cytotechnologists and cytopathologists then stain and examine the specimens for evidence of cancer or precancerous changes. Since its introduction and widespread use, the Pap smear has played a key role in reducing the morbidity and mortality from cervical cancer. (For more on this test, see pages 54 and 279.)

TEST RESULTS AND IMPLICATIONS

Anatomical pathology results are described in a report written by the pathologist; it begins with a detailed description of the gross inspection of the patient's specimen or specimens. The results of microscopic studies may be described more briefly, as the slides are kept indefinitely and may be re-examined at any time. The report includes a diagnosis section; when a malignancy is found, the pathologist describes the type of cancer and may comment on its likely clinical behavior.

Gross and microscopic inspection of biopsied tissues or cells can usually provide a definitive diagnosis in a broad range of disorders. Many tumors can be readily categorized as either benign or malignant; however, some cancers are more difficult to identify than others, and occasionally the biopsy results are ambiguous. For example, a specimen may contain only a small portion of the lesion or show abnormalities that are unreliable indicators that the lesion is malignant. In cases where the diagnosis is uncertain, the pathologist typically consults colleagues in an effort to obtain a consensus opinion among knowledgeable experts. Not infrequently, however, a definitive diagnosis is unachievable, and the report will note that the findings are "suspicious" or "atypical." In such instances, depending upon the specific circumstances, another biopsy or additional tests may be required.

You are entitled to obtain a copy of your pathology report. Requesting one from your doctor can help you become a more educated patient and allow you to make better treatment decisions with your doctor.

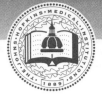

DIAGNOSTIC IMAGING

For centuries, medical science drew almost all of its knowledge about the inner structure and workings of the human body from surgery or autopsy studies. Up until the late 1900s doctors had little more than the thermometer and the stethoscope to help them pinpoint the source of a health problem; medical diagnoses were largely based on a patient's description of symptoms and physical examination. But in 1895 the German physicist Wilhelm Conrad Roentgen made a serendipitous discovery that soon transformed the practice of medicine: He observed that a form of invisible radiation called x-rays could penetrate solid objects, including the human body, to create a photographic image. The subsequent development of x-ray machines allowed doctors to peer inside the human body for the first time without using a scalpel.

Some of the initial uses for x-ray machines were to detect broken bones, lung disorders such as tuberculosis, and foreign objects in the body. As early as 1898, for example, the U.S. Army used x-rays to pinpoint the location of bone fractures and bullets in soldiers wounded during the Spanish-American War. The introduction of contrast dyes in the early decades of the 20th century greatly extended the diagnostic potential of x-rays. These agents are used to fill various body cavities, rendering them opaque to x-rays and bringing specific organs more sharply into view. This advance allowed doctors to view the gastrointestinal tract, gallbladder, kidneys, and urinary tract for the first time.

Continued refinements to x-rays, as well as the numerous other imaging techniques that are currently available, have provided ever more sophisticated information about the structure and function of our internal organs, enabling physicians today to diagnose many health problems earlier and in a noninvasive or minimally invasive fashion. In addition, these imaging techniques have revolutionized treatment by allowing doctors to assess patients before surgery, perform less invasive operations guided by images of internal structures transmitted to a television screen, and monitor the effects of therapy on the course of an illness. This chapter will review all of the major techniques used to visualize the body's internal structures.

RADIOGRAPHY

Radiography is the medical term that describes the use of x-rays to visualize the internal structures of the human body. Like light and radio waves, x-rays are a form of electromagnetic radiation; because of their high energy and short wavelength, they can easily penetrate body tissues.

Diagnostic radiography is a noninvasive procedure using a machine that produces x-rays by passing an electrical current under high voltage in a vacuum tube. The body region being examined is positioned between an x-ray tube and a sheet of photographic film. As the x-rays pass through body tissues, they form an image on the film in varying degrees of dark and light, depending on the amount of radiation absorbed by each tissue. Denser tissues, such as bone, block more of the rays and appear white on x-ray film. Conversely, tissues filled with air or gas, such as the lungs or intestines, allow x-rays to pass through easily and thus appear very dark or black on the film. Muscles, tendons, nerves, blood vessels, and intestines and other inter-

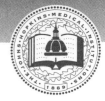

nal organs of intermediate density are seen as varying shades of gray.

Different views of anatomic structures can be obtained by changing the orientation of the x-ray machine relative to the body part being examined. The most common angles are the anteroposterior view, in which the x-rays enter the body from the front and exit through the back, and the lateral view, in which the x-rays penetrate the body from the side. X-rays are also sometimes passed through the body from back to front (posteroanterior view) or from an oblique angle.

Major uses. Plain x-ray films—that is, films taken without the use of contrast dyes—can provide valuable information about the bones, skull, abdomen, and chest. For example, a bone fracture or spinal deformity, such as scoliosis (curvature of the spine), can be seen clearly on a plain x-ray. Also, x-ray pictures of the lungs are easy to interpret because the air spaces within the lungs are more transparent to radiation than denser lung tissues. The presence of a lighter shadow on the dark region of the lungs, for instance, can reveal a lung disorder such as a tumor or tuberculosis.

Refinements. *Contrast dyes* are employed to enhance the images of internal organs that are not readily viewed on plain x-ray films. These agents are not precisely dyes, but rather materials which are opaque to x-rays. Barium sulfate, for example, is introduced directly into the gastrointestinal tract to visualize the esophagus, stomach, and intestine. Iodine-based contrast dyes are administered by injection to delineate structures such as the kidneys, gallbladder, and blood vessels (the latter is a procedure termed angiography, described on page 42). Computed tomography (see page 43) also greatly expands the applications of radiography by using computers to combine several x-ray images and translate this information into two-dimensional, cross-sectional views of the body.

In addition, advances in digital technology have greatly enhanced the information provided by conventional x-rays, such as mammograms (see page 255). Digital images can also be easily sent to other computers so that many experts can share the information rapidly and assist in diagnosis.

Risks and drawbacks. The major disadvantage of x-rays—and other imaging techniques based on x-rays, including fluoroscopy, angiography, and computed tomography—is that they expose patients to ionizing radiation, which poses some health risks. Since the introduction of the first x-ray machines, however, significant advances in technology have markedly reduced the amount of radiation emitted during routine x-ray examinations. For example, x-rays of the head currently expose patients to only about 2% of the radiation delivered during similar tests in the early days of their use.

Although the amount of radiation from plain x-rays is considered harmless for most patients, there are some significant exceptions. For instance, exposing a developing fetus to x-rays can cause birth defects, and radiation can damage the male sperm and female eggs, leading to genetic defects in offspring. In general, women should not have an x-ray exam during pregnancy unless it is absolutely essential for medical reasons. If an x-ray is deemed necessary, a lead apron is placed over the woman's abdomen to shield her fetus from radiation. To prevent radiation damage to the reproductive organs during various x-ray procedures, a lead shield may be placed over the ovaries in women or testicles in men. In addition, because frequent exposure to ionizing radiation over a period of time has a cumulative effect that raises the risk of cancer, certain routine x-ray screening tests, such as an annual chest x-ray exam, are no

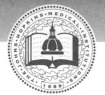

longer recommended. Others, such as mammography, are still recommended because the important information yielded by the test is considered worth the radiation risk.

The contrast dyes used during certain x-ray examinations may pose additional risks. People allergic to seafood, which is rich in iodine, may experience a serious allergic reaction to the iodine-based contrast agents used in some x-ray studies. In addition, excretion of the contrast dye may cause kidney damage in individuals who already have impaired kidney function. These potential risks must be balanced against the valuable information that x-rays can yield; in most cases, the possible benefits clearly outweigh the risks.

FLUOROSCOPY

The variation of x-ray technology known as fluoroscopy was developed soon after Roentgen's initial discovery. With subsequent refinements, it has evolved into an essential diagnostic tool. In this noninvasive procedure, a continuous beam of x-rays is passed through the body and projected onto a television screen to provide real-time images of internal structures in motion. These images may also be recorded on film or videotape for later analysis

Major uses. Fluoroscopy may be performed alone to observe the function and movement of the lungs, diaphragm, or other structures in the chest during breathing. It may also be used to assist in a wide variety of diagnostic or therapeutic procedures that require placement of a needle or catheter. For example, fluoroscopic guidance helps to ensure accurate tissue sampling during needle biopsies. Doctors may also use fluoroscopy to accurately guide a catheter into selected arteries, and then to track the flow of contrast dye as it circulates through the vessels, during angiography. In addition, fluoroscopy may be employed to track contrast agents during

studies of the upper and lower gastrointestinal tract, spinal cord, uterus, or joints.

Refinements. When first introduced, fluoroscopy required the use of fluorescent screens and special glasses so a doctor could view the images in real time, and both doctor and patient were exposed to somewhat high doses of radiation during the test. By the 1960s, the old fluorescent system was largely replaced by a combination of an x-ray image intensifier, which allows a reduction in radiation exposure, and a television camera and monitor. A more recent modification is a high-speed version of the technology called *cinefluorography,* which allows doctors to image the working heart and its blood vessels once a catheter has been inserted using standard fluoroscopy.

Risks and drawbacks. Although x-rays are generated constantly during fluoroscopy, this radiation is emitted at a lower intensity compared to conventional x-rays. Nonetheless, in certain procedures—specifically, invasive medical tests that take more than one hour—patients may be exposed to a significant amount of radiation. If contrast dyes are used during fluoroscopy, they may pose additional risks (which are discussed above, under radiography).

ANGIOGRAPHY

Because arteries and veins are not readily observed with standard radiography, a contrast dye must be injected to opacify them on x-ray film. This technique, called angiography, permits examination of blood vessels throughout the body; it is also known as arteriography (when used to view the arteries) and venography (when used to view the veins). Angiography is more invasive and carries more risk than plain x-rays because it requires inserting a thin tube, or catheter, into a blood vessel (a procedure called catheterization) in order to introduce the contrast dye. Once the material has entered the bloodstream, the vessels are

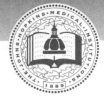

visualized by fluoroscopy and the images recorded digitally or on x-ray film.

Major uses. Angiography can be used to examine blood vessels in the heart, liver and spleen, kidney, lungs, brain, and lower extremities. In one common procedure, coronary angiography (see page 140), a catheter is threaded into an artery in the groin or arm and carefully guided to the coronary arteries of the heart. After the injection of a contrast dye, fluoroscopy is used to study these vessels. This test provides valuable information about coronary blood flow, including the location and extent of artery-blocking plaques (atherosclerosis), and is now considered the definitive test for coronary artery disease. A similar procedure, cerebral angiography, is used to help detect plaques or other lesions in the major arteries supplying blood to the brain.

Refinements. A recently developed procedure, called *magnetic resonance angiography,* offers much promise as a potential noninvasive alternative to x-ray-based angiography. This technique is discussed on page 44, under magnetic resonance imaging.

Risks. Although angiography is generally considered a safe and accurate technique for evaluating blood vessel disease, the procedure does carry certain risks. These include bleeding or infection at the site of catheter insertion; allergic reaction to the contrast dye (see page 42); kidney damage caused by excretion of the contrast agent; abnormal heart rhythms (arrhythmias); blood clot formation; and catheter-induced damage to a blood vessel. Certain procedures—particularly cerebral or coronary angiography—carry a small risk of provoking a stroke or a heart attack (and thus are always performed in a hospital room where emergency equipment is available). Because of these risks, doctors usually reserve angiography for situations in which they cannot derive the necessary information from other, less invasive procedures. For example, coronary angiography is essential for evaluating blockages in the arteries that supply blood to the heart prior to coronary bypass surgery.

COMPUTED TOMOGRAPHY

Computed tomography—known as CT or CAT scanning—is a powerful, noninvasive imaging test that was invented in 1972 by applying computer technology and digital imaging techniques to traditional x-ray studies. In this test, an x-ray tube revolves around the patient and directs x-rays through internal structures at many different angles. A computer then combines the information derived from the multiple x-rays to construct highly detailed, two-dimensional, cross-sectional images of particular organs or regions of the body (which appear as slices through the structure being studied). A contrast dye—either oral or intravenous, depending on the area being examined—is sometimes used to help distinguish between different tissues or organs.

Major uses. CT scanning can detect lesions or other abnormalities that cannot be seen with plain x-rays. It is considered the method of choice for examining the chest and area between the lungs (mediastinum), the upper abdomen, and the peritoneal cavity (which surrounds the organs of the abdomen), and is also useful for studying the brain and spine. In particular, CT scanning is considered highly accurate for detecting tumors, abscesses, accumulations of fluid, and organ injury. It is also a preferred imaging technique for guiding needle biopsies and introducing tubes that are used to drain abscesses.

Refinements. The speed and resolution of CT scanners have improved significantly since their introduction. Faster scanning can eliminate artifacts on the x-ray film caused by patient movement and produces excellent images with small amounts of radiation. A

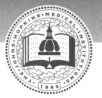
newer CT technology, dubbed *electron-beam or ultrafast CT scanning,* can even visualize moving organs (such as the beating heart) by taking pictures so quickly that the image distortion caused by motion, a problem with conventional CT scans, is avoided. This test is particularly useful for detecting calcium associated with plaques in the coronary arteries of the heart (see page 179). The role of ultrafast CT scanning in screening for early coronary artery disease is now being evaluated.

Helical or spiral CT scanning, a refinement that was introduced in 1989, allows for continuous imaging as the examining table slides through the scanning unit, dramatically cutting the amount of time needed for the procedure. This approach permits radiologists to fully scan the lungs and other body structures in 20 to 30 seconds as you hold your breath. Because it is quick and easy and can identify very small abnormalities in the lungs, helical CT scanning is currently being investigated as a possible screening test for lung cancer.

Risks and drawbacks. Because a large number of images are taken during a CT scan, the total amount of radiation delivered to the patient is typically greater than that delivered by a conventional x-ray (though it may sometimes be less). As with x-rays, the contrast dyes used during certain CT procedures may pose additional risks (see page 42). And, since CT scanning takes place in a narrow, tunnel-like structure, people who are claustrophobic may find it difficult to undergo this procedure.

MAGNETIC RESONANCE IMAGING

Magnetic resonance imaging (MRI)—a potent imaging tool that came into general use in the mid-1980s—is a noninvasive procedure that takes advantage of the fact that the body is filled with small biological magnets, including the proton in the nucleus of the hydrogen

atom. When a person lies inside an MRI unit, a strong magnetic field causes protons in the body to align themselves in a particular direction. The MRI machine then stimulates the body with radio waves to alter the protons' orientation. When the radio-wave stimulation stops, the protons return to their original state, emitting weak radio signals that reflect the properties of the organ or other internal structures being studied. A computer then translates these signals into highly detailed, cross-sectional images (which, like CT images, appear as slices through the organs).

Major uses. Like CT scans, MRI provides superior detail compared to conventional x-rays—and MRI is significantly better than CT for delineating soft tissues in the body, particularly in organs that are not in constant motion. (X-rays and CT scans may be better for imaging bones.) Thus, MRI is an excellent method for studying the brain, spinal cord, and the cartilage and ligaments in large joints such as the knee, hip, shoulder, and temporomandibular joint in the jaw.

Refinements. A refinement of MRI termed *magnetic resonance angiography* (MRA) was introduced in the early 1990s and has since evolved into a promising noninvasive test for imaging the coronary arteries and evaluating heart disease. Unlike standard angiography, MRA does not require the insertion of a catheter: The weakly magnetic contrast dyes used in this procedure, such as gadolinium, can be injected into a vein in your arm. In addition, these agents are not toxic to the kidneys, as are the iodine-based contrast dyes typically used in angiographic studies. Besides visualizing the coronary arteries, MRA can also be used to image arteries in the brain, chest, abdomen, and lower extremities. While it is not yet widely available, MRA is the subject of intense research and its use will likely grow in the future.

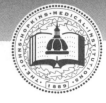

Another form of MRI, called *functional MRI* (fMRI), can furnish information about microscopic changes in blood flow to different areas within an organ as the organ performs its normal functions. In particular, fMRI may help to determine which regions of the brain are involved as a person performs a certain task or is exposed to particular stimuli. With fMRI and positron emission tomography (see page 47), imaging technology has moved beyond simply visualizing organs and tissues to offer a glimpse of how they work.

Risks and drawbacks. People who experience claustrophobia may find it difficult to undergo an MRI exam, which takes place in a narrow, tunnel-like structure. Severely overweight individuals (over 300 lbs) may also be unable to undergo the test. In some cases, a larger unit that is open on several sides (open MRI scanner) may be used as an alternative; however, open MRI units are associated with poorer image quality than standard MRI scanners. Because the MRI scanner generates a strong magnetic field, the exam cannot be performed on people who have certain types of internally placed metallic devices, such as pacemakers, inner ear implants, or intracranial aneurysm clips. In addition, MRI is more costly than CT scanning. It is not commonly done in pregnant women because the long-term effects of MRI on the fetus are unknown.

ULTRASONOGRAPHY

Ultrasonography is a noninvasive technique that uses high-frequency sound waves, or ultrasound, to examine various internal structures in the body. Arising out of the sonar technology that was originally developed to detect enemy submarines and other underwater objects, ultrasound was first used for medical purposes shortly after World War II.

In a typical ultrasound study, a small device called a transducer is placed against the skin near the organ or structures being examined. As the physician moves the transducer over the area, it emits high-frequency sound waves that penetrate the region. The sound waves are then reflected back to the transducer, where they are electronically converted by a computer into detailed, two-dimensional pictures that are displayed on a viewing monitor. In some cases, a series of images may be obtained to show an organ in motion over a period of time. The images may then be recorded on film or video as a permanent record.

Major uses. Although ultrasound is essentially risk free and is much less expensive than either CT or MRI, it is not always as accurate as these other techniques. It is most useful for examining soft tissue that cannot be easily seen on x-rays—particularly organs that are uniform and solid (such as the liver) or fluid-filled (such as the gallbladder); other common sites include the abdominal and reproductive organs, urinary tract, heart, and thyroid gland. Ultrasound is especially helpful for studying the heart, because it allows a physician to evaluate its thickness, size, and function, as well as the motion and structure of the four heart valves. It is commonly used for guidance during needle biopsies and the introduction of drainage catheters, and also has an essential role in pregnancy because it avoids exposing the fetus to ionizing radiation.

Refinements. Doppler technology has significantly extended the applications of conventional ultrasound by allowing doctors to examine blood flow in various blood vessels, such as the carotid arteries. In *Doppler ultrasound,* the movement of red blood cells through a vessel distorts the frequency of the ultrasound waves; this change in frequency corresponds to the velocity of blood flow. The reflected sound waves are then converted into audible sounds and graphic wave recordings. An enhancement of this technique, called

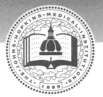

color Doppler ultrasound, uses different colors to demonstrate the speed and direction of blood flow. *Duplex ultrasound,* which combines Doppler and standard imaging ultrasonography, provides the most detailed information about the blood vessels. It is increasingly being used to screen major arteries for blockages and to detect aneurysms (abnormal outpouchings of a blood vessel wall).

Intracavitary ultrasound procedures—which introduce an ultrasound transducer inside a body cavity—are being used with growing frequency. For example, transvaginal ultrasound (see page 285) can evaluate pelvic malignancies in women, while transrectal ultrasound is valuable for assisting in prostate biopsy (see page 300). In a modification called transesophageal echocardiography (see page 365), a transducer is passed down the esophagus and placed directly behind the heart to assess its function.

Risks. There are no known risks associated with ultrasonography itself, but some slight risks may be associated with placing a transducer within the body; for example, transesophageal echocardiography may cause a sore throat or esophageal bleeding.

NUCLEAR SCANNING

Nuclear scans are imaging studies performed after a small amount of radioactive material—which may be referred to as a radioisotope, radionuclide, radiopharmaceutical, or radiotracer—has been injected into a vein or taken orally. First used during the 1950s to study thyroid disease, nuclear scans provide important insights into an organ's function as well as its anatomy. This functional information allows nuclear scans to detect certain medical disorders much sooner than other imaging exams, which provide primarily anatomic information.

In a typical nuclear scan, a trace amount of a radioisotope (such as technetium or thallium) is injected into a vein, and the gamma rays emitted by the radioactive material are measured by a special detector called a gamma scintillation camera. A computer is used to translate this information into two-dimensional images, which are recorded on film. Nuclear scanning relies on the fact that particular radioisotopes are normally absorbed and concentrated in specific tissues at a known rate over a designated time period. Changes in the normal rate of absorption can indicate possible disease, such as a tumor, inflammation, infection, or injury. Different radiotracers are used to image different organs.

Major uses. Nuclear scans have numerous applications, including the detection of cancer (both primary tumors and metastases) in various organs; evaluation of heart function; diagnosis of gallbladder disease, pulmonary embolism (a blood clot in the lungs), and gastrointestinal bleeding; and determining the life span of red blood cells. Among the organs that can be examined by nuclear scanning are the bones, heart, lungs, kidneys and bladder, thyroid, and gallbladder.

Refinements. Over the years, the development of additional radiotracers that target specific organs has extended the range of nuclear scanning. Today, there are almost 100 different nuclear scanning procedures that provide information about nearly every major organ system in the body. In the future, more radiotracers should become available to target, and aid in the early diagnosis of, specific cancers.

A refinement of nuclear scanning called *single photon emission computed tomography* (SPECT) uses the single gamma rays emitted by certain radionuclides, such as technetium-99m, iodine-123, and indium-111. In this study, the scanning camera is rotated around the body, and computer methods similar to those used in CT scanning are employed to produce enhanced images of tracer distribution in multiple organ sections.

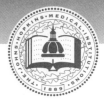

SPECT studies are used to examine the heart and blood flow in the brain.

Risks and drawbacks. In general, nuclear scanning is safe and often avoids the need for more dangerous and invasive procedures. For most people, exposure to the small amount of radioactive material used in these procedures poses no significant risks. Radioactive tracers, however, should not be given to pregnant women because of possible risks to the fetus. In extremely rare cases, patients may be hypersensitive to the radiopharmaceutical and experience an adverse reaction.

POSITRON EMISSION TOMOGRAPHY

First employed as a research tool, positron emission tomography (PET) has been used for medical diagnosis since the mid-1980s, and is steadily becoming more commonplace. Like nuclear scanning, PET measures the uptake and distribution of radioactive material by specific regions of the body—but the radioisotopes employed in PET scans emit positrons, or positively charged electrons. By incorporating these radioisotopes into a chemical compound such as glucose, oxygen, or certain drugs, PET scans are able to assess chemical functions in body tissues and organs—particularly body processes such as blood flow and metabolism. Thus, like functional MRI, PET scans can provide information not only about the structure of organs or tissues, but also about how they work.

In this noninvasive procedure, the radioactively tagged chemical is administered by injection, and you enter a PET scanner (which resembles a CT scanner). Special radiation detectors are used to record the pattern of distribution of the radioactive material. (In some cases, when the brain is being scanned, you may be asked to perform certain cognitive activities, such as math problems, during the test.) This data is then sent to a computer, which generates two-dimensional, color-coded images that reveal which areas of the organ are active.

Major uses. While PET can track biochemical changes and visualize any region of the body, it is currently used only on a limited basis because it is costly and requires sophisticated laboratory facilities and a team of highly trained specialists. As yet, the added value of the information provided by PET in most cases is not clear. Most often, the technique is used to help doctors examine how specific areas of the brain work, detect certain types of cancer, evaluate the amount of muscle damage after a heart attack, and assess the effectiveness of chemotherapy drugs on specific tissues.

Refinements. PET is a developing technology that will undoubtedly become more commonplace as improved techniques become less costly and more convenient. Researchers hope one day to use the test as an aid in the diagnosis of disorders such as transient ischemic attacks ("mini-strokes"), Alzheimer's disease, Parkinson's disease, multiple sclerosis, and various psychiatric disorders that may produce altered patterns of glucose metabolism in the brain.

Risks. For most people, exposure to the trace amount of radioactive material used in this test poses no significant risks. Radioactive isotopes, however, should not be given to pregnant women because of possible risks to the fetus. In extremely rare cases, patients may be hypersensitive to the radiochemical and experience an adverse reaction. Because the scan takes place in a narrow, tunnel-like structure, people who experience claustrophobia may find it difficult to undergo this procedure.

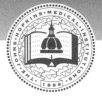

SCREENING FOR DISEASE

In recent years, both medical practitioners and the public have become increasingly aware of the importance of preventive medicine. Research has repeatedly confirmed an association between lifestyle and health and shown the benefits of adopting healthy habits—such as regular exercise, good nutrition, avoidance of smoking, and stress reduction. The evidence is unquestionable: These lifestyle measures can reduce your risk of developing chronic diseases and help you live a longer, healthier life.

An equally prevalent, if more controversial, issue is the role of screening tests for the early detection of disease. A screening test can be defined as any type of health evaluation—including labwork, physical exams, and imaging procedures such as x-rays—that is intended to identify potential health problems in people who have no signs or symptoms of disease. (Diagnostic tests, on the other hand, are performed to identify the problem in people who are already experiencing symptoms—for example, dizziness, abdominal discomfort, or chest pain.)

While an increasing number of screening tests have been developed in the past several decades, these tests have brought a new understanding of the potential costs and harms associated with their overuse. For example, some screening interventions themselves have slight but definite risks. Sigmoidoscopy—a procedure that involves the insertion of a viewing instrument into the rectum and colon so a doctor can look for abnormalities—can identify and remove precancerous polyps or early-stage tumors before colorectal cancer has spread and become life-threatening; however, this invasive procedure carries a small risk of

bowel perforation that requires surgical repair. Whether or not this test is appropriate depends on a number of factors—your age, risk factors, and family history of colorectal cancer, to name a few. While periodic sigmoidoscopy would make good sense in a 50-year-old man with a family history of colorectal cancer, it would be inappropriate for a woman in her 30s with no family history of the disease.

In fact, the usefulness of many screening tests is a matter of continuing debate: Is the test accurate? Does it improve outcomes, reduce suffering, and save lives? Or does the test cause more harm than good? These questions must be resolved by experts before any screening test can be widely accepted as valuable. This chapter discusses the current issues surrounding screening tests—including their limitations, potential benefits and risks, and when they are worth having.

THE IDEAL BEHIND SCREENING

The ultimate goal of any screening test is to catch a disease in its earliest and most treatable stages—and thus to increase the likelihood of effective therapy, forestall the complications associated with advanced disease, and even provide a cure in some cases. To be useful, a screening test must accurately detect a disease; there must be effective treatments available; and early intervention must be able to either reduce suffering or save lives.

One example of a widely successful screening test is blood pressure measurement with a device called a sphygmomanometer. When performed correctly, this simple test can accurately identify people with high blood pressure (hypertension)—which often causes no symptoms—in a timely manner. Prompt

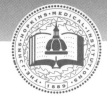

management with lifestyle modifications and antihypertensive medications may then help to ward off potentially life-threatening complications, such as stroke, heart disease, and vision loss. Another example, the Pap smear—a simple test to detect abnormal cells in the lower part of the uterus, or cervix—can identify early-stage cervical cancer, which is almost always curable by surgery. This simple and inexpensive test can certainly save lives. Despite these benefits, however, experts still disagree on how often a Pap smear should be done.

THE POTENTIAL DRAWBACKS OF SCREENING

Even the most valuable screening interventions have limits. To begin with, even highly reliable tests can never be 100% accurate. Screening tests typically produce a certain number of *false-negatives,* meaning that the disease is present, but the test result falls within the normal range. The main danger in these cases is that you may be falsely reassured and lulled into making uninformed medical decisions, such as postponing a doctor's visit when symptoms do appear. For example, a resting electrocardiogram or ECG (see page 174) cannot detect most cases of coronary artery disease. It would be a mistake, however, to ignore chest pain just because a recent resting ECG was normal. Another possibility is a *false-positive,* meaning the test result is abnormal even though you do not have the disease. Such false alarms may cause a great deal of anxiety and lead to further unnecessary testing to exclude the diagnosis. (For more on false-negatives and false-positives, see page 35.)

Indeed, it is important to remember that screening tests alone are usually insufficient to provide a diagnosis—in general, a positive result will lead to additional, and often more invasive, diagnostic tests. For example, many cancer screening tests (such as a Pap smear) are designed to identify the possible presence of cancer, but further procedures, such as a biopsy to obtain tissue samples for microscopic examination, are needed to confirm or rule out a diagnosis and to determine the extent of the problem. Even if the screening test itself is risk-free, these follow-up procedures may pose some risks.

Finally, it is important to remember that even the most accurate screening tests offer little benefit if early diagnosis and treatment do not influence the outcome of a disease. For example, early detection of some cancers (when they are still localized and can be surgically excised) may lead to a cure; in other types of cancer, survival rates are similar whether the disease is identified promptly or in its later stages. Advancing the diagnosis of such conditions would only lead to earlier stress and worry for the patient. And certainly, there is no advantage to early diagnosis for a disease that has no effective therapy (such as Huntington's disease).

WHEN IS A SCREENING TEST APPROPRIATE?

Before the usefulness of any screening test can be considered decisive, it must be examined in a large-scale scientific study known as a randomized clinical trial. These studies are designed to prove that a test is accurate and that its use can reduce disability and prolong life. Carrying the most weight are well-designed trials that randomly assign people either to be screened or not to be screened with a specific test; results indicating an improved outcome in the screened group provide the best support for widespread use of the test. Unfortunately, however, such large-scale studies have yet to be performed for screening tests commonly used for many disorders.

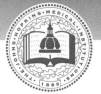

In addition, study results suggesting that a particular screening test improves survival may be misleading, especially when available therapy cannot markedly alter the course of a particular illness. For example, if the average period between diagnosis and death for a specific disorder is four years, and screening detects the condition three years earlier than usual, the results could be interpreted as indicating that the screening test had extended survival from four to seven years. However, in such cases the apparent impact of the screening test on survival would be illusory—screening just allowed the disease to be detected earlier than usual, but the end result is the same.

In the absence of reliable clinical trial data, the following criteria are generally accepted to establish the utility of a screening test:

• The test should screen for a common condition that produces significant disability and mortality.

• It must be able to detect the disease before symptoms appear.

• It must detect a condition for which early intervention can improve the outcome.

• It must be accurate: It should be both highly sensitive (few false-negative results) and highly specific (few false-positive results).

• It should be generally safe and preferably noninvasive.

• It should be widely available and have a reasonable cost.

At present, only a limited number of screening tests are recommended for use in the general population. These include blood pressure and blood lipid measurements, vision and hearing exams, and certain screening tests for colon, breast, and prostate cancer. Many other tests are considered beneficial when they are targeted at selected individuals in certain groups, primarily people at high risk for a particular disease. For example, the test for uri-

nary cystine levels, though highly accurate, is not used in the general population because cystinuria, the disorder it detects, is quite rare. Rather, this screening test is reserved for people who are more likely to have the disease because of their family history. In general, groups that may be targeted for more aggressive screening measures include those with a family history of a particular disease; environmental exposure that increases the risk of developing a disease (for example, workers who have been exposed to asbestos are at increased risk for lung cancer); and pregnant women.

In certain cases, widespread screening may be recommended for a rare disease—despite a lack of scientific evidence for the benefit of screening—if the disease has severe consequences and effective treatment is available. For example, most infants are now screened at birth for the rare disorder phenylketonuria for two reasons: the disorder can be identified simply with a blood test, and treatment during the first days of life (by excluding the amino acid phenylalanine from the diet) can prevent irreversible mental retardation.

If you have any questions about whether you need or might benefit from a particular screening test, consult your physician. He or she will be able to help you make informed decisions that are tailored to your particular circumstances.

GENERAL SCREENING GUIDELINES

Many different health organizations and groups of experts have issued their own guidelines for various screening tests. Among the recommendations that have received the most attention are those of the U.S. Preventive Services Task Force, the American Cancer Society, the American College of Physicians, the National Cholesterol Education Program, and the Canadian Task Force on the Periodic Health Exam-

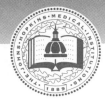

ination. The U.S. Task Force is a government-sponsored group of experts who have reviewed evidence on the usefulness of different measures, including screening, for preventing various illnesses. With the stated goal of preventing disease while avoiding unnecessary testing, this group issued its first report in 1989 and an updated version in 1996.

The guidelines provided by these organizations often differ, particularly regarding the age at which screening should begin and the frequency of testing. In general, a group with a primary focus on a particular disease is apt to issue more far-reaching screening recommendations for that disorder. For example, the American Cancer Society, whose principal goal is to detect the greatest number of cancers, is more aggressive in some of its cancer screening guidelines than other organizations. The U.S. Task Force, on the other hand, tends to use the most stringent criteria to evaluate the effectiveness of various screening tests.

In general, doctors use their clinical judgment when applying these screening recommendations to individual patients. Doctors consider such factors as your age, risk factors, any coexisting disorders, and your attitude about various outcomes and potential side effects of different screening tests. As a rule, screening is more important in older adults and in those at high risk for a disease. For example, you are more likely to benefit from a screening test if you have a family or personal history of a particular disease; have known risk factors; or carry a particular genetic mutation that increases your susceptibility to the illness.

COMMONLY PERFORMED SCREENING TESTS

The following are the screening tests most often performed in the general population. Included are the current recommendations issued by various major organizations regarding when and how often they should be performed.

Blood pressure measurement. Hypertension—usually defined as a blood pressure value higher than 140/90 millimeters of mercury (mm Hg)—is a leading risk factor for stroke, coronary artery disease, congestive heart failure, kidney disease, and vision problems—serious disorders that account for substantial morbidity and mortality. Approximately 1 in 5 Americans have hypertension, and the disorder is more common in African Americans and older adults. Lowering high blood pressure with dietary measures, exercise, and antihypertensive drugs clearly decreases the risk of death from stroke, kidney disease, and heart disease. Thus, screening people without symptoms for hypertension can produce important benefits.

Measuring blood pressure with a sphygmomanometer is simple and highly accurate when performed correctly. However, such factors as equipment error, misreading of values by the doctor, and patient anxiety or changes in posture can all produce inaccurate results. It is generally recommended that hypertension should only be diagnosed based on the average of two or more readings taken at each of two or more visits after an initial screening.

The U.S. Task Force and the American Heart Association recommend screening of all children and adults for hypertension. Most guidelines advise that people with normal blood pressure have their pressure rechecked at least every two years. Those with elevated values should have their blood pressure measured more frequently, ranging from monthly to annually depending on the specific reading.

Blood cholesterol measurement. The accumulation of cholesterol in artery walls plays a primary role in the buildup of plaques that block arteries and decrease blood flow to major organs (a process called atherosclerosis). Abnor-

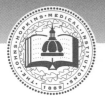

mal blood cholesterol is considered a major risk factor for coronary artery disease (CAD), and research shows that middle-aged and older men who lower their cholesterol levels with lifestyle modifications and/or medications can significantly reduce their risk of CAD and heart attack. While there are less data regarding women and younger men, most experts agree that keeping cholesterol levels in the normal range is the prudent course for all individuals.

Blood lipids (or fats) such as cholesterol are carried on several lipoproteins, each with a different effect on CAD risk. For example, low-density lipoprotein (LDL or "bad") cholesterol and triglycerides both promote atherosclerosis. High-density lipoprotein (HDL or "good") cholesterol, on the other hand, protects against CAD by removing cholesterol deposits from artery walls; a high HDL cholesterol level can help to counteract the negative impact of elevated LDL cholesterol and triglycerides. Page 238 covers a complete lipid profile and the target levels recommended by the National Cholesterol Education Program (NCEP).

Although the incidence of CAD is low in men younger than 35 and in premenopausal women, it climbs rapidly during middle age for both men and women. The NCEP recommends periodic cholesterol screening for all adults starting at age 20. Most experts advise having your cholesterol checked every five years; screening may be performed more frequently if the cholesterol level is elevated in you or your family members, or in the presence of CAD, peripheral vascular disease, diabetes, or a history of stroke. Because heart disease risk is determined not only by total cholesterol levels but also by the levels of HDL and LDL cholesterol and triglycerides, the NCEP now recommends that the initial screening test for all healthy adults should measure these important cholesterol components as well as total cholesterol levels.

Blood glucose measurement. Diabetes mellitus is a disorder marked by chronically high levels of blood sugar (glucose). According to the American Diabetes Association (ADA), type 2 diabetes—which usually develops in individuals over age 30—is nearing epidemic proportions because of the increasing number of older Americans and the greater prevalence of obesity and sedentary lifestyles. Some experts believe that earlier diagnosis and treatment (with dietary changes, exercise, and, if necessary, glucose-lowering medications) may help to prevent or forestall long-term complications of diabetes, which include damage to the kidneys, eyes, nerves, and heart.

The ADA currently recommends that physicians consider testing blood glucose levels (see page 210) in all adults age 45 and older every three years to screen for diabetes. More frequent screening, starting at a younger age, should be considered for those at especially high risk for the disease. (Major risk factors for type 2 diabetes include a family history of the disease, obesity, physical inactivity, and being in high-risk ethnic groups, including African Americans, Hispanics, and Native Americans.) At present, however, the U.S. Task Force believes there is insufficient evidence to recommend routine diabetes screening in adults without symptoms of high blood glucose (such as excessive thirst and urination).

Vision examination. An eye exam by an optometrist or ophthalmologist will check your eye movements, peripheral vision, and visual acuity (or sharpness of vision). An instrument called an ophthalmoscope enables the examiner to view the interior structures of the eye. In addition, a device called a tonometer (see page 362) may be used to measure the pressure inside the eyeball as a test for glaucoma, a condition marked by increased pressure within the eye that can lead to vision loss.

Common vision problems in adults include

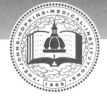

presbyopia (an inability of the eye to focus sharply on nearby objects), glaucoma, macular degeneration (a deterioration of the retinal cells that leads to progressive loss of vision), and cataracts (clouding of the lens that produces blurred vision). The U.S. Task Force recommends that all older adults receive regular screening with the Snellen visual acuity chart (see page 387). Most experts advise that adults without symptoms have eye exams every five years and more frequently after age 50. The exam should be conducted by an eye care specialist who can detect early changes of glaucoma before irreversible vision loss begins.

Hearing examination. In older adults, the U.S. Task Force recommends that primary care physicians screen for hearing impairment by interviewing patients during regular check-ups, counseling them about the availability of hearing aid devices, and referring them to hearing specialists when abnormalities are detected.

Colon cancer screening. Colorectal cancer is the second leading cause of cancer-related deaths in the U.S. Early detection is critical because a full recovery is likely if precancerous polyps and early-stage cancers are detected and removed before they produce symptoms. (Cancer discovered while it remains confined to the top layer of the colon or rectum is 95% treatable.) At present, the two major screening tests for early detection of colorectal cancer are the fecal occult blood test (FOBT) and flexible sigmoidoscopy.

• **Fecal occult blood test.** The FOBT (see page 199) checks for blood in a sample of your stool, since bleeding from cancerous growths or precancerous polyps in your colon may lead to stools containing trace amounts of blood that cannot be seen with the naked eye. The FOBT is most often performed using a home test kit with simple instructions; you will bring the stool specimens to your doctor or a testing laboratory. In the laboratory, the specimens are examined for the presence of blood with a chemical test. The American Cancer Society, American College of Physicians, and the U.S. Task Force all recommend annual testing with the FOBT for all adults starting at age 50.

• **Flexible sigmoidoscopy.** In this test (see page 323), a flexible sigmoidoscope—a slender, flexible viewing tube—is inserted through the rectum and into the lower part of the large intestine (colon). The doctor can then inspect the lining of the colon and rectum for signs of any abnormality, such as polyps or cancer. Although this screening procedure is unpleasant, it is highly accurate and research has indicated that it may significantly decrease the risk of dying from colorectal cancer by detecting cancers at a treatable stage. Sigmoidoscopy permits the doctor to view only about half of the colon, however; if abnormalities are found, you may need to undergo a follow-up procedure called colonoscopy (see page 159) to examine the entire length of the colon.

The American College of Physicians and the American Cancer Society recommend screening with flexible sigmoidoscopy every three to five years for all adults beginning at age 50. The U.S. Task Force also advises screening with sigmoidoscopy for all people aged 50 and older, but does not specify a particular interval between tests.

Breast cancer screening. Breast cancer is the second leading cause of cancer-related deaths among women; only lung cancer is more common. Screening for breast cancer is critically important because the likelihood of long-term survival and cure is highest when the disease is detected in its early stages. In fact, the death rate from breast cancer declined significantly during the mid-1990s, probably as a result of earlier detection and improved treatments. The three major screening tests for breast cancer are

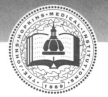

breast self-examination, clinical breast examination, and mammography.

• **Breast self-examination.** Breast self-examination is a simple, 5-minute procedure that women can perform monthly to detect any unusual lumps, discharge, or other changes in their breasts. (For more on the specifics of this test, see page 57.) Any abnormality you find should be brought to your doctor's attention for further evaluation.

Studies reviewing the effectiveness of breast self-examination as a screening test for breast cancer have produced inconclusive results. As a result, the U.S. Task Force maintains that there is insufficient evidence at this time to recommend for or against the teaching of breast self-examination. By contrast, the American Cancer Society advises all women over the age of 20 to perform monthly breast self-exams.

• **Clinical breast examination.** In a clinical breast exam, your physician visually inspects your breasts for nipple inversion, dimpling of the skin, unusual lumps, or any other changes that might indicate breast cancer. He or she also manually examines the breasts using a circular motion. Further testing is performed if any abnormalities are found.

The American Cancer Society recommends that all women between the ages of 20 and 39 have a clinical breast exam every three years; starting at age 40, the exam should be conducted annually. By contrast, the U.S. Task Force concludes that there is insufficient evidence to recommend for or against the use of this screening test alone. The task force does, however, recommend that the clinical breast exam be used in combination with mammography for breast cancer screening in women between the ages of 50 and 69.

• **Mammography.** Mammography (see page 255)—a special x-ray procedure used to visualize tissue inside the breasts—can detect small tumors that would be impossible to feel by either self- or clinical examination. More than 75% of women diagnosed with breast cancer are age 50 or older, and there is general agreement that mammography reduces the risk of dying from breast cancer by one third for women in this age group. All experts now advocate regular mammography screening for older women. The U.S. Task Force recommends that all women aged 50 to 69 undergo routine mammography every one to two years, either alone or combined with a clinical breast exam. The American Cancer Society and the American College of Radiology recommend annual mammograms in women older than 50.

The value of mammography in younger women has been the subject of controversy, however. Some groups have questioned whether mammograms can save lives in younger women or just lead to unnecessary treatment. Because they have more dense breast tissue than older women, young women tend to experience a higher rate of false-negatives as well as false-positives and unnecessary biopsies. Several studies appearing in the late 1990s, however, strongly suggested that regular mammograms could also lower breast cancer mortality among women in their 40s. The American Cancer Society and the American College of Radiology now recommend that routine screening with mammography begin at age 40 and continue annually thereafter. For women at high risk for breast cancer (those with a mother or sister with the disease, for example), screening may begin sooner. The National Cancer Institute recommends that women in their 40s undergo mammography every other year. The U.S. Task Force, however, still concludes that there is insufficient evidence to recommend for or against routine mammography for women between the ages of 40 and 49.

Pelvic examination and Pap smear. Cervical cancer was previously one of the most

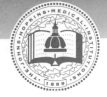

common causes of cancer death for American women, but between 1955 and 1992, the number of deaths from the disease declined by 74% in the U.S. The main reason for this dramatic change is believed to be the increased use of screening with the Papanicolaou (Pap) smear (see page 279). In this test, a sample of cells taken from the cervix is specially stained and examined under a microscope to detect precancerous changes and early invasive cancer.

While all expert groups uniformly advocate that women start having Pap smears to test for cervical cancer once they become sexually active, there is some disagreement on how often the test should be done. The U.S. Task Force recommends that Pap smears be repeated every one to three years. The American Cancer Society advises that all women begin having Pap tests annually at age 18 (or when they become sexually active, whichever occurs earlier). If a woman has three negative annual Pap tests in a row, her physician may decide to perform the test less frequently. In addition, regular testing may be discontinued after age 65 in women whose previous Pap smears have been consistently normal, since the risk of cervical cancer drops dramatically at around this age.

The Pap smear is typically taken during a pelvic exam, in which a physician inspects the vaginal tissues and cervix, palpates the reproductive organs, and may also take a sample of a vaginal discharge for analysis. The pelvic exam can be used to diagnose various abnormalities affecting the uterus, cervix, and ovaries, and may also aid in the detection of certain sexually transmitted diseases. The American Cancer Society recommends that women between 18 and 39 years of age have a pelvic exam every three years and that women over age 40 have an annual exam.

Prostate cancer screening. Prostate cancer is the second most common cancer among men in North America (after skin cancer) and the second leading cause of cancer-related deaths in men (after lung cancer). Screening tests have the potential to detect cancer while it is still confined to the prostate and may be curable with surgical removal of the gland (surgery is not advised if cancer has spread beyond the prostate). However, routine screening for prostate cancer remains controversial for several reasons. First, prostate cancer is frequently a very slow-growing cancer: For example, men with cancer that has not spread beyond the prostate gland have a five-year relative survival rate of nearly 100%, whether or not they receive treatment. Thus, it remains unclear whether treatment will extend the survival of all men with prostate cancer. And treatment for prostate cancer can produce troubling side effects, such as incontinence and impotence, in a significant percentage of men. In addition, available screening tests, such as the digital rectal exam and prostate specific antigen (PSA) assay, generate a significant number of false-positive results, which require a biopsy to rule out cancer. For these reasons, many groups of experts, including the U.S. Task Force, American College of Physicians, and National Cancer Institute, do not currently advocate mass screening for prostate cancer.

Other organizations, such as the American Cancer Society and the American Urological Association, however, believe the benefits outweigh the risks and recommend offering prostate cancer screening tests to older men. These groups recommend that both the PSA test and digital rectal examination be offered annually, beginning at age 50, to men who have at least a 10-year life expectancy, and to younger men who are at high risk for the disease. They also advise that doctors discuss the risks and benefits of early detection and treatment of prostate cancer with their patients at the time of screening.

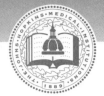

• **Digital rectal exam.** In the digital rectal exam (DRE), the doctor inserts a gloved finger into the rectum and feels the prostate gland through the rectal wall to check for enlargement, bumps, and any other abnormalities. The DRE is less effective than the PSA test in detecting prostate cancer but can sometimes find cancers in men who have normal PSA levels. If an abnormality is detected, a biopsy is recommended.

• **PSA test.** The prostate specific antigen is a protein produced by cells in the prostate. Higher-than-normal blood levels of PSA may signal the presence of prostate cancer cells. However, PSA levels may also rise in men who have noncancerous prostate conditions, including infection (prostatitis) and benign enlargement, known as benign prostatic hypertrophy (BPH).

PSA levels lower than 4 nanograms per milliliter (ng/ml) are usually considered normal. Results over 10 ng/ml are classified as high, while values between 4 and 10 ng/ml are regarded as borderline. Men with an elevated PSA that cannot be explained by other conditions are advised to undergo a biopsy. When the PSA result is borderline, new types of PSA tests, including the percent free PSA test, PSA velocity, and PSA density, are sometimes performed to help determine whether a biopsy should be done. Abnormal results on these tests would indicate a greater likelihood of cancer and support the need for a biopsy.

Testicular self-examination. Testicular self-exam is a simple procedure you can perform at home to detect any lumps or changes in the texture of the testes (for more on the specifics of this test, see page 59). Any abnormality should be brought to your doctor's attention for further evaluation. Since the risk of testicular cancer declines with age, self-exams are considered unnecessary in men after age 40. While the practice may be useful for younger men, there have been very few well-designed studies (because testicular cancer is relatively rare). For this reason, the U.S. Task Force does not recommend routine screening of asymptomatic men for testicular cancer by self-examination. The American Cancer Society does not currently advocate monthly testicular self-exams for men at average risk, but suggests that those with an increased risk for testicular cancer should seriously consider doing the monthly checks. Risk factors for testicular cancer include cryptorchidism (an undescended testicle), a positive family history of the disease, and a previous germ cell tumor on one side.

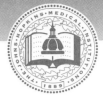

HOME TESTING

Many medical tests that were once performed only in a doctor's office can now also be done at home. Home testing can provide a valuable adjunct to your regular medical check-ups for a variety of reasons. It allows you to screen for potential health problems in their earliest and most treatable stages and to seek prompt medical attention. In addition, certain home tests—such as blood pressure and glucose monitors—offer a way to keep track of the effectiveness of your prescribed medical therapy and lifestyle modifications. Plus, home testing is convenient.

A wide array of home testing equipment is available today, from thermometers to pregnancy tests to a test for hepatitis C infection. In general, these products are accurate, relatively inexpensive, pose little risk, and cause little or no discomfort. Most can be obtained at pharmacies, health stores, and supermarkets, by mail order, and over the Internet. Others require a prescription from a physician. When properly used, home tests can save time and enable you to take a more active role in maintaining your own health. However, self-testing is *not* intended to take the place of regular examinations by a doctor.

GENERAL PRECAUTIONS

When buying a home test kit or device, always look at the expiration date first to check that it is still valid. Read all the instructions carefully to ensure that you understand the test and how to use it. Follow these directions precisely in order to obtain the most accurate results. Note any special precautions, and be sure to perform the test at the recommended time. If you are color-blind, ask someone else to interpret the results of tests that use color indicators. Finally, if some of the directions seem confusing or you have any questions, check with your doctor, pharmacist, or another health professional before performing the test.

Because the results of home tests are generally not as reliable as those performed by a medical professional, any positive findings should be confirmed by a doctor. In addition, if results are negative on a home test but you experience persistent symptoms or other signs of a health problem, be sure to schedule a visit to your doctor because false-negative findings (see page 35) are fairly common with some of these tests.

SELF-EXAMINATIONS

The most basic of all home tests, self-examinations can help you to spot potential problems and bring them to your doctor's attention.

Breast self-examination. Breast self-exam (BSE) is a simple procedure that can help women detect breast cancer earlier and seek prompt treatment. The American Cancer Society recommends that all women perform breast self-exams monthly starting at age 20. Only with practice can you expect the exams to be useful in finding early breast cancers: By doing it regularly, you will become familiar with how your breasts feel and learn to distinguish between what is normal and abnormal for you. Thus, if a change does occur in texture or appearance, you will be able to spot it right away. (Another tip: The next time your doctor does a breast exam, ask her to teach you what are normal and abnormal lumps in your breasts.)

Most breast lumps found during self-examination are not cancerous, but any unusual

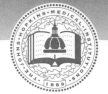

findings should be reported to your doctor for further evaluation. Although BSE is useful, it is not intended to replace regular breast exams by your doctor or routine mammography (see pages 54 and 255).

Because your breasts change with the monthly hormonal cycle, you should examine them at the same time each month. The best time is about two or three days after the end of your menstrual period, when the breasts tend to be least swollen. If you are postmenopausal, perform the exam on the same day, such as the 1st or 10th of the month, every time. The following are common guidelines for the BSE.

1. Stand in front of a mirror with your arms at your sides. Observe each breast in turn, including the areola (the colored area surrounding the nipple) and the nipple itself. Check for any change in the size or contour of the breast, dimpling of the skin, skin discoloration, or spontaneous nipple discharge.

2. Clasp your hands behind your head and press them forward, and again inspect each breast as in step 1.

3. Lean slightly toward the mirror with your hands on your hips and your shoulders and elbows pulled forward. Repeat the inspection as in step 1.

4. Raise your left arm over your head. Use three or four fingers from your right hand to examine your left breast for any unusual lump or mass. Beginning at the outside edge of the breast, press down firmly and carefully with the pads of your fingers (not the fingertips). Feel for lumps while using a circular, rubbing motion. Rotate these circles along the outer edge of the breast, and then make a slow, gradual spiral toward the nipple. After you have inspected the entire breast thoroughly, examine the area between the breast and underarm and the underarm itself.

5. Squeeze the nipple gently, checking for any type of discharge. Now perform steps 4 and 5 while examining your right breast with your left hand.

6. Repeat step 4 on the left breast while lying down with your left arm extended over your head and a small pillow or rolled towel placed under your left shoulder. Now repeat this inspection on your right side.

Skin self-examination. Regular skin self-exams are the best way to spot potentially cancerous skin conditions in their early stages. The earlier skin cancer is detected, the greater the chances for successful treatment. Early detection and treatment are particularly crucial for malignant melanoma, the most dangerous type of skin cancer with the fastest growing incidence of any cancer.

The American Academy of Dermatology recommends that people at high risk for skin cancer (including those with blond or red hair, blue or green eyes, an outdoor occupation, a family history of skin cancer, or a personal history of several blistering sunburns before age 18) should perform a skin self-exam monthly. Those at lower risk should do it once every six months.

In general, when examining your skin you should look for any changes in existing moles or freckles. Also check for any new spots that are asymmetrical (meaning one half is unlike the other); are more than one color; have a diameter larger than that of a pencil eraser; or have uneven borders. Perform the examination in a well-lighted room with the aid of both a full-length mirror and a hand-held one. The American Academy of Dermatology offers the following guidelines for performing skin self-exams.

1. Examine your body front and back in the mirror and then check your right and left sides with your arms raised.

2. Bend your elbows and look carefully at your forearms, upper underarms, and palms.

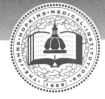

3. Look at the backs of your legs and feet, the spaces between your toes, and the soles of your feet.

4. Examine the back of your neck and scalp with a hand mirror. To obtain a better look at your scalp, you should part your hair. You can use a blow dryer if needed.

5. Finally, check your back and buttocks with a hand mirror.

If you detect any abnormalities during the self-exam, schedule an appointment with a doctor as soon as possible.

Testicular self-examination. Many doctors recommend that men between the ages of 15 and 40 perform monthly testicular self-exams to help identify testicular cancers in their early stages (with early treatment, more than 90% of these cancers can be cured). However, after age 40, testicular cancer is so rare that self-exams are no longer necessary. The American Cancer Society currently suggests that men under 40 decide whether to perform monthly self-exams on an individual basis in consultation with their doctors, but recommends that those with an increased risk for testicular cancer (such as men who had undescended testicles at birth) seriously consider them.

The best time for testicular self-examination is after a warm bath or shower, because heat causes the skin of the scrotum to relax, making it easier to detect a lump or mass. To perform the test, look and feel for any hard lumps or nodules (smooth rounded masses) or any change in the size, shape, or consistency of the testes. If you detect any irregularity, schedule an appointment with your physician as soon as possible.

HOME MONITORING TESTS
The following tests may be useful for assessing the effectiveness of ongoing therapy for chronic conditions, such as hypertension and diabetes mellitus.

Blood pressure measurement. High blood pressure, or hypertension, usually causes no symptoms at first. If untreated or inadequately treated, however, the condition can eventually damage organs throughout the body, including the heart, blood vessels, kidneys, and eyes.

Monitoring blood pressure at home is often helpful in the management of hypertension. Regular self-testing supplements your doctor's measurements and can provide a more complete picture of your blood pressure levels under various circumstances. For example, some people's blood pressure rises when recorded by a doctor, nurse, or physician's assistant, even though their pressure may be normal or close to normal at other times (a phenomenon called "white-coat hypertension"). With home testing, you can obtain several readings over the course of a day or a week in a stress-free setting. Averaging these values together provides another gauge of your blood pressure levels and the effectiveness of any lifestyle measures or antihypertensive medications during real-life situations.

The two basic types of home blood pressure monitors are manually operated aneroid devices and automated electronic units. Traditionally, the best way to measure blood pressure at home has been the aneroid monitor, which typically includes an arm cuff, a squeeze bulb to inflate the cuff, a stethoscope, and a mechanical gauge to measure blood pressure. To use this device, you wrap the cuff snugly around your upper arm (over the brachial artery); use two fingers to locate your pulse over the crease of your elbow joint; and place the flat part of the stethoscope on this spot. Next, you squeeze the bulb rapidly to inflate the cuff until it blocks the brachial artery, and then slowly loosen the valve on the bulb to release air from the cuff. Carefully listen for thumping sounds through

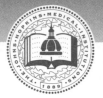

the stethoscope, which indicate reentry of blood flow through the brachial artery. Record the numbers on the dial when the thumping sounds first begin and when they disappear; these numbers correspond to your systolic and diastolic blood pressures, respectively. Because correct use of aneroid monitors requires good hearing, eyesight, and manual dexterity, certain individuals may not be able to use them.

Electronic monitors were once considered inferior, but their technology has improved so that they now generally give accurate and consistent readings. To operate these devices, you simply wrap a cuff around your upper arm or wrist. Some models have a cuff that inflates automatically when you press a button, and even the manually inflated cuffs deflate automatically. After the unit measures your blood pressure (using a tiny microphone that can detect blood pulsing in your artery), it displays the numbers on a digital screen. The monitor also records your pulse rate.

While the electronic blood pressure monitors are easier to use, they are more expensive than the manually operated ones. In general, the electronic models equipped with an arm cuff are more accurate than those using a wrist cuff. All blood pressure monitors should be checked annually against the one used at your doctor's office to ensure continuing accuracy. In addition, keep in mind the following tips to maximize the accuracy of home blood pressure monitoring.

1. Avoid caffeine, cigarettes, and alcohol for at least 30 minutes before a blood pressure measurement.

2. Sit down and relax for 3 to 5 minutes before performing the test.

3. While taking a reading, sit in a comfortable position, with your legs and ankles uncrossed and your back supported.

4. Place your wrist or upper arm inside the cuff. The bottom edge of the arm cuff should be 1 inch above the crease of your elbow. Be sure to remove any jewelry or constrictive clothing that might interfere with placement of the cuff.

5. Place your arm on a table so that the arm cuff will be at heart level. If you are using a wrist model, it is essential that you position your wrist at heart level to obtain an accurate reading.

6. Take 2 readings at each sitting, at least 2 minutes apart, and average them. If the difference between the 2 readings is 5 millimeters of mercury (mm Hg) or more, take an additional reading and average the 3.

7. Keep track of your blood pressure readings and bring this record with you on your next visit to the doctor. If your blood pressure monitor is equipped with a memory function, you can use this feature to keep a record of your blood pressure and pulse measurements.

Blood glucose monitoring. Diabetes is characterized by chronically elevated blood sugar (glucose) levels. Most physicians recommend that all patients with type 1 diabetes (which usually develops before age 30) regularly measure their own blood glucose levels. Self-monitoring is also recommended for almost all individuals with type 2 diabetes (which usually develops after age 30).

The goal of home blood glucose testing is to determine how effectively your treatment regimen—which may include diet, exercise, oral medications, and insulin injections—is controlling your blood glucose levels. When performed correctly, home glucose monitoring allows changes in your diet and medication to achieve the best possible blood glucose control. Recommendations for the frequency and timing of self-testing range from once a day or less in people with well-controlled type 2 diabetes to multiple times (2 to 4) daily in those with type 1 disease.

Blood glucose monitoring begins with a

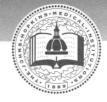

puncture device to obtain a drop of blood, usually from a fingertip. The blood is placed on a testing strip that contains an enzyme called glucose oxidase. The strip is then inserted into a glucose meter, which scans the strip and displays the result as a digital readout in about 15 to 45 seconds. Some devices are equipped with data management systems that can store hundreds of glucose readings, thereby simplifying your record keeping.

The Food and Drug Administration (FDA) recently approved several new alternatives for measuring blood glucose levels at home. Some of these devices (such as the AtLast Blood Glucose System) use a tiny drop of blood drawn from the forearm. This method is less painful than pricking the fingertip with a lancet. Another new monitor (the Precision Xtra) measures not only blood glucose levels, but blood ketone levels as well. Testing ketone levels can help prevent diabetic ketoacidosis, a serious complication that can occur in people with type 1 diabetes when blood glucose levels rise above 300 mg/dL.

Another recent development, called the GlucoWatch Biographer, is a wristwatch-like device that sends out tiny electric currents to extract glucose-containing fluid through your skin. While it is currently of unproven value, this technology permits you to take glucose measurements through your skin every 20 minutes for up to 12 hours at a time. The watch is not intended to replace finger-stick glucose measurements. Rather, it's designed to provide additional information on glucose trends and patterns to help you and your doctor better manage your diabetes. The watch has received FDA approval for use in adults age 18 and over; however, it is not yet available to the general public. (Updated information on its availability can be obtained online at www.glucowatch.com or by phoning toll-free at 866-GLWATCH.)

Home cholesterol testing. High blood cholesterol is one of the major risk factors for heart disease. Several home test kits—which involve measuring the cholesterol level in a drop or two of blood obtained by pricking your finger with a lancet—are now available for monitoring cholesterol levels. However, these products are currently considered to be of limited usefulness for a variety of reasons. First, they can only measure your *total* cholesterol levels, but not levels of the key components HDL ("good") cholesterol, LDL ("bad") cholesterol, and triglycerides, which are very important for assessing your overall risk for heart disease (see page 238). Thus, a normal result on these tests may be deceptive and falsely reassuring to people who are, in fact, at heightened risk for heart disease (due to a low HDL cholesterol level, for example). If you have risk factors such as diabetes, obesity, physical inactivity, or a family history of heart disease, it is essential that you have your cholesterol levels measured by a doctor. And, for people who are already diagnosed with high cholesterol levels, regular visits to the doctor are the only safe and effective way to evaluate the success of dietary changes, exercise, and/or cholesterol-lowering medications.

Prothrombin time. Many individuals—including those with artificial heart valves, certain abnormal heart rhythms, or blood clotting disorders—receive long-term therapy with anticoagulant drugs, most often warfarin (Coumadin, Panwarfin). These medications reduce the risk of abnormal blood clots that can lead to a heart attack or stroke. To be effective, blood levels of anticoagulant drugs must be maintained within a certain specified range. When anticoagulant levels are too low, the risk for clot formation persists; levels that are too high can cause bleeding.

To keep anticoagulant levels within the proper range and reduce the chances of

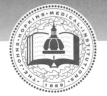

bleeding or clotting complications, a laboratory test called prothrombin time (PT) should be performed frequently—once or twice a month, or more often if the anticoagulant dose has just been changed. This test (described in more detail on page 157) measures how long it takes for a blood clot to form. If the PT results are significantly higher or lower than the normal range, your doctor may adjust your dose of medication.

While regular PT testing once required visits to a doctor or laboratory, two portable, battery-operated instruments (ProTime and AvoSure PT) recently became available for the self-measurement of PT values at home. These devices, which require a doctor's prescription, allow easier, more frequent monitoring of PT values. The test is performed by collecting a blood sample from your fingertip and running the sample through a small, hand-held electronic device that displays the results on a screen in several minutes. Some devices can store multiple PT test results in memory. Home PT monitoring is especially valuable for individuals who travel frequently, are homebound, or live in a rural area that is far from a testing laboratory.

However, self-monitoring is not always appropriate. For example, people with liver disease are prone to inaccurate results (since prothrombin is a protein produced by the liver), and are better off maintaining their regular schedule of laboratory visits. In addition, home PT testing devices are expensive—ranging from $750 to $1,500 for the initial investment, in addition to the continuing cost of test supplies. For now, home PT testing is considered most appropriate for high-risk patients: those who need high warfarin doses, have had bleeding problems in the past, have medical conditions that make them more susceptible to bleeding, or take drugs known to interact with warfarin.

OTHER HOME TESTS

A wide range of other home test kits and devices are available for a variety of purposes—and their number is expanding rapidly in today's environment of self-advocacy in health care. The following are a few examples.

Lyme disease. The tests that are used to determine whether a person has been infected with the bacterial organism that causes Lyme disease are performed in a doctor's office or a medical laboratory. A service called TICK-ITT is available, however, which allows you to mail in a tick that has been removed from a person or an animal to a laboratory, where tests will be performed to determine if it was carrying the Lyme disease bacterium and thus had the potential for transmitting the infection. You will receive an interim report of the test results after two weeks, and are notified of the final results after four weeks. If the test is positive, you will be contacted immediately by phone. (For more information on this test, which costs about $80, call 1-877-842-5488.)

Hepatitis C testing. Chronic infection with the hepatitis C virus may lead to cirrhosis (scarring of the liver) and liver cancer. Early detection of the infection is important for initiating appropriate therapy and counseling. People at increased risk for hepatitis C may want to consider using a home test, called the Hepatitis C Check, that was recently approved by the FDA. (Risk factors include the use of intravenous drugs or sharing needles; blood transfusion or solid organ transplant before July 1992; occupational exposure to blood or blood products, for example, during healthcare work or military service; long-term kidney dialysis; and evidence of liver disease.) This test can only determine whether you have contracted a hepatitis C infection, but not whether the infection is active. In addition, it is not able

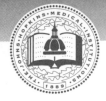

to detect the infection until six weeks to six months after it was contracted.

Home testing for hepatitis C uses a spring-loaded device to prick your finger and obtain a few drops of blood that are placed on a blotter. This blotter is then sent to a laboratory to be tested for antibodies to the hepatitis C virus (see page 111). After 10 days, you call a toll-free number and obtain the test results anonymously using an assigned numerical code. If your results are positive, you will receive professional counseling and medical referrals. The home test kit, which costs about $70, is available at many pharmacies and can also be ordered directly (by phone at 1-800-211-6636 or online at www.hepatitisctesting.com).

Fecal occult blood. Regular screening with a fecal occult blood test (see pages 53 and 199) is an important measure to help detect colorectal cancer in its early and most treatable stages. This test involves obtaining stool samples at home and bringing them to your doctor or a testing laboratory to be analyzed for trace amounts of blood (or "occult" blood). These periodic screenings may now be supplemented with a new home test, called EZ Detect. To perform the test, you simply drop a test tissue into the toilet bowl and wait for two minutes. If blood is present in the stool, a blue-green color will appear. (Call 1-800-854-3002 or check online at http://ezdetect.com for more information.)

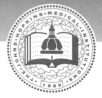

GENETIC TESTING & SCREENING

One of the most exciting, rapidly expanding, and controversial areas of medical science and research today is genetic testing and screening. The clinical practice of genetics involves the collection and analysis of a person's genetic material, or DNA, in order to identify particular changes associated with disease. Genetic testing can be used to detect a disorder that is already present, or to screen individuals in order to determine the likelihood that they or their offspring will develop a disorder in the future.

Inherited genetic abnormalities are already known to be responsible for over 4,000 diseases, and genetic alterations are a factor in most cancers, heart disease, and many other common disorders. While genetic testing is still a relatively new field with many current limitations, it has the potential to one day save a multitude of lives through prevention or early detection of treatable diseases. For now, the controversy over the psychological impact and the legal and ethical issues surrounding genetic testing continues to grow even more heated as these tests become increasingly available.

GENES AND CHROMOSOMES

Genes are units of information inside each cell in the body. They contain hereditary material that ordains a person's physical characteristics, such as hair color and height. Genes also play a critical role in all body functions, for example, the processing of food and the activity of the immune system. Thanks to recent findings by the Human Genome Project, which has completed mapping of the entire human genome, scientists now know that the human body contains approximately 30,000 genes. (Until recently, the estimated number was 100,000.)

With the exception of eggs and sperm, each cell in the body contains an identical set of genes. They are organized in linear strands, called *chromosomes,* located in the cell nucleus. Every cell has 23 pairs of chromosomes; 1 in every pair is inherited from the mother, and 1 from the father. All but 1 of these 23 chromosomes is a matching pair. The 23rd pair is matching in women (known as the XX chromosomes) but not in men (XY chromosomes).

Chromosomes are made up primarily of DNA (deoxyribonucleic acid), an immense database of chemical information that contains instructions for making the proteins required for the metabolism, structure, and growth of all cells in the body. Proteins determine all body processes, and nearly every protein has a different function. For example, one protein regulates the amount of salt in sweat; another carries oxygen in the blood; a third forms the major component of skin and hair. Each gene contains a specific set of instructions for making a particular protein. When a cell reproduces, it divides into two replicas—this is how the body creates new cells for growth, repair, and replacement of older cells—and a complete copy of its DNA is given to each daughter cell.

Different genes play different roles. Some genes are active in many kinds of cells, making proteins that are needed for basic functions. Many genes are active only in cells with specialized functions, such as the production of particular hormones. Other genes perform one job, such as supporting the early development of the embryo, and then become permanently inactive. A normal cell activates only the genes it needs at any given time.

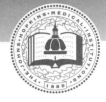

HOW GENES ARE LINKED TO DISEASE

For the body to be healthy, thousands of proteins must interact correctly, performing their functions in exactly the right amounts and at the right places. Normal functioning requires intact genes, but often genetic changes, or mutations, occur. These mutations can be inherited or acquired.

Hereditary mutations. Hereditary mutations are genetic alterations that come from one or both parents. They can be passed from generation to generation and are copied every time the body's cells divide. An inherited mutation can be found in all cellular DNA.

All genes come in pairs, called *alleles,* one on the chromosome inherited from the mother and one on the chromosome inherited from the father. Genes can be considered as "dominant" or "recessive." Only one allele of a dominant gene is required for the expression of its protein product. Expression of a recessive trait requires both alleles of a recessive gene. Thus, the inheritance pattern of a genetic mutation for a certain disease depends on whether the allele is dominant or recessive. If a mother carries an allele for a dominant disorder, each of her children has a 50 percent chance of inheriting it. If both parents have a single allele for a recessive trait, their children have a 25 percent chance of inheriting both of the recessive alleles—one from each parent—and developing the disease. If only a father has an allele for a recessive disorder and passes it on to his offspring, it will not be detected in the presence of the mother's normal allele, and their children will not develop the disease. However, these children will become "carriers," meaning they have a 50 percent chance of passing the recessive allele to each of their own children.

The mere presence of an abnormal gene does not always have the last word, however. Even a dominant mutated gene will not necessarily result in illness. The detection of an abnormal dominant gene is determined by its *penetrance*—the probability that it will be expressed and produce disease. A mutation with complete penetrance will always cause the associated disease; most mutations have incomplete penetrance and are linked to variable degrees of disease severity.

Acquired mutations. Acquired mutations are flaws in DNA that occur during a person's lifetime. Unlike hereditary mutations, these abnormalities develop only in the DNA of individual cells, and are copied only by direct descendants of those cells. Acquired mutations can be caused by mistakes that take place during cell division, or they can result from factors such as radiation, toxins, or other environmental stresses.

Acquired mutations occur frequently. Fortunately, cells are normally able to detect these changes and fix them before they are passed on to the next generation of cells. But this repair mechanism can be overwhelmed, or it can fail to recognize a mutation. And as the body ages, repair can become less efficient and mutations are more likely to slip through to the daughter cells.

Mutations and disease. Most genetic mutations and variations are harmless and have little or no important effect on the structure of the related protein or the job it performs. Some mutations, however, result in a seriously abnormal protein. The protein may be completely disabled and no longer able to perform its function, or it may still function, but not correctly. An example of the latter is sickle-cell anemia, which is caused by abnormal hemoglobin (the oxygen-carrying protein in the blood).

Whether your health is affected by a gene mutation depends on how the affected protein's function is changed, and how important

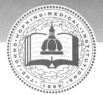
that protein is to body function and survival. In some cases, the disease may not develop for a long time and it may progress slowly; in others, the illness occurs at a young age or you may become severely ill.

Different mutations in the same gene can lead to a variety of effects in different individuals. In cystic fibrosis, for example, the gene responsible for mucus production can have over 300 different types of mutations. Depending on the particular mutation, a person may have no symptoms or very severe ones. On the other hand, in many cases, mutations in different genes can result in the same problem. The lack of eye, skin, and hair color in albinism can be due to mutations in several genes that are required to make pigment.

In many cases, an increased genetic risk is only one factor that determines the development of a disease; whether the disease manifests itself may also depend on environmental factors such as diet, exercise, smoking, stress levels, exposure to toxins and radiation, and access to health care. For example, a woman with a genetic risk for type 2 diabetes mellitus is much more likely to develop the disorder if she is overweight, because excess weight is a major risk factor for diabetes.

THE MAJOR TYPES OF GENETIC DISORDERS

Genetic disorders fall into several broad categories. Although scientists have linked a large number of diseases to specific genetic mutations, only a few examples are mentioned here.

Single-gene disorders. Single-gene (or Mendelian) disorders are the result of mutations in a single gene or pair of genes. They are relatively rare, and their effect can range from mild to severe. Symptoms may not appear until late in life. The three types of single-gene disorders include autosomal dominant, autosomal recessive, and sex chromosome-linked disorders.

- **Autosomal dominant disorders** develop when one dominant gene is abnormal (its partner gene may be normal). Examples include: early-onset Alzheimer's disease (AD), which typically causes symptoms of dementia in the 40s and 50s; certain breast cancers; familial adenomatous polyposis (FAP), a disorder characterized by the formation of polyps in the colon and rectum that eventually leads to colorectal cancer (unless the colon is surgically removed); and Huntington's disease, characterized by progressive mental and physical decline that first appears in middle age.

- **Autosomal recessive disorders** occur only when both genes in a pair are abnormal. The parents of an affected child are "carriers" who do not have the disorder because, in their case, the abnormal gene is paired with a normal one. These disorders include: cystic fibrosis, which causes the body to produce thick mucus that interferes with the functioning of the lungs and pancreas; hemochromatosis, a disorder resulting from the storage of excessive amounts of iron; and sickle-cell anemia, in which distorted red blood cells damage vital organs.

- **X-linked disorders** are caused by genes located on the X chromosome. They produce symptoms only in males, while females are asymptomatic carriers. Examples include Duchenne's muscular dystrophy (a group of disorders that cause muscle degeneration) and the bleeding disorder hemophilia A.

Chromosomal disorders. These are defects in the structure or number of chromosomes, and usually result in severe disease. The most common one is Down syndrome, characterized by mental retardation and a number of physical abnormalities.

Multifactorial genetic diseases. Multifactorial (or polygenic) genetic diseases are the most common genetic disorders, but unfortunately are the most poorly understood. They include, among others, heart disease, type 2 dia-

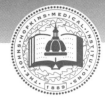

betes, and schizophrenia. In these conditions, the inheritance of one or more mutated genes results in an increased risk of developing a particular disorder, but whether or not the disease appears depends in part on environmental factors. For example, the gene for APOE4, on chromosome 19, may contribute to over 60 percent of late-onset Alzheimer's disease cases. However, APOE4 is a susceptibility gene; it is not as strongly predictive of Alzheimer's disease as the genetic mutations that are associated with the early-onset form of the illness. Researchers are currently working to determine the role of genetics in many polygenic diseases.

Somatic gene disorders. Somatic gene disorders are diseases caused by genetic defects that are not inherited, but instead occur during a person's lifetime. In these diseases, genetic abnormalities develop only in certain cells. An example is cancer, in which only genes in the diseased tissue are abnormal. All cancers are triggered by altered genes; in the vast majority of cases, however, these are random mutations that occur either during cell division or as a result of environmental stresses, such as exposure to carcinogens. Several types of genes are involved in cancer:

• **Oncogenes** normally promote cell growth, but when mutated, they can become a permanent green light that instructs cells to keep dividing.

• **Tumor-suppressor genes** normally limit cell growth, but if they are missing or disabled by a mutation, they allow uncontrollable cell growth.

• **DNA-repair genes** (also known as "proofreader" genes) work by fixing errors that occur when DNA copies itself; failure to perform this function may contribute to cancer by allowing mutations to slip through to newly formed cells.

Research studies are currently under way to identify other somatic gene mutations involved in cancers of the colon and rectum, prostate, thyroid, eye, skin, kidney, and other organs.

HOW GENETIC TESTS ARE PERFORMED

To perform a genetic test, a person's DNA is taken from cells in a blood sample—or occasionally from urine, other body fluids, or a tissue specimen—and examined for one or more mutations previously recognized as contributing to a particular disorder. When the protein formed by a gene and its function are known, this protein, called a *gene product,* can be measured. If a gene contains a mutation, its gene products may be abnormal or present in unusual amounts.

Certain diseases can be detected by *direct testing,* which involves analyzing a specific gene for known mutations. When a particular gene has not been identified as the cause of a disorder, but the gene is known to be located within a certain region of a chromosome, doctors use linkage analysis, or *indirect testing.* In this type of test, researchers look for variations in DNA that do not cause the disease but are located near (linked) to the mutation being examined. DNA is taken from family members with the disorder and used as a basis for comparison. Indirect testing has been used successfully even when the gene mutation is unknown, the gene product cannot be identified, or the gene can be identified but the mutation in a specific family is unknown.

WHY GENETIC TESTS ARE DONE

In practice, genetic tests are done in adults when there is a strong family history of a specific disease, such as a certain type of cancer, or when a person has symptoms of a genetic disorder. Genetic tests may also be done if a couple is concerned about passing on a genetic disorder to their children. In general, medical professionals might recommend genetic testing for any of the following reasons:

To predict genetic disorders. If you have a known risk for a hereditary disease, but no

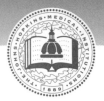

symptoms, a genetic test can determine if you carry the gene or genes that will cause or increase the risk of the disease when you are older. This information can help your doctor decide on the need for regular monitoring or initiation of treatment to prevent serious complications.

To diagnose a genetic disease that has already occurred. If you have symptoms of a genetic disease, genetic testing can help to make a specific diagnosis. For example, in people with a progressive inability to remember events and facts, a genetic test may help to diagnose Alzheimer's disease (though such testing is often considered unnecessary).

To test newborns for inherited diseases. The most common use of gene testing is for newborn screening, which is done on four million newborn infants every year in the U.S. Doctors test for phenylketonuria, sickle-cell anemia, Tay-Sachs disease, metabolic disorders, and other conditions. In some cases, such as phenylketonuria—a rare disorder for which treatment in the first few days of life can prevent irreversible mental retardation—early intervention can avoid serious health problems or even prevent a disease.

To screen couples for genetic disorders. Carrier testing is done so couples who are considering having children can learn if they have—and risk passing on—a recessive gene for a range of inherited disorders. These include sickle-cell anemia, Tay-Sachs disease, cystic fibrosis, hemophilia, and Huntington's disease.

To help detect cancer. Genetic tests may be used to identify DNA changes in cancerous or precancerous cells. This information can help doctors to detect the early stages of cancers, identify different types of a particular cancer, establish how aggressive a cancer is likely to be, and determine the best treatment.

To increase the success of organ transplantation. A close match between the genetic types of an organ donor and a recipient reduces the risk of organ rejection.

To perform prenatal screening for genetic disorders. Prenatal diagnostic tests can be done on the fetus for Down syndrome and certain other genetic diseases.

WHAT GENETIC TESTING CANNOT TELL YOU

Genetic testing can be a useful diagnostic tool, but it has limitations. A predictive genetic test can only tell you whether or not you have a genetic mutation known to be linked to a certain disease. A positive test means that you have the mutation, and therefore have a greater risk of developing the disease than those in the general population—but it does not *guarantee* that you will ever get the disease. For example, a woman with a mutation in either the BRCA1 or BRCA2 breast cancer susceptibility gene has a greater than 50 percent chance of developing breast cancer by age 70. Despite this high risk, she may never develop breast cancer. And, if breast cancer does occur, a genetic test cannot predict when or how severe it will be.

In addition, an inherited disease may be due to a genetic mutation that has not yet been identified. (For example, only about half of the families with hereditary breast cancer have a BRCA gene mutation.) Thus, a negative genetic test for a disorder cannot rule out the possibility that you will develop it. Your risk may be no greater than that for the general population, or you may have inherited a different, as yet unidentified, gene that increases your risk for the disease.

Probably the greatest limitation of gene testing is that the availability of effective diagnostic and therapeutic measures lags behind the genetic testing technology for many diseases. A genetic test may show a predisposition to a certain type of cancer, but that

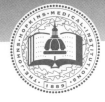

information is of limited value if the diagnostic tools are not sophisticated enough to detect that cancer at an early stage or if there are no effective treatments.

WHAT TESTS ARE AVAILABLE?

Today, at least 400 genetic tests are being offered to the public. Predictive tests are available for some two dozen diseases, including early-onset Alzheimer's disease (some tests are only available by joining a research study), breast cancer (for the BRCA1 and BRCA2 susceptibility genes), cardiovascular disease, familial adenomatous polyposis (this condition can also be diagnosed without the gene test), and sickle-cell anemia, to name just a few.

In addition, scientists are now working to identify genes that predispose people to many types of cancer, including cancers of the prostate, breast, ovary, colon, thyroid, skin, and eye. Genetic mutations have also been reported for melanoma, leukemia, and renal cell cancer. Researchers expect to soon isolate the gene that causes autism, and a recent discovery is a gene linked with type 1 diabetes. New tests are also being developed to identify a predisposition to other forms of Alzheimer's disease and extremely high cholesterol levels.

THE POTENTIAL BENEFITS OF GENETIC TESTING

Genetic testing can provide great benefits for people with an increased risk of developing a specific inherited disease. Most notably, a negative test can bring peace of mind for you and your children by determining that you don't carry the mutated gene despite a strong family history of a disorder. A negative result also eliminates the need for frequent checkups and diagnostic tests.

A positive genetic test may also be beneficial. A positive result can be an early warning that allows you to take preventive measures and have careful follow-up in order to maximize your chances for early detection and treatment. A positive gene test for colon cancer, for example, indicates the need for regular colonoscopy (see page 159) to detect precancerous polyps or early-stage cancers, and to maintain a healthy lifestyle. And in a few cases, a positive test can allow preventive surgery, such as removal of the ovaries (oophorectomy) when the risk for ovarian cancer is very high. In the case of carrier testing, a positive result can help expectant parents decide whether to continue a pregnancy.

For some people, knowing with certainty that they are at increased risk for—or already have—a disease is better than the uncertainty of not knowing. If you are experiencing symptoms, a genetic test may be able to identify their cause. Such tests also allow you to give family members useful information, if you choose to share your results. Even when there is no treatment for a disease, a genetic test can enable you to make informed choices about your future.

In coming years, scientists hope that genetic testing and research will provide even more significant benefits, such as contributing to improved cancer diagnosis and treatment. For example, the effectiveness of cancer-preventing drugs is likely to be determined more easily when they can be tested on groups who are at high risk for developing the disease. Ultimately, scientists hope to treat disease with gene therapy—by inactivating, repairing, or replacing abnormal genes.

THE RISKS AND CONTROVERSIES OF GENETIC TESTING

While the physical risks of genetic testing are minimal, the psychological implications can be considerable. In addition, the practice is asso-

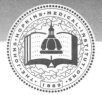

ciated with a number of potentially harmful legal and ethical ramifications.

Psychological impact. The news that you have tested positive for a disease—especially a serious one for which there is no treatment—can be devastating. In addition to being distressed about your own health, you may be concerned about family members with the same genetic legacy. Moreover, doctors may want to test your close relatives, and it can be difficult to ask your family to submit to screening tests. They may feel pressured to take part, even if they don't wish to, and feel guilty if they refuse. A gene test can also inadvertently disclose secret adoptions or issues of paternity.

Even people who test negative for a disorder can have difficulty coping with the results; they sometimes experience "survivor's guilt" if other family members have not been so fortunate. Negative test results can also cause a false sense of security. A woman who tests negative for genetic mutations linked to breast cancer may decide that she no longer needs to perform breast self-exams or to have regular mammograms (see pages 57 and 255), even though she still carries the same risk for breast cancer as the general population.

Finally, waiting for test results can take weeks or months, and the tests are often expensive. Genetic testing may not be covered by health insurance, or you may not want your health insurance company to know about the test for fear of losing your coverage.

Health insurance. You could be denied health insurance, or charged higher premiums, because of a positive genetic test—even if you had no symptoms of the disease when the test was performed. Currently, legislation in most (but not all) states bars health insurance discrimination based on the results of genetic tests. In 1996, the federal government passed the Health Insurance Portability Act and

Accountability, which prohibits insurance companies from using genetic information to refuse group health insurance coverage or to charge higher rates.

Workplace discrimination. The 1990 Americans with Disabilities Act (ADA) makes it illegal to discriminate against disabled employees as long as they can perform the basic functions of the job. The federal Equal Employment Opportunity Commission has ruled that the ADA also prohibits employers from discriminating based on workers' genetic profiles. Nonetheless, there have been reports of people who were fired from jobs or refused promotions based on the results of genetic testing.

Genetic testing also has the potential for bias in hiring. An employer might decide not to hire a qualified job applicant who has a genetic marker that indicates an increased risk for the future development of a disease, reasoning that the person may eventually need more sick days and require higher insurance premiums.

Ethical issues. Medical ethicists have raised several concerns regarding genetic testing. Some people might feel pressured to undergo a genetic test before they are fully prepared for the psychological impact of the result. Another question is what should be done when a person's genetic information also applies to their relatives' risk of future disease. Current law says that you should be advised to share information with such relatives; however, if you do not wish to do so, your decision should be respected.

WHO IS A GOOD CANDIDATE FOR GENETIC TESTING?

For now, genetic testing is useful only for the relatively small percentage of people who may have a disease caused by a single mutant gene. Thus, the best candidates for predictive genetic testing are members of families in

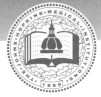

which several relatives have been affected by the disease over at least two generations. People with a less profound family history of a genetic disorder—for example, one or two relatives who developed it at a young age—may also be good candidates.

Some couples planning a pregnancy may also be good candidates for genetic testing. These include couples who have suffered two or more miscarriages and those who already have a child with an inherited disorder. Genetic testing may also help couples with concerns about disorders that affect their race or ethnic group. For example, family origins in Greece or Italy may suggest a test for thalassemia, a blood disorder that afflicts mainly people of Mediterranean ancestry.

Genetic experts generally agree that widespread testing is not warranted. Most common diseases are caused by increased genetic risk combined with environmental factors. Only 5 to 10 percent of cancers, for example, are thought to be due to inherited genes. Even in diseases where genetics plays a significant role, such as late-onset Alzheimer's disease, environmental factors and lifestyle choices are thought to be equally important.

In addition, genetic testing still involves a relatively new technology. Current facilities for testing DNA are limited, and only a small number of well-trained medical professionals can accurately perform the tests, interpret the results, and counsel the affected individuals. Widespread testing would overwhelm testing facilities, and the results would be of no use to most people.

GENETIC COUNSELING AND INFORMED CONSENT

The decision to undergo genetic testing is a personal one, and should be made only if you decide you want the information—not because you feel pressure from family members or health care providers. Genetic counseling is vital to enable you to give your informed consent for this type of testing.

Genetic counselors are doctors, technicians, or nurses who are specially trained to help people make choices about genetic testing and assist them once the test results are known. If you are considering a genetic test, it is essential to discuss the idea with a genetic counselor beforehand. You should receive information—both verbally and in writing—about the risks and benefits involved, the effectiveness of the proposed test, what the results can and cannot tell you, and whether the disorder can be prevented, detected early, or treated. You should also be made aware of any alternatives to genetic testing before you can make an informed decision about proceeding. If you do decide to go through with the test, your counselor should help prepare you to cope with the emotional impact of a positive result.

After your genetic test is completed, your counselor should interpret the test for you, help you come to terms with the results, and assist you in arranging for appropriate prevention, screening, and treatment measures. To learn more about genetic counseling, you can contact the National Society of Genetic Counselors at 610-872-7608 (press 7) or www.nsgc.org, or the National Cancer Institute at 800-4CANCER.

INDEX OF TESTS
BY SUBJECT

This section of the book is designed to help you find information about the medical tests that are used to evaluate specific organ systems and diagnose different types of disorders. Beneath each major category, such as The Brain and Nervous System, you will find a list of the tests that relate to that category. If you would like to read more about a particular test, simply look it up in the main list of tests (which is organized alphabetically) or locate its page number in the general index at the end of the book.

1 ASTHMA & ALLERGY

2 THE BLOOD

3 THE BRAIN & NERVOUS SYSTEM

4 CANCER

5 THE DIGESTIVE SYSTEM

6 THE EARS, NOSE, & THROAT

7 THE ENDOCRINE SYSTEM

8 THE EYES

9 THE HEART & BLOOD VESSELS

10 INFECTIOUS DISEASE

11 THE KIDNEYS & URINARY TRACT

12 THE LUNGS & RESPIRATORY SYSTEM

13 MEN'S HEALTH

14 THE BONES

15 RHEUMATOLOGY

16 THE SKIN

17 WOMEN'S HEALTH

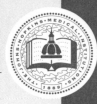

Head and Neck CT Scan
Head and Neck MRI
Hearing Tests
Laryngoscopy
Modified Barium Swallow
Nasal or Sinus Endoscopy
Smell and Taste Testing
Video Stroboscopy

7 THE ENDOCRINE SYSTEM

Adrenal Hormone Tests
Bone Densitometry
Calcium Tests
Glucose Tests
Lipid Profile
Octreotide Scan
Pituitary Hormone Tests
Sex Hormone Tests
Thyroid Biopsy
Thyroid Hormone Tests
Thyroid Nuclear Scan
Thyroid Ultrasound

8 THE EYES

Electroretinography
Fluorescein Angiography
Ocular and Orbit Ultrasound
Oculoplethysmography
Ophthalmodynamometry
Schirmer Tearing Test
Tonometry
Vision Tests
Visual Field Testing

9 THE HEART & BLOOD VESSELS

Arteriography
Cardiac Blood Tests
Cardiac Catheterization

Cardiac MRI
Cardiac Nuclear Scan
Cardiac Stress Test
Doppler Studies of the Extremities
Electrocardiography
Electron-Beam CT Scan
Electrophysiology Studies
Holter Monitoring
Magnetic Resonance Angiography
Pericardiocentesis
Plethysmography
Pulmonary Angiography
Pulmonary Artery Catheterization
Renal and Mesenteric Doppler Ultrasound
Stress Echocardiography
Tilt Table Test
Transesophageal Echocardiography
Transthoracic Echocardiography
Venography
Venous Doppler Studies

10 INFECTIOUS DISEASE

Antigen/Antibody Tests
Cultures and Microscopic Exams
HIV and AIDS-related Blood Tests
Tuberculin Test

11 THE KIDNEYS & URINARY TRACT

Abdominal CT Scan
Abdominal Ultrasound
Antegrade Pyelography
Blood Chemistry Screen
Cystography
Cystoscopy
Intravenous Pyelography
Kidney, Ureter, Bladder X-ray
Renal and Mesenteric Doppler Ultrasound
Renal Biopsy
Renal Function Tests

Abdominal CT Scan
(Computed Tomography Scan of the Abdomen)

Abdominal CT Scan *(side tab)*

Description

• In this test, a body scanner delivers x-rays to the abdominal cavity at many different angles. A computer compiles this information to construct highly detailed, cross-sectional images of tissues and organs, which are displayed on a TV monitor and recorded on x-ray film. In some cases, a contrast dye may be used to help define the major blood vessels and various abdominal structures on the images. Abdominal CT scans are useful for detecting abnormalities in the liver, pancreas, spleen, gallbladder and bile ducts, kidneys and urinary tract, adrenal glands, gastrointestinal (GI) tract, uterus, fallopian tubes, ovaries, prostate, peritoneum (the membrane lining the abdomen), and retroperitoneum (the space behind this lining). (For more on how CT scans work, see Chapter 2.)

• **Spiral CT scanning,** a variation that improves the visibility of blood vessels, may be used to evaluate patients suspected of having an aneurysm (abnormal outpouching) in the abdominal aorta, the largest artery in the body. After contrast dye is injected, the spiral CT scanner provides highly detailed three-dimensional constructs of the abdominal aorta, yielding accurate measurements of the size and extent of aortic aneurysms.

• **CT portography** is a variation that may be used in patients suspected of having very small liver tumors. Contrast dye is injected through a catheter inserted into the femoral artery in the groin and threaded to the splenic artery, and a newer, faster type of CT scanner is used to examine the liver.

Purpose of the Test

• To detect cysts, abscesses, tumors, inflammation, obstructions, bleeding, and other abnormalities in various abdominal and pelvic organs—particularly when other, less invasive tests, such as ultrasound, have failed to yield a diagnosis.

• To identify blood clots or an aneurysm in the abdominal aorta and its branches.

• To stage and monitor tumors before and after treatment for cancer.

• To detect enlarged lymph nodes in the abdomen.

• To guide the placement of biopsy needles and other instruments for various medical procedures.

Who Performs It

• A radiologist or a qualified technician.

Special Concerns

• Pregnant women should not undergo this test because exposure to ionizing radiation may harm the fetus.

• Barium retained in the GI system from recent contrast x-rays, such as an upper GI series (see page 373), may interfere with the results.

• People with allergies to iodine or shellfish may experience an allergic reaction to iodine-based contrast dyes.

• Elderly individuals with chronic dehydration or kidney impairment are at risk for renal failure induced by the contrast dye. To determine whether the dye can be administered safely, your doctor may perform a blood test to assess kidney function before the test.

Results

▼

➡ A physician will examine the CT scans and other test data for evidence of abnormalities.

➡ If a definitive diagnosis can be made based on the findings, appropriate medical or surgical treatment will be initiated.

➡ In some cases, additional diagnostic tests may be needed to further evaluate abnormal results.

• People who experience claustrophobia may find it difficult to undergo a CT scan, which takes place in a narrow, tunnel-like structure.

• This test may not be possible for severely overweight individuals (over 300 lbs).

Before the Test

• Inform your doctor if you have an allergy to iodine or shellfish. You may be given a combined antihistamine-steroid preparation to reduce the risk of an allergic reaction.

• Tell your doctor if you suffer from claustrophobia. He or she may prescribe a sedative that can help you tolerate the procedure.

• If you are to undergo CT portography, be sure to inform your doctor if you are taking any anticoagulants. It may be necessary to discontinue these drugs prior to the procedure.

• If a contrast dye is to be used, you should fast for 4 hours before the test and drink large amounts of fluids on the day before the test to prevent dehydration. If a dye is not being used, avoid eating for 2 hours before the test.

• Just before the test, remove your clothes and any metal objects, including watches, hair clips, and jewelry, and put on a hospital gown.

What You Experience

• You are asked to lie on your back on a narrow table that is then advanced into the CT scanner.

• The scanner, which encircles you, takes pictures of your abdomen at different intervals and from various angles. The resulting images are then recorded on x-ray film.

• Remain still because any movement can distort the image on the scan. The examiner may advise you on how to control your breathing at several points during the procedure.

• If a contrast dye is used, it is either administered orally before the test or given during the test through an intravenous (IV) catheter inserted into a vein in your arm. (Upon injection of the dye, you may experience a brief flushing sensation and a metallic taste in the mouth.)

• The procedure usually takes about 45 minutes to 1 hour.

Risks and Complications

• Although radiation exposure is minimal, you will receive a higher dose of radiation than during standard x-ray procedures.

• Some people may experience an allergic reaction to the iodine-based contrast dye, which can cause symptoms such as nausea, sneezing, vomiting, hives, and occasionally a life-threatening response called anaphylactic shock. Emergency medications and equipment are kept readily available.

• Patients who are dehydrated or those with impaired kidney function may experience acute renal failure from infusion of the contrast dye. Adequate hydration before the test can reduce this risk.

After the Test

• If contrast dye was used, you are encouraged to drink clear fluids to avoid dehydration and help flush the dye out of your system.

• If you underwent CT portography, the catheter is removed and a pressure dressing is applied to the puncture site. A small sandbag is typically placed over the incision site for several hours to prevent bleeding. You will rest in a recovery room for about 4 to 8 hours to allow the arterial puncture site to seal completely; during this time, your vital signs will be monitored and you will be observed for signs of complications.

• You are free to resume your normal diet and activities.

• Blood may collect and clot under the skin (hematoma) at the dye injection site; this is harmless and will resolve on its own. For a large hematoma that causes swelling and discomfort, apply ice initially; after 24 hours, use warm, moist compresses to help dissolve the clotted blood.

• Delayed allergic reactions to the contrast dye, such as hives, rash, or itching, may appear 2 to 6 hours after the procedure. If this occurs, your doctor will prescribe antihistamines or steroids to ease your discomfort.

Estimated Cost: $$$

Abdominal CT Scan continued

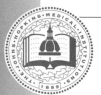

Abdominal MRI
(Magnetic Resonance Imaging of the Abdomen)

Abdominal MRI

Description

• Abdominal magnetic resonance imaging (MRI) uses a powerful magnetic field combined with radiofrequency waves to create highly detailed, cross-sectional images of tissues and organs in the abdomen; these scans are examined for abnormalities. Abdominal MRI is most often performed to visualize the liver, but may also be used to examine other soft tissues, such as the lymph nodes, kidneys, pancreas, or other organs. This imaging procedure is particularly useful when the area to be scanned is blocked by overlying bone or foreign bodies, or when differentiation of soft tissues on the images is required. (For more information on how MRI works, see Chapter 2.)

Purpose of the Test

• To detect and evaluate a variety of abnormalities in abdominal organs such as enlargement, cysts, and tumors.
• To clarify findings from previous abdominal x-rays (see page 82) or CT scans (see page 76).
• To evaluate blood flow in abdominal blood vessels.

Who Performs It

• A radiologist or a qualified technician.

Special Concerns

• People who experience claustrophobia may find it difficult to undergo an MRI, which takes place in a narrow, tunnel-like structure. In some cases, an open MRI—a larger unit that is open on several sides—may be used as an alternative.
• This test may not be possible for severely overweight individuals (over 300 lbs). Some open MRI scanners can accommodate larger patients.
• Because the MRI generates a strong magnetic field, it cannot be performed on people who have certain types of internally placed metallic devices, including pacemakers, inner ear implants, or intracranial aneurysm clips.
• The test should not be done in pregnant women because the long-term effects of MRI on the fetus are unknown.

Before the Test

• Tell your doctor if you suffer from claustrophobia. He or she may administer a sedative to help you tolerate the procedure.
• Before evaluation of some abdominal organs, you may need to clear the colon with a laxative or cleansing enema.
• In some cases, medications may be given to reduce the motion of the intestines (peristalsis), which may blur the MRI images.
• You will be instructed to empty your bladder before the test.
• Remove any magnetic cards or metallic objects, including watches, hair clips, belts, credit cards, and jewelry.

Results

➡ The MRI scans are displayed on a video monitor and then recorded on film. A physician will examine the images for any evidence of abnormalities.

➡ If a definitive diagnosis can be made based on the MRI images, your doctor will recommend appropriate treatment, depending on the specific problem.

➡ In some cases, additional tests, such as a liver biopsy (see page 240), liver or kidney function tests (see pages 111 and 311), or abdominal ultrasound (see page 80), may be required to establish a diagnosis or determine the extent of a problem.

• You may be asked to disrobe and put on a hospital gown.

What You Experience

• You will lie down on a narrow padded bed that slides into a large, enclosed cylinder containing the MRI magnets.
• You must remain still throughout the procedure because any motion can distort the scan.
• There is a microphone inside the imaging machine, and you may talk to the technician performing the scan at any time during the procedure.
• You will hear loud thumping sounds as the scanning is performed. To block out the noise, you can request earplugs or listen to music on earphones.

• The procedure time ranges from 30 to 90 minutes.

Risks and Complications

• MRI does not involve exposure to ionizing radiation and is not associated with any risks or complications.

After the Test

• Most patients can go home right after the scan and resume their usual activities.
• Sedated patients may be monitored for a short period until the effects of the sedative have worn off.

Estimated Cost: $$ to $$$

Abdominal MRI continued

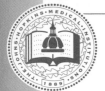

Abdominal Ultrasound
(Abdominal Ultrasonography)

Abdominal Ultrasound

Description
• In this test, a device called a transducer is passed lightly over your abdomen, directing high-frequency sound waves (ultrasound) at abdominal structures or organs. The sound waves are reflected back to the transducer and electronically converted into real-time images displayed on a viewing monitor. (These images may also be recorded on film or video and reviewed for abnormalities.) Abdominal ultrasound may be used to examine the liver, gallbladder, bile ducts, spleen, pancreas, kidneys, ureters, bladder, and abdominal aorta. It is most helpful for visualizing organs that are uniform and solid, such as the liver, or fluid-filled, such as the gallbladder. (For more on how ultrasound works, see Chapter 2.)
• A technique called Doppler ultrasound may be used to evaluate blood circulation through abdominal blood vessels including the abdominal aorta, the largest blood vessel in the body. In duplex scanning, this data is combined with standard ultrasound imaging to provide detailed information about abdominal blood vessels.

Purpose of the Test
• To determine the size, shape, and position of organs in the abdominal cavity.
• To detect tumors, abscesses, cysts, organ enlargement, and other abnormalities affecting tissues and organs in the abdomen.
• To detect stones in the gallbladder, bile ducts, or kidneys.
• To detect an enlarging aneurysm (abnormal outpouching) in the abdominal aorta.
• To diagnose the presence of excess fluid in the abdomen (ascites).
• To evaluate the spleen after trauma to the abdomen.
• To monitor a transplanted kidney.
• To guide the placement of biopsy needles or other instruments in various medical procedures.

Who Performs It
• A radiologist or a technician who is trained in ultrasound.

Special Concerns
• Because residual barium in the stomach or colon can distort sound waves and affect the test results, this exam should be done before any barium contrast x-rays are performed.
• The presence of gas or feces in the bowel can prevent adequate visualization of some regions of the abdomen.
• Ultrasound may fail to accurately show the boundaries between organs and tissue structures in dehydrated patients because of deficient body fluids.
• This test may be difficult in very obese patients, since fat may interfere with transmission of sound waves.

Before the Test
• If you are having an ultrasound exam of the gallbladder, liver, pancreas, spleen, or abdominal aorta, you must fast for 8 to 12 hours before the procedure; in addition, the evening meal before a gallbladder ultrasound test should be fat-free.

Results
▼
➡ A physician reviews the recorded images and video for evidence of any abnormality.
➡ If a definitive diagnosis can be made, appropriate treatment will be initiated.
➡ If ultrasound fails to yield a definitive diagnosis, other, more invasive diagnostic tests may be needed to provide more specific information or to further evaluate abnormal findings.

• No fasting is required before an ultrasound exam of the kidney.

• Just before the test, you will be asked to disrobe and put on a hospital gown.

What You Experience

• You will lie on an examination table, either on your back or on your stomach, depending on the organ to be studied.

• A water-soluble gel is applied to your skin to enhance sound wave transmission.

• The examiner then moves the transducer back and forth over your abdomen to obtain different views of the targeted organs.

• You may be asked to hold your breath and to assume different positions during the test.

• Once clear images are obtained, they are recorded on film or video for later analysis.

• The procedure takes up to 30 minutes.

Risks and Complications

• Ultrasound is painless, noninvasive, and involves no exposure to radiation. There are no associated risks.

After the Test

• The examiner removes the conductive gel from your skin.

• You are free to resume your normal diet and activities.

Estimated Cost: $$

Abdominal Ultrasound continued

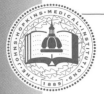

Abdominal X-ray
(Obstruction Series, Abdominal Radiography)

Description
• X-ray beams are passed through the abdomen, producing images of the internal structures on a special type of film. This basic imaging test is used for the quick evaluation of patients with acute abdominal pain. (For more on how x-rays work, see Chapter 2.)

Purpose of the Test
• To help determine the cause of acute abdominal pain in cases of suspected abdominal obstruction, perforation of the stomach or another abdominal organ, kidney stones, appendicitis, or ingestion of a foreign object.
• To monitor the progression or resolution of a chronic gastrointestinal disorder (for example, in patients with an obstruction of the small bowel).

Who Performs It
• A radiologist or an x-ray technician.

Special Concerns
• Pregnant women should not undergo this test because exposure to ionizing radiation may harm the fetus.

Before the Test
• Remove your shirt, belt, and any jewelry or metal objects and put on an x-ray gown.

What You Experience
• You will be positioned, either standing or lying down, in front of an x-ray machine.
• You are asked to take a deep breath and hold it while the x-ray is being taken, in order to provide a clear view of the abdomen. It is important to remain still throughout the procedure because any motion can distort the image. Several views from different angles will be taken.
• A chest x-ray (see page 156) may also be taken because pain in the lower part of the lungs may be mistaken for abdominal pain.
• The procedure takes several minutes.

Risks and Complications
• Radiation exposure is minimal.

After the Test
• Depending on the cause of the pain, you may return home and resume your usual activities.

Estimated Cost: $

Results
▼

➡ X-ray films are usually ready shortly after the test is completed. A doctor will examine the images for abnormalities, such as an obstruction, foreign body, or free air (air that is present in the abdominal cavity when there are holes along the digestive tract).

➡ If the doctor can make a definitive diagnosis, appropriate treatment will be initiated, depending on the specific problem.

➡ In many cases, additional tests—such as contrast x-rays to better visualize the digestive tract (see pages 104, 106, and 373), abdominal CT scan (see page 76), sigmoidoscopy (see page 323), or colonoscopy (see page 159)—may be required to establish a diagnosis and determine the extent of the problem.

Adrenal Hormone Tests

Description

• The body has two adrenal glands, one located above each kidney (see page 18). Hormones secreted by these endocrine glands help to regulate many body processes. Measuring blood and urine levels of adrenal hormones, including the following, is often the first step in diagnosing a variety of disorders associated with adrenal gland dysfunction.

• **Aldosterone** controls salt, potassium, and water balance in the body and helps to regulate blood pressure. Overproduction (hyperaldosteronism) or underproduction (hypoaldosteronism) of this hormone may be caused by tumors or other abnormalities within the adrenal glands (primary) or may result from problems outside the adrenals (secondary). Both blood levels and urinary excretion of aldosterone may be measured.

• **Cortisol** is a glucocorticoid hormone that helps to control the metabolism of carbohydrates, proteins, and fats; mediate the body's response to stress; and regulate the immune system. Oversecretion of cortisol, most often caused by a benign adrenal tumor, results in Cushing's syndrome. Undersecretion may indicate a form of adrenal insufficiency known as Addison's disease. Both blood levels and urine levels (known as free cortisol) are usually measured.

• **18-Hydroxycortisol,** a product of cortisol metabolism, is an unusual steroid produced in excessive amounts in patients with primary hyperaldosteronism. Measuring blood levels of this hormone can help to determine whether primary hyperaldosteronism is caused by a tumor called adrenal adenoma, or by overgrowth (hyperplasia) of adrenal tissue; levels are significantly higher in people with an adenoma.

• **DHEA-S,** or dehydroepiandrosterone-sulfate—a sex hormone (androgen) synthesized by the adrenal gland—is a precursor to testosterone. In women, the adrenal glands are the major, and sometimes only, source of androgens. Elevated DHEA-S levels are associated with virilism (male body characteristics), hirsutism (excessive hair growth), amenorrhea (absence of menstruation), and infertility. Adrenal abnormalities such as tumors may lead to abnormally high DHEA-S levels.

Purpose of the Test

• To evaluate patients with suspected dysfunction of the adrenal glands.

• To aid in the diagnosis and evaluation of adrenal abnormalities, such as Cushing's syndrome, Addison's disease, adrenal adenoma, or adrenal hyperplasia.

• DHEA-S may be measured to determine the cause of hirsutism, amenorrhea, or infertility in women and to evaluate precocious puberty in children.

Who Performs It

• A doctor, a nurse, or a technician.

Special Concerns

• A nuclear scan performed within the last

Results
▼

➡ Your blood and/or urine samples are sent to a laboratory for analysis. The doctor will review the results for evidence of any adrenal hormone disorder. (For more on laboratory testing, see Chapter 1.)

➡ In many cases, abnormal results on one or more of the adrenal hormone tests will necessitate additional tests to establish a definitive diagnosis.

➡ If an abnormality is found and the doctor can make a definitive diagnosis, appropriate treatment will begin.

week may affect the results of adrenal hormone tests, because these hormones are often measured with a laboratory technique that utilizes a radioactive isotope (radioimmunoassay).

• Certain medications and nutritional supplements may alter the results.

• Cortisol and aldosterone levels vary at different times during the day and are also affected by diet, physical activity, and stress.

• Pregnancy can alter the levels of aldosterone, cortisol, and DHEA-S.

• Posture and excessive licorice ingestion can affect aldosterone levels.

• Home kits are now available to monitor cortisol levels through periodic saliva samples (which you send to a laboratory for analysis). They may be useful to selected individuals. Ask your doctor for a recommendation.

Before the Test

• You may be asked to fast, observe certain dietary restrictions, limit your physical activity, and reduce stress levels for variable periods before these tests.

• Report to your doctor any medications, herbs, or supplements you are taking. You may be advised to discontinue certain of these agents before the test.

• Tell your doctor if you've had a recent nuclear scanning procedure.

What You Experience

Blood tests:

• A sample of your blood is drawn from a vein, usually in your arm, and sent to a laboratory for analysis. (For more on this procedure, called venipuncture, see page 32.)

Urine tests:

• To accurately assess urinary excretion of aldosterone, cortisol, and 18-hydroxycortisol, timed urine specimens are collected in a special container over a 24-hour period (for specific instructions, see page 34).

• Once urine collection is complete, label the container with your name, date, and time of completion and return it as instructed by your doctor.

Risks and Complications

• None.

After the Test

• Immediately after blood is drawn, pressure is applied (with cotton or gauze) to the puncture site.

• Resume your normal diet and any medications that were withheld before the test, according to your doctor's instructions.

• Blood may collect and clot under the skin (hematoma) at the puncture site; this is harmless and will resolve on its own. For a large hematoma that causes swelling and discomfort, apply ice initially; after 24 hours, use warm, moist compresses to help dissolve the clotted blood.

Estimated Cost: $

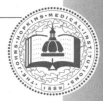

Anorectal Manometry
(Anal Rectal Motility)

Description
• In this procedure, a thin tube, called a manometry probe, is inserted into the anal canal and slowly withdrawn. The probe is attached to a pressure transducer that measures the pressures exerted by the rectal and anal sphincter muscles, which relax and contract to control bowel movements.
• An alternative method uses another type of probe—a metal cylinder equipped with three balloons (known as a three-balloon manometry system)—to measure the anal and rectal sphincter pressures.

Purpose of the Test
• To evaluate functioning in the anal canal and determine the cause of chronic constipation or fecal incontinence.
• To confirm the diagnosis of Hirschsprung's disease (a defect in the nerves of the colon that causes chronic constipation).
• Sometimes, this procedure is used as a treatment to retrain anal muscle contraction in people who experience fecal incontinence.

Who Performs It
• An experienced gastroenterologist or a specially trained assistant.

Special Concerns
• Anorectal manometry is not necessary for many cases of fecal incontinence. It is performed only in carefully selected patients, including those with suspected anorectal muscle or nerve damage caused by surgical trauma or systemic disease (such as diabetes or scleroderma) and those suspected of having Hirschsprung's disease.
• This test should not be performed in individuals with active lower gastrointestinal (GI) bleeding.
• The test is not possible in people who are allergic to latex or rubber.

• Anorectal manometry may be done in a hospital procedure room or in a doctor's office.

Before the Test
• You may be given a cleansing enema to clear the rectum.
• If you are very anxious prior to the test, the doctor may administer a sedative.
• You will be asked to disrobe and put on a hospital gown.

What You Experience
• You will lie down on an examining table.
• The examiner inserts a gloved, lubricated finger into your rectum to perform a manual examination.
• The manometry probe—a narrow tube of soft plastic or rigid metal—is gently inserted about four inches into the rectum.
• As the manometer is slowly withdrawn, it measures the pressure exerted by the rectal and anal muscles. This procedure may be repeated several times to confirm the results.
• Next, a balloon at the tip of the probe is

Results
▼
➥ Your doctor will review the test findings.
➥ In general, high pressures in the anal canal may cause constipation, while low pressures may lead to fecal incontinence. Analysis of muscle and nerve function at different points along the length of the anal canal may indicate specific conditions, such as Hirschsprung's disease.
➥ Based on the test findings, your doctor should be able to recommend an appropriate course of treatment, depending on the specific problem.

Anorectal Manometry

inflated slowly, and you are asked to tell the doctor when you experience the sensation of rectal fullness and the urge to defecate.

• Pressure may also be measured as you squeeze the anus as hard as possible.

• Alternatively, three-balloon manometry uses another type of probe—a hollow, metal cylinder equipped with three special manometry balloons. When the probe is positioned in the rectum, the balloons are inflated and the pressure readings are noted. You will be asked to tell the doctor when you experience the sensation of rectal fullness and the urge to defecate.

• The probe is withdrawn.
• The procedure time ranges from 30 to 90 minutes.

Risks and Complications

• Anorectal manometry is considered a safe procedure, but you will experience some discomfort as the probe is inserted and removed.

After the Test

• Most patients may return home immediately and resume their usual activities.

Estimated Cost: $$

Antegrade Pyelography

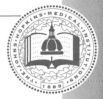

Description

• In this test, a contrast dye is injected directly into one of the kidneys, and a series of x-ray films is taken to visualize the flow of dye through the ureter, which connects the kidney to the bladder (illustrated on page 26). Because the dye is more dense than urine, it will settle in the ureter on top of any obstruction, thereby revealing its location. Antegrade pyelography is performed when intravenous (see page 225) and retrograde (see page 315) pyelography cannot be done or fail to provide an adequate picture of the ureter. (For more on contrast x-rays, see Chapter 2.)

Purpose of the Test

• To determine the site of a known or suspected ureteral obstruction caused by a stricture, stone, or tumor.
• To aid in the placement of a nephrostomy tube, a catheter that is surgically positioned in the kidney for drainage.
• To assess the function of the upper collecting system of the kidney after surgery.

Who Performs It

• A physician.

Special Concerns

• People who have an allergy to shellfish or iodine may experience an allergic reaction to the contrast dye.
• Pregnant women should not undergo this test because exposure to ionizing radiation may harm the fetus.
• This test may not be safe for people with bleeding disorders.

Before the Test

• Tell your doctor if you regularly take anticoagulant drugs. You may be instructed to discontinue them for some time before the test.
• Be sure to tell your doctor if you have a known shellfish or iodine allergy or have ever had an adverse reaction to x-ray contrast dyes.
• Do not eat solid food for 8 hours before the test; you may drink clear fluids until 3 hours before the test.
• You will be asked to disrobe and put on a hospital gown.

What You Experience

• You are asked to lie on your stomach on an examination table.
• The doctor locates the position of the renal pelvis (the area at the center of the kidney where urine collects) by means of ultrasound, fluoroscopy, or CT scanning (see Chapter 2).
• The skin over this site is marked and cleansed with an antiseptic solution. A local anesthetic is then injected into the area; this injection may cause brief discomfort.
• You will be asked to hold your breath as the doctor, using fluoroscopy or ultrasound as a guide, inserts a hollow needle into your kidney.
• If necessary, a syringe may be used to drain urine through the needle. (Urine samples may be sent to a laboratory for analysis.)

Results

▼

➡ Your doctor will examine the x-rays and other test data to locate any obstruction or blockage of urine flow or other abnormalities.
➡ If a definitive diagnosis can be made, appropriate treatment will be initiated, depending on the specific problem.
➡ In some cases, additional tests, such as a CT scan (see page 76), a nuclear scan (see page 313), or ureteroscopy (see page 375), may be needed to establish a diagnosis and determine the extent of the problem.

Antegrade Pyelography

• A contrast dye is injected through the needle into the kidney. You may feel a brief burning or flushing sensation as the dye is injected.
• X-ray films are obtained to visualize the kidney and ureter. Remain still as each x-ray is taken.
• A catheter (nephrostomy tube) may be left in place for further drainage of urine, if necessary.
• The test takes about 60 to 90 minutes.

Risks and Complications

• X-ray exams involve minimal exposure to radiation.
• Possible complications include bleeding at the site of needle insertion.
• Some people may experience an allergic reaction to the iodine-based contrast dye, which can cause symptoms such as nausea, sneezing, vomiting, hives, and occasionally a life-threatening response called anaphylactic shock. Emergency medications and equipment are kept readily available.

After the Test

• A pressure dressing is applied to the site of needle insertion.

• You will rest in a recovery room for 15 to 30 minutes. Your vital signs will be monitored, and pain medication will be provided if necessary.
• If no complications develop, you are usually free to leave the testing facility.
• You will be instructed to keep track of your urine output and report any urinary retention. Your urine may contain blood at first, causing a slight pink tinge; this should resolve after voiding a few times. If blood persists or you see bright red blood or blood clots, notify your physician.
• Delayed allergic reactions to the contrast dye, such as hives, rash, or itching, may appear 2 to 6 hours after the procedure. If this occurs, your doctor will prescribe antihistamines or steroids to ease your discomfort.
• You may be given prophylactic antibiotic drugs for several days to prevent infection.
• You may resume your normal diet and any medications withheld before the test.
• Report to the doctor any signs of infection, such as chills, fever, rapid breathing, or a feeling of faintness.

Estimated Cost: $$

Antibody Tests for Autoimmune Disorders

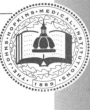

Description

• In autoimmune disorders, the immune system mistakenly recognizes a natural body constituent as "foreign" and begins to attack healthy cells, causing tissue destruction. This immune attack—which may be generalized and take place in a number of tissues, or may focus on a single organ—is executed by substances called autoantibodies, which target specific components of cells such as the nucleus or cell receptors. Blood tests for the following autoantibodies are often performed to aid in the diagnosis of autoimmune disorders:

• **Antinuclear antibody** is present in almost all people with systemic lupus erythematosus (SLE)—a generalized autoimmune condition that attacks a number of different tissues. It is also found in some individuals with rheumatoid arthritis, scleroderma (which destroys connective tissue), Sjögren's syndrome (which causes dry mouth and eyes), polymyositis (which affects the nerves and muscles), and certain forms of chronic active hepatitis (a nonautoimmune liver disease).

• **Anti-DNA antibody** may be found in people with SLE, but is typically not present in other autoimmune diseases.

• **Antiphospholipid antibody,** which is associated with blood clot formation and miscarriages, may be present in SLE and certain other autoimmune conditions.

• **Anti-smooth muscle antibody,** frequently present in patients with chronic active hepatitis, aids in distinguishing between this and other forms of liver disease.

• **Antimitochondrial antibody** is present in most patients with primary biliary cirrhosis (an autoimmune liver disorder) and is found rarely in other types of chronic liver disease.

• **Acetylcholine receptor antibodies**—which are present in the majority of patients with myasthenia gravis (an autoimmune disorder affecting the nerves and muscles)—are tested to aid in the diagnosis of this disease, and also to help monitor the effectiveness of immunosuppressive therapy for the condition.

Purpose of the Test

• To assist in the diagnosis of autoimmune disorders.
• To monitor the course and treatment of an autoimmune disorder.

Who Performs It

• A doctor, a nurse, or a lab technician.

Special Concerns

• False-positive and false-negative results (see page 35) are possible.

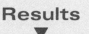

Results

➡ Your blood sample is sent to a laboratory and analyzed for the presence of autoantibodies. Your doctor will review the test results in conjunction with your symptoms, medical history, and physical exam for evidence of an autoimmune disorder. (For more on laboratory tests, see Chapter 1.)

➡ If results are positive and your doctor can make a definitive diagnosis, appropriate therapy will begin.

➡ In many cases, one or more positive results on these blood tests will necessitate additional procedures—for example, a biopsy of the lip (see page 242), liver (see page 240), or muscle (see page 261)—to confirm a diagnosis.

➡ The absence of autoantibodies suggests you may have a condition other than an autoimmune disorder, and other tests may be scheduled.

Antibody Tests for Autoimmune Disorders continued

• Certain medications may alter the results of some of these tests.

• A radioactive scan performed within 1 week before the anti-DNA antibody test may alter the results of this test.

• Antinuclear antibodies may be found in the blood of healthy older people and occasionally in some healthy younger individuals.

Before the Test

• Report to your doctor any medications you are taking. You may be advised to discontinue certain of these agents before the test.

What You Experience

• A sample of your blood is drawn from a vein, usually in your arm, and sent to a laboratory for analysis. (For more on this procedure, called venipuncture, see page 32.)

Risks and Complications

• There are no known risks or complications.

After the Test

• Immediately after blood is drawn, pressure is applied (with cotton or gauze) to the puncture site.

• Resume your normal diet and any medications withheld before the test.

• Blood may collect and clot under the skin (hematoma) at the puncture site; this is harmless and will resolve on its own. For a large hematoma that causes swelling and discomfort, apply ice initially; after 24 hours, use warm, moist compresses to help dissolve the clotted blood.

Estimated Cost: $

Antigen/Antibody Tests for Infectious Disease

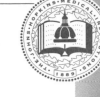

Description

• Infectious diseases are caused by tiny microorganisms such as bacteria, viruses, fungi, and parasites. Proteins, called antigens, are carried on the cell surface of all infectious organisms; the immune system recognizes these foreign invaders, and in response forms proteins called antibodies to destroy or control them. Antigen/antibody tests rely on the fact that there is a specific antibody for each antigen—thus, each one can be used to detect the presence of the other. For example, a known antigen may be added to a blood sample; if the corresponding antibody is present in the specimen, the two proteins will bind together. These tests are usually performed on serum (the liquid portion that remains when blood clots and the cells are removed); but occasionally, samples of other body fluids, tissue, or stool may be used. Several different techniques may be employed, including the following:

• **Precipitation reaction.** When an antigen-antibody reaction takes place, the antigens and antibodies cross-link to form a latticelike structure that precipitates out of the solution, settling on the bottom of the beaker. Observation of this precipitate can confirm the presence of a specific infectious agent.

• **Agglutination reaction.** Agglutination refers to a clumping that occurs when an antigen comes into contact with its corresponding antibody. This process mimics what happens in the body when antibodies cause antigens to agglutinate, promoting easy removal of the infectious organism. Observation of an agglutination reaction aids in the detection of specific antibodies, such as those produced in syphilis or *salmonella* infections.

• **Complement fixation** refers to a reaction in which an antigen binds with an antibody, forming a combination that causes complement (a complex group of blood proteins) to become fixed at the same site. Detection of this complement fixation reaction leads to identification of the original antigen.

• **Immunofluorescent assay** is a technique in which specific antibodies are tagged with a fluorescent dye. When these antibodies bind to antigens from a particular organism, they appear as green, glowing particles under a fluorescent microscope, thereby revealing the presence of the infectious agent.

• **Enzyme-linked immunosorbent assay (ELISA)** uses tagging to identify unknown antibodies or antigens in a serum sample. In this technique, the antibodies are tagged with certain enzymes (proteins that speed up chemical reactions in the body). When an antigen and antibody bind to each other, the enzyme causes a reaction that produces a color change, thereby identifying the unknown microorganism.

• **Radioimmunoassay** is a similar technique to ELISA that tags antibodies with radioactive material.

Purpose of the Test

• To aid in the diagnosis of viral, bacterial, fungal, and parasitic infections.

Results

▼

➡ The blood specimen or other sample is sent to a laboratory for analysis. (For more on laboratory tests, see Chapter 1.)

➡ Your doctor will make a diagnosis based on these results, as well as your medical history, symptoms, physical exam, and findings from any other tests, such as a culture (see page 166). Appropriate treatment will be initiated, depending on the specific infection.

Who Performs It
• A doctor, a nurse, or a laboratory technician draws the blood sample.

Special Concerns
• Cross-reactions can occur, in which one antigen reacts with antibodies developed against another antigen, leading to false-positive results.
• False-negative results can occur in the early stages of certain infections, prior to the development of antibodies. (For more on false-positives and false-negatives, see page 35.)

Before the Test
• No special preparation is needed for a blood test. Preparation varies for other procedures according to what type of tissue or fluid sample is required; your doctor will provide specific instructions.

What You Experience
• In most cases, a sample of your blood is drawn from a vein, usually in your arm, and sent to a laboratory for analysis. (For more on venipuncture, see page 32.)

• Occasionally, a sample of another body fluid, tissue, or stool is obtained and sent to a laboratory for analysis. These procedures may be noninvasive or invasive, depending on what type of sample is needed.

Risks and Complications
• Possible risks vary according to what type of tissue or fluid sample is required.

After the Test
• Post-test care varies according to what type of tissue or fluid sample is required.
• Immediately after a blood sample is drawn, pressure is applied (with cotton or gauze) to the puncture site. Blood may collect and clot under the skin (hematoma) at the puncture site; this is harmless and will resolve on its own. For a large hematoma that causes swelling and discomfort, apply ice initially; after 24 hours, use warm, moist compresses to help dissolve the clotted blood.

Estimated Cost: $

Arterial Blood Gases

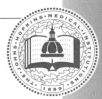

Description
• In this test, the concentrations of various gases in the blood are measured. Arterial blood gas levels can provide important information about the respiratory function of the lungs and metabolic status. This test is used to analyze oxygen and carbon dioxide levels, as well as the acidity of the blood.
• **Oxygen** is necessary for cellular function; it is inhaled and absorbed into the blood via the lungs. Abnormal levels may result from a variety of disorders, including nearly all forms of lung disease, anemias, and oversedation from certain drugs.
• **Carbon dioxide (CO_2)** is a waste product of cellular metabolism that passes out of the blood in the lungs and is then exhaled. Carbon dioxide also acts as a buffer system to help maintain the acid-base balance of the blood. Abnormal levels can be caused by certain medications or by lung or kidney disease, severe vomiting, diabetic ketoacidosis (a life-threatening complication of type 1 diabetes mellitus), and other disorders.
• **pH levels** give an indication of the acid-base balance of the blood. Abnormal levels can be caused by lung disease, kidney failure, severe vomiting or diarrhea, chronic heart failure, diabetic ketoacidosis, and other disorders.

Purpose of the Test
• To evaluate how efficiently the lungs deliver oxygen to and remove carbon dioxide from the blood.
• To provide clues as to possible causes of shortness of breath.
• To determine the acidity of the blood.
• To monitor respiratory treatments, such as oxygen therapy or a ventilator.

Who Performs It
• A doctor or a trained nurse or technician.

Special Concerns
• This test requires drawing blood from an artery. Thus, it may cause more discomfort than most routine blood tests (which use blood from a vein), since arteries are deeper and have more nerves than veins.
• This test should not be performed in people with severe bleeding disorders.

Before the Test
• Report to your doctor any medications, herbs, or supplements that you regularly take. You may be advised to discontinue certain of these agents before the test.

What You Experience
• The person performing the test will select an artery in your arm, usually in the wrist, and check for adequate circulation by placing brief pressure on it, cutting off blood flow, and seeing how quickly color returns to the hand when the flow returns. If your palm does not turn pink within a few seconds, blood flow is

Results
▼
➡ Your blood sample is analyzed in the office or is sent to a laboratory for analysis. The doctor will consider the test results together with your physical signs and symptoms. (For more on blood tests, see Chapter 1.)
➡ Abnormal blood gas levels may indicate a wide variety of potential health problems. Additional tests, such as pulmonary function tests (see page 306), are often necessary to establish a definitive diagnosis.
➡ If lung function is severely reduced, the doctor may recommend treatment, such as oxygen therapy.

insufficient, and the procedure will be repeated in your other arm. If blood flow is inadequate in both arms, an artery in your leg will be used.

• Blood is drawn from the selected artery. (For more on arterial puncture, see page 33.)

Risks and Complications

• Arterial puncture carries a significant risk that blood will collect and clot under the skin (hematoma) at the puncture site, causing swelling and discoloration. This is harmless but may cause some discomfort.

• In rare cases, the puncture may damage the artery or nearby structures, such as a nerve.

After the Test

• After the needle is removed, the person drawing blood will apply firm pressure on the puncture site for several minutes (or longer in patients who tend to bleed excessively, such as those who take anticoagulants or have a bleeding disorder).

• A gauze bandage will then be firmly taped to the area.

• If a large hematoma develops at the puncture site, apply ice initially; after 24 hours, use warm, moist compresses to help dissolve the clotted blood.

• Inform your doctor if you experience any pain, numbness, tingling, or bleeding in the limb used for the puncture.

Estimated Cost: $

Arteriography
(Angiography)

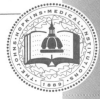

Description

• In this test, a contrast dye is injected through a thin, flexible tube (catheter) into selected arteries, and a series of x-rays is obtained. Filled with the dye, these vessels are differentiated from other bodily structures on the x-ray film. Arteriography is commonly used to evaluate arteries in the abdomen, kidneys, brain, lower extremities, and adrenal glands, as well as to visualize the coronary arteries (see page 140) and the pulmonary arteries (see page 302).

• Digital subtraction angiography is a technique that is currently used to enhance arteriographic images. Continuous x-ray imaging, or fluoroscopy (see page 205), records images of arteries before and after a contrast dye is injected. A computer converts these images into digital information, and then subtracts the preinjection from the postinjection images, removing bone and soft tissue and leaving an enhanced picture of the contrast-filled blood vessels.

Purpose of the Test

• To identify and evaluate narrowing, blockages, and other abnormalities in various arteries, including the femoral arteries in the legs, the carotid arteries in the neck, and the arterial systems of the brain, kidneys, and adrenal glands.

• To obtain an accurate picture of the anatomy of specific blood vessels prior to vascular surgery.

Who Performs It

• A radiologist or another physician.

Special Concerns

• Pregnant women should only undergo this test in extreme circumstances because exposure to ionizing radiation may harm the fetus.

• People with allergies to iodine or shellfish may experience an allergic reaction to iodine-based contrast dyes.

• In people with kidney disorders or chronic dehydration, the contrast dye can worsen kidney function and may cause renal failure. To determine whether the dye can be administered safely, your doctor may perform a blood test to assess your kidney function (see page 311) before the test.

• This test may not be safe in people who have bleeding disorders or unstable cardiac disorders. Coagulation studies (see page 157) may be performed prior to the procedure to ensure that your blood will clot normally.

Before the Test

• Inform your doctor if you regularly take anticoagulants or nonsteroidal anti-inflammatory drugs (such as aspirin, ibuprofen, or naproxen). You may be advised to discontinue these drugs for some time before the test.

• Be sure to inform your doctor if you have a known shellfish or iodine allergy or have ever had an adverse reaction to x-ray contrast dyes. You may be given preventive medication before the test, or a noniodinated dye may be used.

• Do not eat anything for 8 hours before the test. You may consume clear liquids.

• At the testing facility, remove any metal objects, including watches, hair clips, or jewelry.

• An intravenous (IV) line is inserted into a vein in your arm so that any necessary medications can be administered during the procedure.

• Empty your bladder before the procedure

Results

▼

➡ The doctor will examine the recorded images for signs of significantly narrowed or blocked arteries and any other abnormalities.

➡ This test usually establishes a definitive diagnosis. Based on the findings, your doctor will recommend a course of medical or surgical treatment.

Arteriography continued

begins. (Because iodinated dye can act as a diuretic, your bladder may feel uncomfortably full during the test. For more prolonged studies, this may require the insertion of a temporary catheter into the bladder.)

• You will be given a sedative to help you relax during the test.

What You Experience

• You will lie on your back on an x-ray table. If blood vessels in the head or neck are being examined, your head is immobilized in a brace (but your face is left uncovered).

• Electrocardiogram (ECG) leads (see page 174) may be taped to your arms and legs to monitor your heart during the test.

• The area where the catheter is to be inserted—usually the femoral artery in the groin—is cleansed with an antiseptic solution and (if necessary) shaved. A local anesthetic is injected to numb the site.

• A needle is inserted into the femoral artery, and a guide wire is passed through the needle. A thin catheter is then inserted over this wire and into the artery, and the wire is withdrawn.

• Under the guidance of fluoroscopic imaging, the catheter is directed to the artery being examined. (To examine the cerebral blood vessels in the brain, the catheter is threaded to arteries of the neck.)

• Next, a contrast dye is injected through the catheter. You may experience a flushing or burning sensation, headache, or a metallic taste briefly after the injection; rarely, some people experience nausea and possibly vomiting.

• As the contrast agent spreads through the arteries, serial x-ray films are obtained in a timed sequence.

• The procedure time varies, ranging from less than 1 hour to 3 hours.

Risks and Complications

• Possible serious risks include blood clot formation, bleeding or infection at the catheter insertion site, blood vessel damage, abnormal heart rhythms, and, in rare cases, stroke.

• Some people may experience an allergic reaction to the iodine-based contrast dye, which can cause symptoms such as nausea, sneezing, vomiting, hives, and occasionally a life-threatening response called anaphylactic shock. Emergency medications and equipment are kept readily available.

• Renal failure may occur as a result of exposure to the contrast dye, especially in elderly patients with chronic dehydration or mild kidney impairment.

After the Test

• The catheter is removed, and pressure is applied until the bleeding stops (up to 30 minutes). A pressure bandage is applied, and a small sandbag may be placed over the puncture site for several hours to prevent bleeding.

• You will rest in a recovery room for about 6 to 8 hours. During this time, you should not move the limb where the catheter was inserted. Nurses will check you periodically to ensure there is no bleeding at the puncture site or other complications.

• You are encouraged to drink clear fluids to avoid dehydration and help flush the contrast dye out of your system.

• Most people may return home after about 5 to 6 hours, though some may require overnight hospitalization. Before you leave, a doctor or nurse will demonstrate how to apply pressure to stop any bleeding at the puncture site.

• Blood may collect and clot under the skin (hematoma) at the puncture site; this is harmless and will resolve on its own. For a large hematoma that causes swelling and discomfort, apply ice initially; after 24 hours, use warm, moist compresses to help dissolve the clotted blood.

• You may resume your normal diet and medications, according to your doctor's instructions. Avoid heavy lifting and strenuous activities for a few days.

• If bleeding or any other complications develop, call your doctor or emergency medical service immediately.

Estimated Cost: $$$

Arthrocentesis
(Synovial Fluid Analysis, Joint Aspiration)

Description
• In this procedure, a needle is used to withdraw (aspirate) synovial fluid, which is the viscous liquid that helps to lubricate and nourish bones and cartilage within the joints. The fluid sample is then sent to a laboratory for analysis. The most common site for arthrocentesis is the knee, but it can be performed on any major joint, including the shoulder, elbow, hip, ankle, and wrist. Arthrocentesis may also be done therapeutically to relieve pain and swelling caused by accumulation of fluid in a joint.

Purpose of the Test
• To aid in the diagnosis of certain joint disorders such as infection, rheumatoid arthritis, and gout.
• To determine the cause of joint inflammation or effusion (excessive accumulation of fluid inside the joint).
• To monitor the effectiveness of antibiotic medication used for the treatment of infectious arthritis.
• Performed therapeutically to relieve the discomfort caused by joint effusion or to administer medications, such as corticosteroids, into the joint.

Who Performs It
• A physician.

Special Concerns
• Arthrocentesis should not be performed in areas with a skin or wound infection.
• This procedure may be done in a hospital or in an outpatient setting.
• Sometimes a blood sample is taken from a vein in the arm (a procedure called venipuncture that is described on page 32) to compare chemical test results with analyses of the synovial fluid obtained during arthrocentesis.

Before the Test
• Your doctor may ask you to avoid food and fluids for 6 to 12 hours if glucose levels in the synovial fluid are to be measured. If not, fasting is unnecessary.
• You will be instructed to remove whatever clothing is covering the joint to be aspirated.

What You Experience
• The skin at the site of needle insertion is cleansed with an antiseptic solution, and a local anesthetic is injected to numb the area.
• The area around the joint may be wrapped in elastic bandages to compress the maximum amount of fluid into the joint space.
• A needle is quickly inserted through the skin and into the joint space. You will feel pressure or slight pain as it is inserted.

Results
▼

➡ The specimen containers may be sent to several different laboratories for examination, and the fluid is analyzed for the presence of abnormal components. For example, bacteria may be present in cases of infectious arthritis, elevated white blood cells suggest an inflammatory disorder such as rheumatoid arthritis, and uric acid crystals indicate a diagnosis of gout. (For more on microscopic examination and fluid analysis, see Chapter 1.)

➡ If a definitive diagnosis can be made, the doctor will recommend an appropriate course of treatment.

➡ In some cases, additional tests may be required to establish a diagnosis or determine the extent of a problem.

Arthrocentesis

• Fluid is withdrawn through the needle and placed into multiple specimen containers.

• If a corticosteroid or another medication (such as an antibiotic) is administered, the syringe is detached, leaving the needle in the joint. Another syringe is then attached, and the medicine is injected.

• The procedure takes 3 to 5 minutes.

Risks and Complications

• Serious but rare complications include infection or bleeding in the joint area.

After the Test

• The needle is withdrawn and pressure is applied to the puncture site with sterile gauze pads for 3 to 5 minutes.

• A pressure bandage is then applied to avoid re-collection of fluid or accumulation of blood underneath the skin (hematoma).

• Apply ice or cold packs to the joint for 24 to 48 hours to reduce any swelling and pain. You may also be given pain-relieving medication.

• You may resume your normal activities, but try to avoid excessive use of the affected joint for several days.

• Contact your doctor immediately if you develop increased pain or fever.

Estimated Cost: $$

Arthroscopy

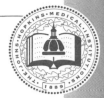

Description
• In this procedure, a thin, flexible viewing tube (called an arthroscope) is inserted through a small incision and into the interior of a joint, most often the knee. Fiberoptic cables permit the surgeon to visually inspect the internal joint structures. In addition, surgical instruments may be inserted, either through the scope or through other small incisions in the area, in order to obtain tissue or fluid samples or to perform therapeutic procedures.

Purpose of the Test
• To examine the interior of a joint (most often the knee, but also the hip, ankle, wrist, elbow, shoulder, or jaw) for the presence of disease or injury.
• To monitor the course of joint disease and the effectiveness of therapy.
• Used therapeutically to irrigate or to perform surgery on a joint.

Who Performs It
• A physician or a surgeon trained in arthroscopic procedures.

Special Concerns
• Arthroscopy is not appropriate if you have fibrous ankylosis (a condition characterized by the stiffening of joints in a fixed position) or a local skin or wound infection.
• This procedure is usually done under local anesthesia but may require spinal or general anesthesia—especially if arthroscopic surgery is anticipated.
• Arthroscopic surgery is associated with fewer risks, less postoperative pain, and faster recovery than open surgery (arthrotomy); however, if bleeding or other complications occur, or the procedure cannot be completed satisfactorily, arthrotomy may be required.

Before the Test
• If general anesthesia is required, do not eat or drink anything after midnight on the day before the procedure.
• You will be asked to disrobe and put on a hospital gown.
• Empty your bladder just before the test.
• If the procedure will be performed under local anesthesia, you may be given a sedative before the test to relax you.
• If general anesthesia is required, an intravenous (IV) catheter is inserted into a vein in your arm, and the medication is administered. A thin tube attached to a breathing machine will be inserted through your mouth and into your windpipe to ensure you breathe properly during the procedure.

What You Experience
• You will either sit or lie down on a table, depending on the joint being examined.
• The hair surrounding the joint is shaved (if necessary) and the area is cleansed with an antiseptic solution. If applicable, a local anesthetic is injected. (This injection may cause brief discomfort.)

Results
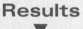

➡ During visual inspection of the joint, the doctor will note any abnormalities. Any tissue or fluid samples are sent to a laboratory for analysis. (For more on laboratory tests, see Chapter 1.) Your doctor will consider these results along with your symptoms, your physical exam, and the results of other tests.

➡ Arthroscopy can often provide a definitive diagnosis. Your doctor will recommend appropriate treatment.

Arthroscopy

Arthroscopy continued

• If the knee is being examined, your leg will be elevated and wrapped in elastic bandages from toe to thigh. A tourniquet may be applied to reduce the amount of blood present within the joint (causing an uncomfortable sensation of pressure), or a fluid mixture containing epinephrine and saline solution may be instilled into the joint to distend the knee and reduce bleeding. These measures will help to improve the doctor's view.

• A small incision is made, and the arthroscope is inserted into the joint. Magnifying devices allow the doctor to directly view the joint interior, and images of the area may also be transmitted onto a TV screen and recorded for later examination. The scope may be moved to different locations as needed.

• Following inspection of the joint, the doctor may insert surgical instruments through small incisions to remove tissue or fluid samples for laboratory analysis or to perform therapeutic measures.

• The scope and other instruments are removed, the joint is irrigated, and all incisions are closed with stitches or adhesive tape. Steroid medications may be injected to reduce any inflammation, and a pressure bandage may be applied to the joint.

• The procedure usually takes 30 to 40 minutes for examination, and up to 2 hours if surgery is required.

Risks and Complications

• Rare complications include infection, thrombophlebitis (a blood clot in a vein in the leg), accumulation of bloody fluid in the joint, joint injury, and excessive swelling.

• If general anesthesia is necessary, the procedure carries the associated risks.

After the Test

• You will rest in bed until you recover from the effects of anesthesia and any sedation. During this time, your vital signs will be monitored and you will be observed for signs of complications.

• The joint that was examined may be wrapped in bandages or (for a shoulder or elbow) placed in a sling.

• If the procedure was performed under general anesthesia, arrange for a ride home.

• Your doctor may ask you to keep the examined joint elevated and to minimize use of the joint for several days (or longer, if surgical treatment was performed). For a knee joint, this may require using crutches.

• The joint may be painful and slightly swollen for several days to weeks, depending on the extent of the procedure. Apply ice to reduce these symptoms. Your doctor may also prescribe pain-relieving medications.

• Call your doctor immediately if you experience severe swelling, fever, or redness or pus at the incision site.

Estimated Cost: $$$

Balance Tests

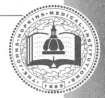

Description

• Your sense of physical balance, or equilibrium, relies on a series of signals that pass from the vestibular organs in the inner ear, through a branch of the 8th cranial nerve (or vestibular nerve), to the brain. The inner ear contains a complex system of fluid-filled chambers and passageways, known as the labyrinth. Changes in body position disturb fluid in the labyrinth and stimulate tiny vestibular hair cells, which then send messages via the vestibular nerve to the cerebellum and brainstem, the balance centers of the brain. This series of cues enables your muscles and eyes to respond almost instantly to changes in position. Abnormalities affecting any part of this system can lead to dizziness, vertigo, and other balance disorders. The following tests may be performed to evaluate balance disorders and determine the origin of the problem:

• **Electronystagmography (ENG)** evaluates nystagmus, or involuntary rapid eye movement, and the muscles that control eye movement. In this test, electrodes are placed on either side of the eye to provide exact measurements of eye movements at rest, after a change in head position, and in response to various stimuli. Analysis of the pattern of eye movements during this test can help distinguish between abnormalities in the vestibular system, brainstem, and cerebellum.

• **Posturography** (or dynamic platform posturography) is a computerized test that assesses your ability to maintain your standing balance under various conditions. In this test, you stand on a computer-controlled platform that moves as your body sways. Your responses are recorded and analyzed to diagnose the origin of your balance problem.

• **The rotary chair test** evaluates vestibular and brainstem function. In this test, you sit in a computer-controlled chair that rotates around a vertical axis. When the chair is rotated in the dark, it induces involuntary rapid eye movement (nystagmus). These movements are recorded, and their speed is compared to the chair rotation at a variety of frequencies to assess vestibular function. The rotary chair test is the most sensitive procedure for detecting loss of vestibular function on both sides (bilateral loss).

• **Electrocochleography (ECOG)** measures electrical activity produced within the cochlea—the primary hearing organ of the inner ear—in response to a sound stimulus. This test is used in the diagnosis of Ménière's disease, a disorder marked by vertigo or severe dizziness, ringing in the ear, fluctuating hearing loss, and pain or pressure in the affected ear.

• **The caloric study** evaluates the function of the vestibular nerve. In this test, cold or hot water is instilled into your ear. This stimulation normally causes characteristic involun-

Results
▼

➡ A physician will review the test results and consider them along with your symptoms and findings from other tests to reach a diagnosis. Possible causes for balance problems include abnormalities affecting the inner ear, cerebellum, brainstem, and vestibular nerve. Treatment and prognosis depend on the nature of the problem.

➡ If your balance tests, symptoms, and physical exam suggest the presence of a growth, the doctor may recommend an imaging test of the head and neck, such as an MRI (see page 214) or a CT scan (see page 212), to determine the precise type and location of the lesion.

Balance Tests

tary movements of both eyes (nystagmus). If the labyrinth is diseased, no nystagmus is induced. This test helps to differentiate between vestibular abnormalities and cerebellar or brainstem disorders.

Purpose of the Test
• To help identify the cause of dizziness, vertigo, or ringing in the ears (tinnitus).
• To evaluate the function of the vestibular system in the inner ear.

Who Performs It
• An ear, nose, and throat specialist (otolaryngologist) or a vestibular technologist.
• A nerve specialist (neurologist) may be involved in the interpretation of the tests.

Special Concerns
• ENG and the caloric study should not be performed in people who have a perforated eardrum because of the risk of ear infection.
• Patients experiencing an acute attack of Ménière's disease should not undergo the caloric study; the test can be performed once the acute episode subsides.
• Drugs such as sedatives, stimulants, and antivertigo agents can alter test results.
• Patients who have pacemakers should not undergo ENG or the rotary chair test because the equipment used in these procedures may interfere with pacemaker function.
• Because hearing problems may also originate in the middle or inner ear, hearing tests (see page 216) are almost always performed in conjunction with balance tests.

Before the Test
• Report to your doctor any medications you are taking. You may be advised to discontinue certain drugs before the test.
• Do not drink caffeine or alcoholic beverages for 24 to 48 hours before balance tests.
• Avoid eating a heavy meal immediately before testing.
• If you use a hearing aid or eyeglasses, bring them with you to the testing facility.

• Women undergoing posturography may want to wear slacks because a safety harness is placed over the clothes during the test.
• Do not apply any facial makeup before ENG or the rotary chair test because electrodes will be taped to the skin around your eyes.
• Prior to ENG and the caloric study, the doctor will examine your ear canal and remove any earwax.
• Before the caloric study, you will be examined for the presence of nystagmus, Romberg's sign (a swaying of the body when your feet are placed close together and your eyes are closed), and past-pointing (an inability to accurately touch the examiner's finger with your index finger when your eyes are either open or closed). This exam will establish certain baseline values for comparison with results obtained during the test.

What You Experience
Electronystagmography (ENG):
• You will sit or lie down on an examining table in a darkened room.
• Electrodes are applied to the skin around your eyes.
• Different procedures are used to stimulate nystagmus, such as asking you to track a pendulum with your eyes, altering the position of your head or your gaze, and caloric studies (see below).
• Several recordings of eye movements are made while you are at rest, changing your head or body position, or responding to various procedures (such as having air blown into your ear).
• The nystagmus response is compared with the expected ranges, and the results are recorded as normal, borderline, or abnormal.
• This procedure takes about 1 hour.

Posturography:
• You will stand barefoot on a special computer-controlled platform and try to keep your balance under various conditions.
• You are surrounded by a 3-sided enclosure with patterns. The enclosure moves as your

body moves, and the grade and angle of the platform are changed to provoke balance reactions.

• Your ability to maintain balance is assessed under increasingly difficult conditions.

• A computer then isolates each of your sensory inputs and identifies where a balance problem exists.

Rotary chair test:

• Electrodes are applied to the skin around your eyes.

• You will sit in a computer-controlled chair that moves very slowly in a full circle. The chair then moves back and forth in a small arc at faster speeds.

• The testing room is dark, but there will be a video camera focused on your face and a microphone mounted at the top of the chair so you can communicate with the examiner.

• As the chair turns to the right and left at varying speeds, your eye movements are recorded by the electrodes.

Electrocochleography (ECOG):

• An electrode is placed inside your ear. In standard ECOG, it is positioned on the eardrum. In transtympanic ECOG, a local anesthetic is used to numb the eardrum and needle electrodes are placed through the drum until they touch the wall of the inner ear.

• A sound stimulus is applied in the form of clicks and tone bursts of varying frequencies.

• Recordings are made of the electrical potentials generated in your inner ear in response to the sound stimulation.

Caloric study:

• Each ear is tested separately. The examiner first places a basin under your ear on the suspected side. Cold water is instilled into your ear canal with a bulb syringe until you complain of nausea and dizziness, or until nystagmus is observed. Nystagmus, which will cause both of your eyes to rapidly turn away from the direction of the cold water and then slowly move back, normally occurs in 20 to 30 seconds.

• If nystagmus fails to occur after 3 minutes, the irrigation is stopped.

• The examiner tests you again for nystagmus, Romberg's sign, and past-pointing (see Before the Test).

• After about 5 minutes, the procedure is repeated on the other side.

• Sometimes hot water is used in addition to cold water. In such cases, nystagmus should occur in the opposite direction (toward the hot water).

• The test usually takes about 15 minutes.

Risks and Complications

• You may experience nausea, vomiting, and dizziness during all the tests except electrocochleography.

• Rarely, excessive water pressure during the caloric study can injure a previously damaged eardrum.

• Transtympanic ECOG has a slight risk of causing otitis media (middle ear infection) or eardrum perforation.

After the Test

• If you experienced nausea, vomiting, or dizziness during the test, you will rest in bed for about 30 to 60 minutes until your symptoms subside.

• Resume your normal diet and any medications withheld before the test, according to your doctor's instructions.

Estimated Cost: $$$

Balance Tests continued

Barium Enema
(Lower GI Series)

Barium Enema

Description
• In this test, the contrast dye barium sulfate is introduced into the lower gastrointestinal (GI) tract, and x-rays are used to visualize the large intestine, or colon. The barium, which is opaque to x-rays, sharply outlines the inner lining of the colon, revealing any structural or tissue abnormalities. In the single-contrast test, barium sulfate alone is used, while in the double-contrast test, both barium sulfate and air are instilled to provide more detailed views. (For more on contrast x-rays, see Chapter 2.)

Purpose of the Test
• To detect polyps and malignant (cancerous) tumors of the colon and rectum.
• To assess the type, extent, and severity of inflammatory bowel disease.
• To detect diverticula (abnormal outpouchings) and other structural changes in the colon.

Who Performs It
• A radiologist.

Special Concerns
• Pregnant women should not undergo this test because exposure to ionizing radiation may harm the fetus.
• This test is not appropriate for people with an extremely dilated colon (megacolon) or those with certain types of abnormal heart rhythms.
• When perforation of the colon is suspected, a water-soluble contrast agent is used instead of barium, and the normal pretest intestinal cleansing is not performed.
• Barium in the abdomen from previous contrast x-rays, such as a barium swallow (see page 106), may interfere with the results. If x-rays of the entire digestive tract are required, the barium enema is usually scheduled first.

Before the Test
• Cleansing your intestine before the test is essential to produce adequate anatomic detail on the x-rays. Your doctor will give you specific instructions.
• Typically, on the day before the procedure you are asked to consume only clear liquids (such as water, bouillon, or gelatin dessert); to drink a glass of water or another clear fluid every hour for 8 to 10 hours; and to take an oral laxative agent at specified times. You should not eat or drink anything after midnight on the day of the test.
• On the morning of the procedure, you may be instructed to self-administer a cleansing enema before leaving your home, or you may be given an enema at the testing facility.

What You Experience
• You are instructed to lie on your side on a table with your knees drawn to your chest.
• The doctor gently inserts the lubricated enema tube into your rectum, and barium is allowed to flow into your colon. A small balloon at the tip of the enema tube may be

Results
▼
➡ The doctor will examine the x-ray images for any abnormality, including polyps, tumor, or signs of inflammatory bowel disease.
➡ If a definitive diagnosis can be made based on the images, appropriate treatment will be initiated.
➡ Additional tests, such as colonoscopy (see page 159), may be needed to obtain a tissue sample (biopsy) for definitive diagnosis of colorectal cancer or inflammatory bowel disease.

inflated to help keep the barium inside.

• The radiologist observes the flow of barium through the colon with the aid of fluoroscopy (see page 205), which transmits continuous, moving x-ray images onto a viewing screen.

• At various points during the examination, you will be instructed to move into different positions as spot x-ray films are taken of any abnormalities. As each x-ray is taken, you should hold your breath and remain as still as possible.

• If you are having a double-contrast x-ray, the doctor instills small amounts of air through the enema tube and additional x-ray films are taken. The air helps the barium adhere to the colon wall, making it possible to visualize small polyps and tumors.

• You may experience mild abdominal cramps or the urge to defecate while the barium or air is being introduced into the intestine. Breathe deeply and slowly through your mouth to help ease this discomfort.

• After all the required x-ray images are taken, you will be escorted to the toilet or provided with a bedpan.

• The procedure lasts about 30 to 45 minutes.

Risks and Complications

• The test involves exposure to low levels of radiation.

• The barium may accumulate and block the intestine if it is not expelled within a day or two; a mild oral cathartic or cleansing enema can resolve the problem.

• A rare complication is perforation of the colon. This risk is higher for the double-contrast than the single-contrast test, and when the colon is weakened by inflammation, tumor, or infection.

After the Test

• Drink extra fluids to prevent dehydration and help eliminate the barium. Your doctor may also give you a mild laxative to help purge the barium from your body.

• Your stool will be chalky and light-colored initially, but should return to normal color in 1 to 3 days.

• Be sure to rest after the procedure; many patients find the test itself and the bowel preparation that precedes it to be exhausting.

Estimated Cost: $$

Barium Enema continued

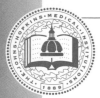

Barium Swallow
(Esophagography)

Description
• In this test, you ingest a liquid mixture containing barium sulfate, a chalky contrast dye that delineates internal structures on x-ray films. The barium, which is opaque to x-rays, sharply outlines the inner lining of the esophagus, revealing any structural or tissue abnormalities. The esophagus—the muscular passage that contracts and relaxes to carry food from the throat to the stomach—is illustrated on page 24 of the body atlas. (For more information about contrast x-rays, see Chapter 2.)

Purpose of the Test
• To detect hiatal hernia, a condition in which a portion of the stomach protrudes upward through the diaphragm.
• To diagnose esophageal diverticula (abnormal outpouchings) or varices (abnormally dilated blood vessels).
• To identify any tumors, strictures, ulcers, or polyps affecting the esophagus, or motility disorders that affect the swallowing function of the esophagus.

Who Performs It
• A radiologist.

Special Concerns
• Patients with an intestinal obstruction should not undergo this procedure. The barium may create a stonelike impaction.
• When esophageal perforation or rupture is suspected, barium is not used because leakage of the dye could worsen any existing infection. A water-soluble contrast agent, diatrizoate (Gastrografin), is usually substituted.
• Pregnant women should not undergo this test because exposure to ionizing radiation may harm the fetus.
• Individuals with a poor swallowing reflex may inadvertently aspirate barium into their lungs. Your swallowing reflex may be assessed before the test.

Before the Test
• Do not eat or drink anything after midnight on the day before the test.
• You will be instructed to remove any metallic objects, such as jewelry, dentures, or hairpins, before the test begins.

What You Experience
• In a radiology room, you are strapped securely to a tilting x-ray table.
• You will be given a thick, milkshake-like liquid containing the barium sulfate. The barium has an unpleasant chalky taste, but it is usually flavored to increase its palatability.
• As you sip the barium mixture, you will be moved through various position changes.
• The radiologist observes the flow of the dye through the esophagus using fluoroscopic imaging (see page 205), which transmits continuous, moving x-ray images onto a viewing screen.
• Spot x-rays are taken of any significant abnormalities. As each x-ray film is obtained,

Results
▼

➡ The doctor will examine the recorded x-ray images for evidence of any abnormality.

➡ If a definitive diagnosis can be made based on the images, your doctor will recommend an appropriate course of treatment, depending on the specific problem.

➡ In some cases, additional tests, such as endoscopic biopsy of the esophagus (see page 194) or esophageal function studies (see page 192), may be needed to further evaluate abnormal results and establish a diagnosis.

you will be instructed to hold your breath and remain perfectly still.

• The test takes about 15 to 30 minutes.

• There is no discomfort associated with this procedure.

Risks and Complications

• Although radiation exposure is still minimal, you will receive a higher dose of radiation during fluoroscopy than during standard x-ray procedures.

• The barium may accumulate and block the intestines if it is not eliminated from your system within a day or two.

After the Test

• Drink plenty of fluids to help eliminate the barium from your system. Your doctor may also give you a mild laxative to purge your body of the contrast agent.

• You are free to resume your normal diet and activities.

• Your stool will be chalky and light-colored initially, but it should return to normal color after 1 to 3 days.

• If diatrizoate was used rather than barium, you may experience diarrhea.

Estimated Cost: $$

Barium Swallow continued

KVCC KALAMAZOO VALLEY COMMUNITY COLLEGE LIBRARY

Blood Chemistry Screen

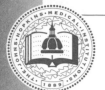

Blood Chemistry Screen

Description

• Analysis of blood chemistry can provide important information about the function of the kidneys and other organs. This common panel of blood tests measures levels of important electrolytes (see page 30) and other chemicals, including the following.

• **Glucose,** or blood sugar, is broken down in the body's cells to provide energy. Elevated levels may be caused by diabetes or medications such as steroids.

• **Sodium** levels in the blood represent a balance between sodium and water intake and excretion. Abnormal blood levels of sodium may indicate heart or kidney dysfunction or dehydration.

• **Potassium** plays a vital role in regulating muscle activity, including contraction of the heart. Kidney failure as well as vomiting or diarrhea may lead to abnormal levels.

• **Chloride** levels may rise and fall in parallel with sodium levels to maintain electrical neutrality. Several disorders may alter chloride levels, including kidney dysfunction, adrenal disease, vomiting, diarrhea, and congestive heart failure.

• **Carbon dioxide (CO_2)** acts as a buffer system to help maintain the acid-base balance of the blood. Respiratory disease, kidney disorders, severe vomiting, diarrhea, and very severe infections can produce abnormal levels.

• **Blood urea nitrogen (BUN)** provides a rough measurement of the glomerular filtration rate, or the rate at which blood is filtered across small blood vessels in the kidney. A high BUN level may indicate kidney dysfunction (see page 311).

• **Creatinine**—which is a breakdown product of creatine, an important component of muscle—is excreted exclusively by the kidneys. The serum creatinine level is considered the most sensitive blood test of kidney function (see page 311).

Purpose of the Test

• To provide general information about how your body is functioning.

• To screen for a wide range of problems, including kidney, liver, heart, adrenal, gastrointestinal, endocrine, and neuromuscular disorders.

Who Performs It

• A doctor, a nurse, or a lab technician draws the blood sample.

Special Concerns

• A variety of medications can alter levels of electrolytes, blood urea nitrogen, and creatinine and interfere with the results of this test.

• Excessive ingestion of licorice or accidental consumption of ethylene glycol or methyl alcohol can affect acid-base balance and alter carbon dioxide levels.

• A diet rich in meats can cause transient elevations of serum creatinine.

• A high-protein diet, gastrointestinal bleeding,

Results

▼

➡ Your blood sample is sent to a laboratory for analysis. The doctor will review the results for evidence of kidney disease or another disorder. (For more on laboratory tests, see Chapter 1.)

➡ A blood chemistry screen is commonly used as an initial test to indicate potential health problems. Abnormal results often necessitate additional tests to establish a diagnosis.

➡ If an abnormality is found and the doctor can make a definitive diagnosis, appropriate treatment will be initiated.

or dehydration elevates blood urea nitrogen levels, while a low-protein diet or overhydration tends to lower them.

Before the Test
• Report to your doctor any medications, herbs, or supplements you are taking. You may be advised to discontinue certain of these agents before the test.
• Avoid a diet rich in meats before a blood urea nitrogen test.
• No special precautions are needed before testing for sodium, potassium, chloride, carbon dioxide, or creatinine.

What You Experience
• A sample of your blood is drawn from a vein, usually in your arm, and sent to a laboratory for analysis. (For more on this procedure, called venipuncture, see page 32.)

Risks and Complications
• There are no risks or complications associated with this test.

After the Test
• Immediately after blood is drawn, pressure is applied (with cotton or gauze) to the puncture site.
• Resume your normal diet and any medications that were withheld before the test, according to your doctor's instructions.
• Blood may collect and clot under the skin (hematoma) at the puncture site; this is harmless and will resolve on its own. For a large hematoma that causes swelling and discomfort, apply ice initially; after 24 hours, use warm, moist compresses to help dissolve the clotted blood.

Estimated Cost: $

Blood Chemistry Screen continued

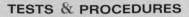
Blood Tests for Allergies

Description

• Allergies are caused by an uncommon immune reaction that occurs upon exposure to a normally harmless substance. This response causes your body to produce antibodies, which are proteins that can trigger the release of chemicals such as histamine. The result is itching, respiratory inflammation, or other allergic symptoms. Blood tests for allergies typically measure levels of the antibody IgE, which is responsible for most allergic reactions. For example, the radioallergosorbent test (RAST) exposes a sample of your blood to a suspected allergen and looks for the presence of the IgE antibody. Total serum levels of IgE may also be measured directly.

Purpose of the Test

• To identify or confirm an allergy to a specific allergen—such as dust mites, animal dander, pollens, certain drugs or foods, or stinging insects—particularly if the results of a skin test (see page 335) are inconclusive or skin testing cannot be done.

Who Performs It

• A doctor, a nurse, or a lab technician.

Special Concerns

• None.

Before the Test

• No special preparation is needed.

What You Experience

• A sample of blood is drawn from a vein, usually in your arm, and sent to a laboratory for analysis. (For more on this procedure, called venipuncture, see page 32.)

Risks and Complications

• None.

After the Test

• Immediately after blood is drawn, pressure is applied (with cotton or gauze) to the puncture site.

• Blood may collect and clot under the skin (hematoma) at the puncture site; this is harmless and will resolve on its own. For a large hematoma that causes swelling and discomfort, apply ice initially; after 24 hours, use warm, moist compresses to help dissolve the clotted blood.

Estimated Cost: $$

Results

▼

➡ Your blood sample is sent to a laboratory for analysis. With RAST, the blood is exposed to small disks, gels, or other materials to which the suspected allergens have been attached.

➡ Different techniques may be employed to assess the presence of IgE antibody. For example, RAST uses a radioactive reagent to quantify IgE levels, while a similar technique called EAST (or ELISA) uses color production by an enzyme that tags the IgE. (For more on laboratory tests, see Chapter 1.)

➡ Your doctor will consider the results along with your symptoms, medical history, and the results of other tests.

➡ If a specific allergy is diagnosed, your doctor may advise you to avoid the allergen, use an antihistamine or other anti-inflammatory medicine, or have a series of allergy shots to increase your tolerance.

Blood Tests to Evaluate the Liver

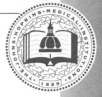

Description

• Analysis of a blood sample can provide essential information about the health of the liver and bile ducts (hepatobiliary system). The following are some of the basic blood tests used to evaluate the liver:

• **Enzyme tests.** The liver is the site of many biochemical reactions that are controlled by numerous enzymes, including alanine aminotransferase (ALT), aspartate aminotransferase (AST), alkaline phosphatase (ALP), and gamma glutamyl transferase (GGT). Elevated levels of liver enzymes in the bloodstream may indicate liver damage; however, they do not necessarily point to a specific liver disease. Although enzyme tests may be ordered individually, they provide more information when performed in combination, since levels of many liver enzymes may be elevated in diseases affecting other organs.

• **Bilirubin,** the main pigment in bile, is a breakdown product of hemoglobin, an iron-containing substance in red blood cells. Normally, only a small amount of bilirubin circulates in the blood. Elevated blood levels may result from many forms of liver and biliary tract disease, including hepatitis and bile duct obstruction. The presence of excess bilirubin in the blood produces a yellowish discoloration of the skin and eyes called jaundice.

• **Albumin** is a major protein that, like most proteins in the bloodstream, is synthesized by the liver. A decreased level of albumin in the serum (the liquid portion of blood that remains after whole blood clots) is an indication of chronic liver disease.

• **Prothrombin time (PT)**—a blood clotting study that is discussed in more detail on page 157—may also be performed to evaluate the function of the liver. Because prothrombin is one of the clotting proteins that is synthesized by the liver, an abnormal PT may reflect liver dysfunction.

• **Viral hepatitis tests** may be done in people with abnormal liver enzymes whose medical history and/or symptoms raise suspicion of the disease. (Symptoms include low-grade fever, malaise, loss of appetite, and fatigue, but are not always present.) The three most common types of this virus found in the U.S. are hepatitis A, B, and C (known as HAV, HBV, and HCV); they are all detected by testing for the presence of specific antigens or antibodies (see page 91) found only in the blood of infected individuals. Different antibody/antigen tests may be performed, depending on which hepatitis type is suspected. In addition, the presence of particular antibodies can signal whether the infection is in an acute or chronic stage.

Results

▼

➥ Your blood sample is sent to a laboratory for analysis. A physician will review the results for any evidence of liver injury or disease. (For more on laboratory testing, see Chapter 1.)

➥ These tests are frequently the first step in assessing potential liver disorders. Abnormal results often necessitate additional tests to evaluate the structure and function of the liver—such as a CT scan (see page 76), ultrasound (see page 80), MRI (see page 78), or liver biopsy (see page 240)—in order to establish a diagnosis.

➥ If antigen/antibody tests indicate the presence of acute or chronic viral hepatitis, a liver biopsy may be required to confirm the diagnosis and assess the degree of damage to the liver.

Purpose of the Test

• Liver enzymes, albumin, and prothrombin time are tested to evaluate liver function, to help diagnose diseases of the liver and bile ducts, and to monitor the progress of known liver disease.

• Viral hepatitis antibodies are used to diagnose viral hepatitis infection, determine the type of the disease (A, B, C, or another variant), and establish the current status of the disease (acute or chronic).

• All blood donors are automatically screened for the presence of hepatitis B and C.

Who Performs It

• A doctor, a nurse, or a technician draws the blood sample.

Special Concerns

• A number of medications and vitamin supplements can alter the levels of bilirubin and liver enzymes and interfere with test results.

• Liver enzyme levels may be affected by a variety of factors other than liver disease, including pregnancy, periods of rapid bone growth, alcohol consumption, obesity, strenuous exercise, consumption of particular foods, trauma, and surgery.

• Even a moderate alcohol intake can raise levels of the GGT enzyme.

• People who have been inoculated with the hepatitis B vaccine may have antibodies in their blood even though they are not infected; this may lead to a false-positive result (see page 35).

Before the Test

• Report to your doctor any medications, herbs, or supplements you are taking. You may be advised to discontinue certain of these agents before a liver enzyme test.

• You are usually asked to avoid eating or drinking for at least 8 hours prior to a liver enzyme test, but fasting requirements vary for different laboratories.

What You Experience

• A sample of your blood is drawn from a vein, usually in your arm, and sent to a laboratory for analysis. (For more on this procedure, called venipuncture, see page 32.)

Risks and Complications

• None.

After the Test

• Immediately after blood is drawn, pressure is applied (with cotton or gauze) to the puncture site.

• Resume your normal diet and any medications withheld before the test, according to your doctor's instructions.

• Blood may collect and clot under the skin (hematoma) at the puncture site; this is harmless and will resolve on its own. For a large hematoma that causes swelling and discomfort, apply ice initially; after 24 hours, use warm, moist compresses to help dissolve the clotted blood.

Estimated Cost: $

Bone Biopsy

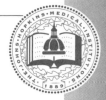

Description

• Bone biopsy removes a small sample of bone for laboratory analysis; several techniques may be used. **Percutaneous core needle biopsy** uses a special drill needle to bore into the bone and withdraw a specimen under the guidance of real-time x-rays (fluoroscopy) or CT imaging (see Chapter 2). **Open biopsy** is a surgical procedure that removes a larger sample through a small incision. Bone biopsy is either performed to analyze a known lesion such as a tumor, or to obtain a representative sample in order to diagnose a systemic bone disease (the pelvic bone is often selected because it is close to the skin's surface).

Purpose of the Test

• To distinguish between benign and cancerous bone tumors.

• To obtain a bone specimen in patients with bone pain and tenderness, particularly if a mass or deformity was detected on an imaging test such as a nuclear scan (see page 329), CT scan (see page 325), or x-ray (see page 331).

• To diagnose systemic bone disease, such as osteoporosis (a decrease in bone mass) or osteomalacia (a disease that causes soft and brittle bones), when the results of imaging tests are inconclusive.

• To identify the microorganism that is causing a bone infection such as osteomyelitis.

Who Performs It

• Core needle biopsy is conducted by an orthopedic surgeon and a radiologist.

• Open biopsy is performed by an orthopedic surgeon and a surgical team.

Special Concerns

• This procedure should be performed with caution in people with blood clotting disorders. Coagulation studies (see page 157) may be needed before the biopsy is done.

• Open biopsy, which requires general anesthesia, is performed less frequently than core needle biopsy. The advantage of this technique is that it provides a larger specimen of bone and improves the chances for a definitive diagnosis.

Before the Test

• Tell your doctor if you regularly take anticoagulants or nonsteroidal anti-inflammatory drugs (such as aspirin, ibuprofen, or naproxen). You will be instructed to discontinue them for some time before the test. Also mention any other medications, herbs, or supplements that you take.

• In some cases (such as a biopsy to detect osteoporosis), you may be given the antibiotic tetracycline for 3 weeks beforehand, including a dose just before the biopsy. The tetracycline binds to the calcium in your blood and can be used to determine the rate at which calcium is absorbed by your bones.

• Do not eat or drink anything for 12 hours before the biopsy. (Fasting is required before core needle biopsy in case there is a need for immediate surgical intervention.)

Results

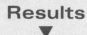

➡ Bone samples are sent to a pathology laboratory and examined under a microscope for unusual cells. They are usually also sent to a microbiology laboratory and cultured (see page 166) for infectious organisms. (For more information on laboratory testing, see Chapter 1.)

➡ This test usually results in a definitive diagnosis. Treatment will be initiated, depending on the specific problem.

Bone Biopsy

- Empty your bladder before the test.
- You will be asked to disrobe and put on a hospital gown.
- An intravenous (IV) needle or catheter is inserted into a vein in your arm immediately before the test begins. A sedative is usually administered before a core needle biopsy, and general anesthesia is given before an open biopsy.

What You Experience

Core needle biopsy:

- The biopsy site is shaved and cleansed with an antiseptic, and a local anesthetic is injected to numb the area. (In some cases, the anesthetic is injected on the surface of the bone itself.) You may still experience some discomfort and pressure as the needle enters the bone.
- The doctor makes a very small incision in the skin and inserts the biopsy needle into the bone. Fluoroscopy (see page 205) or CT scanning may be used to guide placement of the needle.
- The biopsy needle is rotated 180° and then reversed, obtaining a small core of bone, and then withdrawn.
- The procedure takes about 30 minutes.

Open biopsy:

- The biopsy site is shaved and cleansed with an antiseptic.
- The doctor makes a small incision and removes a piece of bone with surgical instruments. The sample is sent to a laboratory for microscopic examination.
- The incision is sutured closed.
- The procedure takes about 30 minutes.

Risks and Complications

- Possible complications include bone fracture, inadvertent needle-induced damage to nearby tissue, and, rarely, infection.
- Open biopsy carries all the risks associated with general anesthesia.

After the Test

- After a core needle biopsy, pressure is placed on the incision site until bleeding has stopped, the site is cleaned, and a small bandage is applied. You may leave in about an hour if there is no bleeding and your vital signs are normal. (You may need to remain in the hospital for at least 24 hours if a biopsy was taken from the spine.)
- After an open biopsy, you will stay in a recovery room for 1 to 2 hours. During this time, your vital signs will be monitored and you will be observed for any signs of complications. You will then be transferred to a hospital room for 24 hours.
- Arrange for someone to drive you home.
- The biopsy site may be sore and tender for several days. Your doctor may prescribe a pain-relieving medication.
- Keep the biopsy site covered and dry for 48 hours following the procedure. You may take showers, but not baths, for 10 days.
- Inform your doctor immediately if you experience bleeding through the bandage or symptoms of infection (such as fever, pain when moving, and redness, swelling, or pus at the biopsy site).

Estimated Cost: $$$$

Bone Densitometry

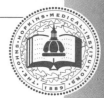

Description

• Bone densitometry is used to assess bone mass by measuring bone mineral density (which is the amount of bone per unit of skeletal area). It is the most sensitive screening tool to detect osteoporosis—a disorder characterized by fragile, weak bones due to a drop in bone mass and increased risk of fracture. The following techniques are used to measure bone mineral density.

• **Dual energy x-ray absorptiometry (DEXA)** is considered the gold standard for quantifying bone mass in the spine and hip bone. In this technique, an x-ray tube emits 2 x-ray beams, which pass through the bone and are picked up by a detector. A computer is used to analyze the resulting images and calculate bone density based on the amount of radiation absorbed by the bone—denser bones absorb more radiation.

• **Peripheral DEXA (pDEXA)** uses a small, portable device that works similar to DEXA but is used to examine bone density in peripheral bones, such as the wrist.

• **Single x-ray absorptiometry (SXA)** also uses a small, portable device that works similar to DEXA, but emits a single x-ray beam. It is used to examine the heel bone or forearm.

• **Quantitative ultrasound (QUS),** the only technique for measuring bone density that does not use x-rays, works by transmitting high-frequency sound waves through the heel bone to a signal receiver.

• **Quantitative computed tomography (QCT)** uses a standard CT scanner—fitted with special equipment and software to measure bone mass—to deliver x-rays to the spine at many different angles. (For more on CT scanning, see Chapter 2.)

Purpose of the Test

• To screen people at high risk for osteoporosis, such as postmenopausal women or individuals on long-term therapy with corticosteroid drugs.

• To detect suspected osteoporosis in people who have experienced recent unexplained bone fractures.

• DEXA is the only method that may be used to make a definitive diagnosis of osteoporosis and to monitor the response to treatment.

• To detect and evaluate other disorders affecting bone mass, such as the inherited disorder osteogenesis imperfecta.

Who Performs It

• A physician or a technician.

Special Concerns

• DEXA is the most accurate method for measuring bone density in the spine and hip bone, the most common sites of fracture. It is of limited use, however, in people with a spinal deformity or those who have had previous spinal surgery. In addition, the presence of vertebral compression fractures or degenerative disease such as osteoarthritis may interfere with the accuracy of the test.

• QCT is only used in selected individuals due to its limited availability, relatively high cost,

Results
▼

➡ A physician reviews the test data to determine your bone mineral status.

➡ If the findings indicate bone loss due to osteoporosis, your doctor will prescribe a treatment program—which typically includes exercise, calcium and vitamin D supplements, and sometimes hormone replacement or other medications—to help forestall further bone loss and fractures.

Bone Densitometry

Bone Densitometry continued

and greater radiation exposure. It is the only method that can evaluate spongy bone tissue in the spine, which may be useful when assessing the response to therapy for osteoporosis.

• Because pDEXA, SXA, and QUS are performed by small, portable instruments and are less expensive than DEXA or QCT, many physicians now use these methods to screen patients in their offices.

• Pregnant women should not undergo x-ray tests because exposure to ionizing radiation may harm the fetus.

• Because residual barium in the gastrointestinal tract can interfere with test results, DEXA should not be performed until about 10 days after an imaging study using this contrast agent.

• Calcium in blood vessels overlying the area being scanned—sometimes found in atherosclerotic plaques—may falsely increase bone density.

• Movement during the scan may alter the test results.

Before the Test

• Do not take calcium supplements for 24 hours before the test.

• Remove all metallic objects (such as belt buckles, zippers, jewelry, coins, and keys) that might obstruct the scanning path.

• You may be able to wear your street clothes, but for DEXA or QCT you may be asked to disrobe and put on a hospital gown.

What You Experience
DEXA:

• You will lie on an padded table with an x-ray generator below and a detector camera above.

• To examine your spine, your legs will be supported on a padded box to flatten your pelvis and lower (lumbar) spine. The detector device is slowly passed over the lumbar area, producing images projected onto a computer monitor.

• To assess the hip, your foot is placed in a brace that rotates the hip inward, and the scanning procedure is repeated.

• The scan may take up to 30 minutes.

pDEXA:

• You place your finger or hand in a small scanning device and a bone density reading is obtained within a few minutes.

SXA:

• You immerse your heel or forearm in a tub of water. A scanning device obtains a bone density reading through the water within a few minutes.

QUS:

• An ultrasound device held next to your heel obtains a reading in about 10 seconds.

QCT:

• You will lie on your back on a narrow table that is then advanced into the CT scanner. The scanner, which encircles you, rotates around you taking pictures at different intervals and from various angles. You will feel the table move during the test.

• You must remain as still as possible because any movement can distort the scan.

• The test typically takes 15 to 30 minutes.

Risks and Complications

• Ultrasound imaging does not expose you to any radiation.

• DEXA, pDEXA, and SXA involve only minimal exposure to radiation. Although radiation exposure is still minimal with QCT, you will receive a higher dose (50 to 100 times greater than DEXA).

After the Test

• You may resume your normal activities immediately after the test.

Estimated Cost: $$

Bone Marrow Aspiration and Biopsy

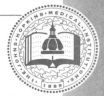

Description

• In this test, a sample of bone marrow—the soft tissue that fills the cavities inside of bone where the majority of blood cells are produced—is obtained and sent to a laboratory for analysis. Two techniques are employed to obtain specimens: Either a fine needle is used to withdraw (aspirate) liquid marrow and marrow fragments, or a larger needle is used to obtain a small core of marrow tissue. Both procedures may be performed consecutively at different sites to yield optimal specimens. There are 4 common sites for bone marrow aspiration and biopsy:

• The preferred site is the rear upper pelvic bone (posterior iliac crest), since no major blood vessels or organs are located nearby.

• A second location is the front upper pelvic bone (anterior iliac crest).

• The central, flat bone at the front of the chest (sternum) is sometimes used because it is close to the surface; however, this location involves a higher risk since it is situated near the heart and major blood vessels.

• The larger shin bone (tibia) is typically used in infants under 1 year of age.

Purpose of the Test

• To help diagnose blood disorders, such as leukemia and myeloma (cancers originating in the bone marrow); granulomatous disorders (in which there is an accumulation of inflammatory cells in the marrow); certain types of severe anemia; leukopenia (low number of white blood cells); thrombocytopenia (decrease in blood platelets); or any combination of these.

• To evaluate the cellularity and architecture of the bone marrow.

• To diagnose primary and metastatic tumors.

• To obtain a specimen for culture in order to identify the cause of an infection.

• To help determine the stage of cancers such as lymphomas and Hodgkin's disease (cancers primarily involving the lymph nodes).

• To evaluate the effectiveness of chemotherapy and monitor one of its major side effects, inhibition of bone marrow function (myelosuppression).

Who Performs It

• A physician specializing in blood disorders (hematologist), a cancer specialist (oncologist), or a trained nurse.

Special Concerns

• This procedure is not appropriate for people taking an anticoagulant medication or those with a bleeding disorder.

Before the Test

• Tell your doctor if you regularly take nonsteroidal anti-inflammatory drugs (such as

---

Results

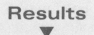

➥ The marrow samples are sent to hematology and pathology laboratories for microscopic examination and other tests. If an infection is suspected, a specimen is cultured (see page 166) in order to identify the responsible organism. Your doctor will review the results for evidence of a blood disorder, infection, or another problem. (For more on laboratory testing, see Chapter 1.)

➥ If an abnormality is found and your doctor can make a definitive diagnosis, appropriate treatment will be initiated.

➥ If bone marrow aspiration alone fails to yield an adequate sample, a needle biopsy will be performed.

Bone Marrow Aspiration and Biopsy

aspirin, ibuprofen, or naproxen) or the anti-coagulants warfarin (Coumadin) or heparin. You will be instructed to discontinue them for some time before the test. Also mention any other medications, herbs, or supplements that you take.

• A blood sample will be obtained and coagulation studies (see page 157) will be performed to ensure you are a proper candidate for this procedure.

• You may request to be given a sedative medication about 1 hour before the procedure.

What You Experience

• You will be positioned differently according to the selected biopsy site—either lying down on your side or stomach (posterior or anterior iliac crest) or on your back (sternum) on a bed or examination table.

• The biopsy site is shaved (if necessary) and cleansed with an antiseptic, and a local anesthetic is injected to numb the area. (You will still feel pressure as the needle enters the bone, and a brief pain as the marrow is removed.)

• You must remain still during the procedure.

• For bone marrow aspiration, a thin needle is inserted and rotated until it penetrates the outer layer of bone. A syringe is attached to the needle and used to withdraw a small amount of marrow. The marrow slides are prepared immediately; if an adequate specimen has not been obtained, the needle is repositioned slightly and the procedure is repeated.

• For a needle biopsy—which may be performed at the same or a different site—a larger needle is inserted through a small skin incision and into the bone using a steady, boring motion. A small core of marrow is sheared off, and the needle is withdrawn.

• Each of these procedures usually takes about 10 minutes.

Risks and Complications

• Minor complications include local bleeding and discomfort at the puncture site.

• Rare but serious complications include infection at the biopsy site and puncture of nearby structures or a major blood vessel.

• In some cases, the procedure does not obtain an adequate marrow specimen.

After the Test

• Pressure is placed on the needle puncture site until bleeding stops. The site is cleansed again and covered with a sterile bandage.

• Unless you were given a sedative, you may leave immediately after the procedure.

• Arrange for someone to drive you home. You may experience some pain or soreness at the biopsy site, but you can resume your usual activities immediately.

• Keep the biopsy site covered and dry for several hours.

• In some cases, you may be instructed to return the following day to have the biopsy site checked by a nurse or doctor.

• You may develop swelling and bruising at the puncture site. Apply pressure and ice to reduce discomfort and inform your doctor.

• Call your doctor immediately if you develop a fever; redness, bleeding, or discharge at the biopsy site; or dizziness.

Estimated Cost: $$

Brain and Spinal Cord MRI
(Magnetic Resonance Imaging of the Brain and Spinal Cord)

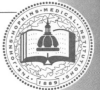

Description
• This test uses a strong magnetic field combined with radiofrequency waves to create highly detailed, cross-sectional images of the brain and spinal cord; these scans are examined for abnormalities. For certain studies, an MRI contrast dye such as gadolinium may be injected to provide better definition of soft tissues and blood vessels and thus enhance the images. (For more on how MRI works, see Chapter 2.)

Purpose of the Test
• To help diagnose disorders affecting the brain, including tumors; infarction (an area of dead tissue due to interruption of blood flow); edema (swelling); abscesses; and leakage of blood (hemorrhage) due to a ruptured blood vessel.
• To assess various abnormalities of the spinal cord and to evaluate the spine before surgery (see also skeletal MRI on page 327).
• To determine the extent of brain or spinal cord tumors before treatment for cancer, and to monitor the area for recurrence after therapy has been completed.
• To identify multiple sclerosis and other similar disorders that cause nerve degeneration in the brain.

Who Performs It
• A radiologist or a qualified technician.

Special Concerns
• Because MRI can define the brain and spinal cord sharply without interference from bone, it is considered the procedure of choice to evaluate these areas (in appropriate candidates).
• People who experience claustrophobia may find it difficult to undergo an MRI, which takes place in a narrow, tunnel-like structure. In some cases, an open MRI—a larger unit that is open on several sides—may be used as an alternative.
• This test may not be possible for severely overweight individuals (over 300 lbs). Some open MRIs can accommodate larger patients.
• Because the MRI generates a strong magnetic field, it cannot be performed on people who have certain types of internally placed metallic devices, including pacemakers, inner ear implants, or intracranial aneurysm clips.
• The test should not be done in pregnant women because the long-term effects of MRI on the fetus are unknown.

Before the Test
• Tell your doctor if you suffer from claustrophobia. He or she may administer a sedative to help you tolerate the procedure.
• Empty your bladder before the test.
• Remove any magnetic cards or metallic objects, including watches, hair clips, belts, credit cards, and jewelry. You may be asked to disrobe and put on a hospital gown.

What You Experience
• You will lie down on a narrow padded bed that slides into the large, enclosed cylinder containing the MRI magnets.

Results
▼
➡ The MRI scans are displayed on a video monitor and then recorded on film. A physician will examine the images for any abnormalities.
➡ If a definitive diagnosis can be made based on the images, appropriate treatment will be initiated, depending on the specific problem.
➡ In some cases, additional tests, such as arteriography of the brain (see page 95) or lumbar puncture (see page 243), may be needed to establish a diagnosis and determine the extent of the problem.

Brain and Spinal Cord MRI

• You must remain still throughout the procedure because any motion can distort the scan. Your head will likely be placed in a cradle to restrict movement.

• In some cases, you will receive an injection of a contrast dye before or during the procedure.

• There is a microphone inside the imaging machine, and you may talk to the technician performing the scan at any time during the procedure.

• You will hear loud thumping sounds as the scanning is performed. To block out the noise, you can request earplugs or listen to music on earphones.

• The procedure can take up to 90 minutes, or longer if a contrast dye is used.

Risks and Complications

• MRI does not involve exposure to ionizing radiation and is not associated with any risks or complications.

After the Test

• Most patients can go home right after the scan and resume their usual activities.

• Sedated patients may be monitored for a short period until the effects of the sedative have worn off.

• If contrast dye was injected, blood may collect and clot under the skin (hematoma) at the injection site; this is harmless and will resolve on its own. For a large hematoma that causes swelling and discomfort, apply ice initially; after 24 hours, use warm, moist compresses to help dissolve the clotted blood.

Estimated Cost: $$$$

Brain CT Scan

(Computed Tomography of the Brain, Intracranial CT Scan)

Description

• A body scanner delivers x-rays to the head at many different angles. A computer then compiles this information to construct highly detailed, cross-sectional images of the brain. In some cases, a contrast dye may be injected to better define tissues and blood vessels on the scans and enhance the images. (For more on how CT scans work, see Chapter 2.)

Purpose of the Test

• To help diagnose disorders affecting the brain, including tumors; infarction (an area of dead tissue caused by interruption of blood flow); bleeding within the brain; hematoma (collection of blood on the brain); and hydrocephalus (accumulation of fluid within the ventricles of the brain).

• To determine the stage of brain tumors and to monitor them after treatment for cancer.

Who Performs It

• A radiologist and/or a trained technician.

Special Concerns

• CT scans are not usually done during pregnancy because exposure to ionizing radiation may harm the fetus.

• People with allergies to iodine or shellfish may experience an allergic reaction to the iodine-based contrast dye.

• People who experience claustrophobia may find it difficult to undergo a CT scan, which takes place in a narrow, tunnel-like structure.

• This test may not be possible for severely overweight individuals (over 300 lbs).

Before the Test

• Inform your doctor if you have an allergy to iodine or shellfish. You may be given a combined antihistamine-steroid preparation to reduce the risk of an allergic reaction to the contrast dye.

• Tell your doctor if you suffer from claustrophobia. He or she may prescribe a sedative to help you tolerate the procedure.

• If a contrast dye is to be used or if sedation is anticipated, you will be instructed to fast for 4 hours before the test and drink large amounts of fluids on the day before the test to prevent dehydration. If a dye is not being used, fasting is unnecessary.

• Just before the test, remove all jewelry and metal objects.

What You Experience

• You are asked to lie on your back on a narrow table. Your head is immobilized in a brace (but your face is left uncovered) and then advanced into the CT scanner.

• The scanner takes pictures at different intervals and varying levels over your head, so you will feel the table move during the test. The resulting images are displayed on a viewing monitor and recorded on x-ray film.

• You must remain still because any movement can distort the image on the scan.

• A contrast dye may be administered through an intravenous (IV) needle or catheter inserted

Results

▼

➡ A radiologist will examine the CT images for evidence of any abnormality.

➡ If a definitive diagnosis can be made based on the images, appropriate treatment will be initiated, depending on the specific problem.

➡ In some cases, additional tests, such as an MRI (see page 119) or a PET scan (see page 298) of the brain, may be needed to establish a diagnosis and determine the extent of the problem.

Brain CT Scan

Brain CT Scan continued

into a vein in your arm. (Upon injection of the dye, you may experience a mild nausea, flushing, warmth, or a salty taste in the mouth.) The scanning process is then repeated.

• The test usually lasts 10 to 20 minutes. If a contrast dye is used, it may take up to 40 minutes because scans are taken before and after the dye is given.

Risks and Complications

• Although radiation exposure is minimal, you will receive a higher dose of radiation than during standard x-ray procedures.

• Some people may experience an allergic reaction to the iodine-based contrast dye, which can cause symptoms such as nausea, sneezing, vomiting, hives, and occasionally a life-threatening response called anaphylactic shock. Emergency medications and equipment are kept readily available.

• Patients who are dehydrated or those with impaired kidney function may experience acute renal failure from infusion of the contrast dye. Adequate hydration before the test can reduce this risk.

After the Test

• If contrast dye was used, you are encouraged to drink clear fluids to avoid dehydration and help flush the dye out of your system.

• You are free to resume your normal diet and activities.

• If contrast dye was injected, blood may collect and clot under the skin (hematoma) at the injection site; this is harmless and will resolve on its own. For a large hematoma that causes swelling and discomfort, apply ice initially; after 24 hours, use warm, moist compresses to help dissolve the clotted blood.

• Delayed allergic reactions to the contrast dye, such as hives, rash, or itching, may appear 2 to 6 hours after the procedure. If this occurs, your doctor will prescribe antihistamines or steroids to ease your discomfort.

Estimated Cost: $$

Brain Nuclear Scan
(Brain Scan)

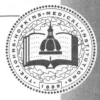

Description

• After injection of a small amount of radioactive material, a special camera records the uptake of the radiotracer within the brain. Normally, the blood-brain barrier—a protective characteristic of blood vessels in the brain that blocks out potentially harmful substances—prevents the radiotracer from being taken up by brain tissues, but if this barrier has been disrupted by disease, the material will concentrate in abnormal regions of the brain. The camera data are translated by computer into two-dimensional images that are recorded on film.

• A variation of nuclear scanning, called single-photon emission computed tomography (SPECT), enhances the sensitivity of the test. It utilizes certain radiotracers that emit single gamma rays to evaluate changes in blood flow and other brain abnormalities. Computer methods similar to those employed in CT scanning are then used to produce images of multiple sections of the brain, which are then recorded on film. (For more on nuclear imaging, CT scanning, and SPECT, see Chapter 2.)

Purpose of the Test

• To detect and evaluate abnormalities affecting the brain, including tumors, infarction (an area of dead tissue caused by interruption of blood flow), infection, bleeding, or blockage of blood vessels.

• To evaluate epilepsy, headaches, and other neurologic symptoms.

• To aid in the evaluation of dementia, cerebrovascular disease, and psychiatric disorders.

Who Performs It

• A radiologist or a nuclear medicine technician.

Special Concerns

• In general, CT scans (see page 121), MRI (see page 119), and carotid artery duplex scans (see page 149) have replaced brain nuclear scans for the diagnosis of neurological disorders. SPECT is rarely used outside of research purposes today.

• This test should not be performed in pregnant or breastfeeding women because of possible risks to the fetus or infant.

• People with allergies to iodine or shellfish may experience a severe allergic reaction if radioactive iodine is used in the test.

Before the Test

• Inform your doctor if you have an allergy to iodine or shellfish.

• You will be asked to rest quietly for 10 to 20 minutes before the procedure is started.

• Remove all jewelry and metal objects.

• Empty your bladder before the test.

• An intravenous (IV) needle or catheter is inserted into a vein in your arm immediately before the test begins.

• Certain medications, called blocking agents, may be administered orally or by injection before the test to prevent excessive uptake of the radioisotope by specific tissues.

What You Experience

• After a radiotracer is injected into the IV line, you lie on your back on a table with your

> ## Results
> ▼
> ➥ A physician will examine the scans for evidence of any brain abnormality.
> ➥ If a definitive diagnosis can be made, appropriate treatment will be initiated.
> ➥ Abnormal results may also necessitate additional tests, such as MRI (see page 119) or MRA of the brain (see page 253).

head under a large scanning camera.

• You will be asked to assume different positions—on your back, side, or stomach—while the scanner records the gamma rays emitted by the radiotracer in a timed sequence to follow the material during its first flow through the brain. (For a SPECT exam, you will lie on your back as a special rotating camera records images from multiple angles.)

• You must remain very still during the scanning process.

• This procedure takes about 35 to 45 minutes. Another scan is then performed 30 minutes to 2 hours later to identify any abnormal areas in the brain.

Risks and Complications

• The trace amount of radioactive material used in this test is not associated with significant risks or complications.

• In extremely rare cases, patients may be hypersensitive to the radiotracer and may experience an adverse reaction.

After the Test

• Drink extra fluids to aid in the excretion of the radioactive material.

• You are free to leave and resume your normal activities.

• Blood may collect and clot under the skin (hematoma) at the IV needle insertion site; this is harmless and will resolve on its own. For a large hematoma that causes swelling and discomfort, apply ice initially; after 24 hours, use warm, moist compresses to help dissolve the clotted blood.

Estimated Cost: $$$

Breast Biopsy

(Needle, Open, or Stereotactic Breast Biopsy)

Description

• A sample of cells or tissue is extracted from the breast for microscopic examination; the specimen is taken from a lump or mass that was detected on an imaging test such as mammography or ultrasound. Several different techniques may be used. Which one is appropriate for you depends on a variety of factors, including the size of the breast mass, its location in the breast, how suspicious it appears, how many abnormalities are present, and your overall health and personal preferences.

• **Fine needle biopsy** uses a thin, hollow needle attached to a syringe to withdraw cells or fluid from a mass. The doctor may feel for the lump to guide the needle or may use ultrasound imaging for guidance.

• **Open biopsy** accesses a breast mass through a surgical incision. Depending on its size, all of the lump may be removed (excisional biopsy) or just part of it (incisional biopsy).

• **Stereotactic biopsy,** a new alternative to open biopsy, uses mammograms taken from two angles to map the precise location of a breast lesion, allowing for a smaller incision. Tissue samples may be removed with a spring-loaded needle (core needle biopsy); a vacuum-assisted biopsy device; or an automated device called Advanced Breast Biopsy Instrumentation (ABBI) that uses a tube, or cannula, to remove an entire lesion.

Purpose of the Test

• To distinguish between benign or malignant (cancerous) tumors that were detected on an imaging test, such as mammography (see page 255), thermography (see page 129), or ultrasound (see page 130).

Who Performs It

• Fine needle biopsy is conducted by a doctor.
• Open biopsy is performed by a surgeon and a surgical team.

• Stereotactic biopsy is usually conducted by a radiologist.

Special Concerns

• Open biopsy may require general anesthesia, but usually is performed using only local anesthesia plus sedation. The fine needle and stereotactic procedures require only local anesthesia.

• Open biopsies obtain larger samples and are therefore more accurate for identifying cancer than the fine needle technique. Stereotactic procedures can be performed at a reduced cost compared to open biopsy and may be cosmetically more appealing.

Results

▼

➡ The tissue samples are sent to a pathology laboratory and inspected under a microscope for unusual cells. This examination usually results in a definitive diagnosis. (For more on laboratory testing, see Chapter 1.)

➡ If the biopsy reveals cancerous cells, surgical treatment to remove the entire malignant tumor will be instituted (unless the mass was already removed completely, as with excisional or ABBI biopsy). Additional tests, including a chest CT scan (see page 152), blood tests, and a bone scan (see page 329), will also be performed to determine if the cancer has spread. If the tissue has been completely removed, radiation therapy or chemotherapy may be initiated.

➡ If no cancer is present, your doctor will recommend a schedule of periodic tests, such as mammography, to monitor your breast health.

Breast Biopsy

Before the Test
All tests:

• Tell your doctor if you regularly take anticoagulants or nonsteroidal anti-inflammatory drugs (such as aspirin, ibuprofen, or naproxen). You will be instructed to discontinue them for some time before the test.

• Do not put talcum powder, lotion, or perfume on your breasts or use deodorant on the day of the test.

Fine needle and stereotactic biopsies:

• You will be asked to disrobe above the waist and put on a hospital gown.

Open biopsy:

• If the procedure will be performed under general anesthesia, do not eat or drink anything after midnight on the day before the test.

• You will be asked to disrobe and put on a hospital gown.

• General anesthesia is administered through an intravenous (IV) line inserted into a vein in your arm before the procedure begins.

• If a local anesthetic is being used, you may receive an IV sedative to help you relax during the procedure.

What You Experience
Fine needle biopsy:

• You will sit in a chair or on a table.

• The skin over the biopsy site is cleansed with an antiseptic solution, and a local anesthetic is injected to numb the area (this injection may cause slight discomfort).

• The doctor inserts a thin biopsy needle and withdraws a small amount of fluid or tissue. In some cases, ultrasound imaging is used to visualize the mass and guide needle placement.

• The needle is withdrawn. Pressure is placed on the biopsy site until bleeding has stopped, and a small bandage is applied.

• The procedure takes less than 15 minutes.

Open biopsy:

• You will lie on your back on a table.

• The skin over the biopsy site is cleansed with an antiseptic solution, and (unless general anesthesia is being used) a local anesthetic is injected to numb the area (this injection may cause slight discomfort).

• The surgeon makes a small incision in the skin over the mass, and removes all or a portion of the lump with surgical instruments.

• The incision is sutured closed and a bandage is applied.

• The procedure takes less than 1 hour.

Stereotactic biopsy:

• The skin over the biopsy site is cleansed with an antiseptic solution, and a local anesthetic is injected to numb the area (this injection may cause slight discomfort).

• You will lie face down on a special table with a hole through which the breast protrudes. The breast is then slightly compressed to keep it immobile.

• Two mammography units positioned at different angles are used to create a three-dimensional image of the breast.

• For core needle biopsy, a biopsy gun is guided to the lesion and fired; the spring-loaded inner needle advances into the lesion and obtains a small core of tissue. The gun is rotated and this process is repeated to obtain multiple samples.

• The vacuum-assisted biopsy device uses a similar technique, except a larger needle is employed and suction is used to remove progressively larger core samples. On average, 10 to 20 specimens are obtained.

• For the ABBI technique, a machine inserts a cannula—a tube that is larger than a needle and designed to remove larger amounts of tissue—through a small incision and guides it to the breast lesion. The entire lump is removed.

• Pressure is placed on the biopsy site until bleeding has stopped, and a small bandage is applied. You may need sutures to close the incision after an ABBI biopsy.

• Stereotactic biopsy takes 1 hour or less.

Risks and Complications

• You may experience some pain or bruising after a breast biopsy.

• A rare complication following an open biopsy is infection.

• If open biopsy was performed under general anesthesia, it will carry all the associated risks.

After the Test
Fine needle and stereotactic biopsies:

• You may return to your normal activities.

• You may experience a small amount of bleeding or bruising around the biopsy site and your breast may be tender for several days. Over-the-counter pain relievers, such as acetaminophen, or ice packs can help to relieve any discomfort.

Open biopsy:

• You will rest in a recovery room until the effects of anesthesia or sedation have subsided. During this time, your vital signs will be monitored and you will be observed for signs of complications.

• You may experience tenderness and bruising around the biopsy site for several days. You may be given pain-relieving medication such as acetaminophen and advised to use ice packs to relieve any discomfort.

• You will be instructed to wear a support bra at all times until the biopsy site has healed. Avoid strenuous activity for 1 to 2 weeks.

• If you develop a fever or you experience increased bleeding, pain, or swelling around the biopsy site, call your doctor.

Estimated Cost: $$

Breast Biopsy continued

Breast Cyst and Nipple Discharge Fluid Analysis

Breast Cyst and Nipple Discharge Fluid Analysis

Description
• In this test, fluid from a breast cyst or nipple discharge is spread on a slide and examined under a microscope.

Purpose of the Test
• To aid in the diagnosis of cancer within a breast cyst.
• To eliminate cancer as a cause of persistent nipple discharge.

Who Performs It
• A physician.

Special Concerns
• Many experts believe these tests are overused and not very helpful for the diagnosis of breast cancer. Since most simple breast cysts are benign, fluid analysis should be done only if a cyst recurs after at least 3 aspirations or if the fluid is bloody. Nonbloody nipple discharge is also seldom caused by breast cancer. In addition, the tests may be unreliable since it can be difficult to distinguish severe inflammatory cells from cancer; this may lead to unnecessary biopsies.
• Nipple discharge is normal during pregnancy and is relatively common in women who have had at least one pregnancy.

Before the Test
• Mammography (see page 255) may be performed before cyst aspiration.
• You will be asked to disrobe from the waist up and put on a hospital gown.

What You Experience
Cyst aspiration:
• You will lie on your back on an examining table.
• The doctor will locate the cyst by palpating the breast or with the aid of ultrasound imaging (see Chapter 2).
• The skin at the site of needle insertion is cleansed with an antiseptic.
• A small needle attached to a syringe is inserted into the cyst, and all of the fluid within the cyst is withdrawn. (Local anesthesia may be used, but is not usually necessary.)
• Pressure is applied to the aspiration site and a bandage is applied.
• The test takes several minutes.

Nipple discharge analysis:
• You will be asked to expose the breast with the persistent discharge.
• The doctor will squeeze the nipple to express fluid.
• The test takes less than 1 minute.

Risks and Complications
• Rare complications of cyst aspiration include bleeding or infection.

After the Test
• You may resume your normal activities.
• Notify your doctor if you develop pain, swelling, or redness at the cyst aspiration site.

Estimated Cost: $$

Results
▼
➡ The fluid is smeared onto a microscope slide, and a laboratory pathologist inspects the specimen under a microscope for the presence of unusual cells. (For more on laboratory tests, see Chapter 1.)
➡ If no abnormalities are found, no further testing is needed.
➡ If suspicious cells are identified, a breast biopsy (see page 125) is required to establish a definitive diagnosis.

Breast Thermography
(Digital Infrared Imaging of the Breast)

Description
• This test uses infrared light waves to measure temperatures across the breasts. Different rates of chemical activity and blood flow can alter tissue temperatures; abnormalities such as breast tumors, may cause minute increases in temperature, or "hot spots." Some research indicates that thermography may be a valuable screening tool to detect early-stage breast cancer; however, large scientific studies have not yet been done. Mammography (see page 255) is still considered the most reliable and cost-effective imaging test for the early detection of breast cancer. Thermography may be used as a complement to regular mammograms and breast exams by a doctor to monitor breast health. (For more on screening tests, see Chapter 3.)

Purpose of the Test
• To screen for precancerous changes of the breast and early-stage breast cancer.

Who Performs It
• A technician trained in thermography.

Special Concerns
• This test has a significant rate of false-positives (see page 35)—meaning that it reveals hot spots when no problem exists—since heat fluctuations can result from a variety of physical changes unrelated to cancer (for example, skin lesions, cysts, or inflammation).

Before the Test
• Avoid sun exposure to your breasts for up to 10 days.
• Avoid alcohol, coffee, smoking, and exercise for 3 to 4 hours before the procedure.
• Do not bathe any later than 1 hour before the test, and do not apply any lotions or powders to your breasts prior to the exam.

What You Experience
• You will enter a temperature-controlled imaging room, where you will remove your clothing above the waist and wait 5 to 10 minutes with your breasts exposed to room temperature. This stabilizes the temperature of your breasts and increases the accuracy of the test.
• You will be instructed to hold your hands above your head or on your knees.
• A special infrared camera takes photographs of your breasts from 3 or 4 angles.
• The test takes less than 15 minutes.

Risks and Complications
• None.

After the Test
• You may be asked to wait while the films are developed to ensure they are readable.

Estimated Cost: $

Results
▼

➡ A physician will examine the thermographic images for evidence of hot spots, asymmetry between breasts, or other abnormalities.

➡ If no abnormality is found, no further testing is necessary. Depending on your age and individual circumstances, your doctor may recommend periodic mammography (see page 255) and physical exams to monitor your breast health.

➡ If a problem is identified, your doctor may recommend further evaluation with mammography or breast ultrasound (see page 130).

Breast Thermography

Breast Ultrasound
(Breast Ultrasonography)

Breast Ultrasound

Description
• For this procedure, a device called a transducer is passed over the breasts, directing high-frequency sound waves (ultrasound) through the underlying tissue. The sound waves are reflected back to the transducer, where they are electronically converted into images of the internal structures that are displayed on a viewing monitor. These images can then be saved on film or video and reviewed for abnormalities. Ultrasound may be performed in addition to or instead of mammography (see page 255) to examine breast tissue in some women. For example, it is more accurate than mammography for detecting abnormalities in the denser breast tissue of younger women. (For more information on how ultrasound imaging works, see Chapter 2.)

Purpose of the Test
• To determine whether a lump or abnormality found on a mammogram is a cyst (fluid-filled) or a solid tumor (which may be benign or malignant).
• To identify and evaluate breast masses in individuals for whom mammography is less effective, including women under the age of 25 (whose breast tissue is too dense for mammography); those with silicone breast implants; and women with masses that are located in the difficult-to-assess area close to the chest wall.
• To monitor a previously detected breast cyst to see if it will enlarge and require treatment or if it will disappear.
• Breast ultrasound is used instead of mammography in pregnant women, since even small amounts of radiation may be harmful to the fetus.

Who Performs It
• An ultrasound technician.

Special Concerns
• None.

Before the Test
• Do not apply any lotions or powders to your breasts prior to the exam.
• Just before the test, you will be asked to disrobe from the waist up and put on a hospital gown.

What You Experience
• You will lie on your back on an examining table.
• A water-soluble gel is applied to your breasts to enhance sound wave transmission.
• The ultrasound technician then moves the transducer back and forth over your breasts to obtain different views while observing the images displayed on a screen.

Results
▼
➡ A radiologist reviews the recorded images for evidence of any abnormalities such as a cyst or a tumor.
➡ If the ultrasound images are normal, your physician will advise you about when to schedule your next breast ultrasound or mammography appointment, depending on your age.
➡ If a fluid-filled cyst is identified, your doctor will recommend appropriate treatment, such as drainage with a needle. Most cysts are benign.
➡ If a solid breast tumor is found by ultrasound, a mammogram or a breast biopsy (see page 125) is usually recommended for further evaluation.

• Once clear images are obtained, they are recorded on film, video, or paper for later analysis.

• Alternatively, you may be asked to lie on your stomach on an examining table that contains a tank of heated, chlorinated water. One breast at a time is immersed in the water; the ultrasound transducer is located at the bottom of the tank.

• Breast ultrasound generally takes from 30 to 45 minutes.

• There is no discomfort associated with this procedure.

Risks and Complications

• Ultrasound is noninvasive and involves no exposure to radiation. There are no associated risks or complications.

After the Test

• The examiner removes the conductive gel from your skin.

• You may leave the testing facility immediately after the test and resume your normal activities.

Estimated Cost: $$

Breast Ultrasound continued

Bronchial Challenge Test
(Bronchial Provocation Test, Methacholine Challenge Test)

Description
• In the bronchial challenge test, your lung function is measured after you inhale methacholine, a chemical that causes the bronchial tubes to constrict; in some cases, the test is performed after inhalation of other allergy-causing substances (allergens). By simulating conditions that may cause asthma symptoms and assessing how your airways react, this test can help to diagnose asthma or to identify whether inhalant allergens provoke a reaction.

Purpose of the Test
• To identify bronchial hyperresponsiveness in people who have normal results on standard pulmonary function tests (see page 306).
• To diagnose mild asthma in some atypical cases, such as persistent cough.
• To diagnose occupational (workplace) asthma caused by certain dusts or chemicals.

Who Performs It
• A physician.

Special Concerns
• Because this test carries a risk of provoking severe airway obstruction, it should not be performed in people who are known to have severe asthma or chronic lung disease.
• The presence of a recent or ongoing chest infection, an upper airway infection, or another respiratory disease may affect the test results.

Before the Test
• Be sure to inform your doctor of all medications you are currently taking. Certain drugs, particularly bronchodilators, may affect the results and should be discontinued before the test.
• Do not smoke or consume products containing caffeine—such as coffee, tea, chocolate, and cola drinks—for 6 hours before the test.
• Avoid exercise or exposure to cold air for 2 hours before the test.
• If you have dentures, you will wear them during the test.
• Wear loose clothing that won't inhibit your breathing.

What You Experience
• First, standard pulmonary function tests are done to establish your pre-test lung function.
• A clip is placed on your nose to prevent air from passing through your nostrils, and you are asked to seal your lips tightly around a mouthpiece that is attached to monitoring equipment.
• You will be asked to inhale aerosolized methacholine through a nebulizer (a device that emits an extremely fine spray for deep penetration of the lungs) for about 2 minutes.

Results
▼

➥ The doctor will calculate how much methacholine or allergen it takes to produce a 20% fall in your lung function. The result is compared to normal values for healthy and asthmatic populations.

➥ Because abnormal airway sensitivity to methacholine (bronchial hyperresponsiveness) may be present in disorders other than asthma, such as chronic obstructive pulmonary disease, your doctor must correlate the test results with your history and symptoms before making a diagnosis.

➥ Based on the test results and clinical findings, your doctor will decide whether to prescribe asthma medication or to adjust your current treatment.

Then, after a 30-second wait, you exhale forcefully through the mouthpiece.

• If occupational asthma is suspected, potential allergens from your workplace may be used in subsequent tests.

• Pulmonary function tests are then repeated to assess how your airways reacted to these substances.

• In some cases, these tests may be performed again with higher concentrations of methacholine or allergens.

• If at any point you feel tired or lightheaded, ask for a chance to rest between test cycles.

• This procedure may take from 1 to 2 hours.

Risks and Complications

• This test may trigger a mild asthmatic episode. Bronchodilator medications are kept available for immediate treatment.

After the Test

• You may resume any medications that were withheld before the test.

• You may experience wheezing or coughing for 30 to 60 minutes after the procedure. You may need to use a bronchodilator to relieve these symptoms.

Estimated Cost: $$

Bronchial Challenge Test continued

Bronchoscopy

Description

• A thin, flexible viewing tube (bronchoscope) is passed through the nose (or less often, the mouth) and into the lungs. Fiberoptic cables permit direct visualization of the vocal cords (larynx), upper airways (trachea), and lower airways (bronchi); these structures are illustrated on pages 22 and 23. In addition, various instruments may be passed through the scope to obtain fluid or tissue samples for laboratory examination. Less commonly, a rigid bronchoscope is used, primarily for the removal of large foreign bodies caught in the airways.

Purpose of the Test

• To visually inspect the airways for tumors, obstruction, narrowing (stricture), inflammation, bleeding, or a foreign body.
• To help diagnose lung diseases, such as inflammatory conditions, infection, or cancer.
• To visualize the larynx and identify possible vocal cord paralysis.
• Used therapeutically to remove foreign bodies, tumors, or excessive secretions from the airways.

Who Performs It

• A pulmonary specialist or a surgeon performs this procedure at your bedside or in an endoscopy room.
• Rigid bronchoscopy must be done in an operating room.

Special Concerns

• While this procedure may be uncomfortable, you will be able to breathe throughout, since the bronchoscope does not block your airways. If needed, extra oxygen may be administered through a special mask or tube.
• Chest x-rays (see page 156) and certain blood tests, such as coagulation studies (see page 157), may be needed before bronchoscopy is done.
• If rigid bronchoscopy is performed, heavy sedation or general anesthesia is required.

Before the Test

• Tell your doctor if you regularly take anticoagulants or nonsteroidal anti-inflammatory drugs (such as aspirin, ibuprofen, or naproxen). You may be instructed to discontinue them before the test. Also mention any herbs or supplements that you take.
• Tell your doctor if you've ever had an allergic reaction to anesthetic medication.
• You will be instructed to avoid food and fluids for 6 to 12 hours before the test.
• If you wear dentures, glasses, or contact lenses, remove them before the test.

Results

➡ During the visual inspection of your airways, the doctor will note any abnormalities, such as inflammation, narrowing, blood, secretions, or tumors. In some cases, this examination is sufficient to provide a definitive diagnosis.

➡ If tissue, cell, or fluid samples were taken, specimen containers may be sent to several different laboratories for examination. For example, biopsied tissue may be inspected under a microscope for the presence of unusual cells, or may be cultured (see page 166) for infectious organisms. (For more on laboratory testing, see Chapter 1.)

➡ If a definitive diagnosis can be made, appropriate treatment will be initiated.

➡ If a definitive diagnosis cannot be made, additional tests, such as a lung biopsy (see page 245), may be needed.

• Immediately before the test, an intravenous (IV) needle or catheter is inserted into a vein in your arm or hand, so that you may be given medications during the test. You may receive a mild sedative to relax you and a drug called atropine to help dry up your saliva.

What You Experience

• You will either lie down on a table or bed, or sit upright in a chair. Remain relaxed, breathing through your nose.

• A topical anesthetic (lidocaine) is applied to the inside of one nostril to minimize discomfort when the scope is inserted. Lidocaine may also be sprayed on the back of your throat to suppress the gag reflex. (If the scope is to be passed through your mouth, a plastic mouthpiece is inserted to protect your teeth and prevent you from biting down on it.)

• Once the lidocaine has taken effect, the doctor inserts the scope into your nose or mouth. When the instrument reaches a certain point, lidocaine is sprayed through it to anesthetize your larynx and trachea and prevent coughing.

• The doctor closely inspects your larynx, trachea, and bronchi through the scope, looking for any abnormalities.

• If appropriate, a tiny brush or other instruments may be passed through the scope to remove samples of tissue or cells from suspicious areas. A suction instrument may be used to remove a foreign object or mucus blockage. (These procedures are painless.) To take deeper samples, the doctor may use fluoroscopy (see page 205) to guide the progress of the instruments.

• If an infection is suspected or there is a buildup of mucus, the doctor may flush saline solution into the lung and suck it back out (bronchoalveolar lavage). This procedure both removes secretions and obtains fluid specimens that will be analyzed for infectious organisms or other abnormalities.

• The procedure takes 30 to 60 minutes.

Risks and Complications

• You may experience temporary hoarseness, loss of voice, a sore throat, or mild fever.

• Less common complications include reduced oxygen concentration in the blood (hypoxemia), aspiration of foreign contents into the lungs, bleeding, infection, and narrowing of the airways (bronchospasm or laryngospasm).

• Rarely, more severe complications such as pneumothorax (leakage of air outside the lungs and into the pleural cavity, resulting in a collapsed lung) and cardiac arrest may occur. Emergency equipment is kept readily available.

• In general, rigid bronchoscopy carries a higher risk of trauma and complications than flexible bronchoscopy.

After the Test

• You will lie down with your head slightly elevated. Your vital signs will be monitored until the sedation wears off, and you will be observed for any complications.

• If a deep biopsy was obtained, a chest x-ray may be performed to ensure that the biopsy did not cause a pneumothorax.

• Flexible bronchoscopy does not usually necessitate an overnight hospital stay. Due to the sedation, you should arrange for someone to drive you home after the procedure. (If you received a general anesthetic, you are more likely to require brief hospitalization.)

• Do not eat or drink until your gag reflex returns, usually in a few hours.

• If a biopsy was performed, there may be a small amount of blood in your sputum, but this should subside within 24 hours.

• If a sore throat develops, lozenges or a warm saline gargle may provide some relief.

• Contact your doctor immediately if you begin coughing up large amounts of blood, develop a high fever, have breathing difficulties, or experience any pain.

Estimated Cost: $$

Bronchoscopy continued

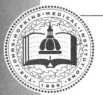

Calcium Tests

Description

• Calcium is a mineral that is necessary for many important body processes, including the building and repair of bones, muscle contraction, heart function, nerve transmission, and blood clotting. Measuring blood levels of calcium—and other substances that affect calcium metabolism through their interactions—can help to evaluate bone diseases, as well as the function of the kidneys and parathyroid glands.

• Calcium in the body is primarily stored in the bones; the remainder travels in the bloodstream. Normally, parathyroid hormone and vitamin D carefully control the amount of calcium (and phosphorus) in the body by regulating the absorption of calcium from food, the amount removed from the body by the kidneys, and the amount mobilized from the bone. Abnormal blood calcium levels may indicate a problem somewhere in this system.

• Parathyroid hormone (PTH) is secreted by the parathyroid glands (illustrated on page 18) when blood calcium levels are low. PTH acts to release calcium reservoirs from the bone into the blood; when blood calcium returns to normal levels, PTH secretion declines. PTH is typically measured to distinguish parathyroid from nonparathyroid causes of abnormal blood calcium. For example, high blood calcium is most commonly caused by elevated PTH due to hyperparathyroidism (overactive parathyroid glands).

• Vitamin D (in its active form, or 1,25-dihydroxyvitamin D) is necessary for the absorption of dietary calcium by the intestine. When blood calcium is low, PTH induces the production of vitamin D to help the intestines to absorb more calcium, and stimulates the bones to release calcium into the blood. Low vitamin D levels—which can be caused by dietary deficiency, impaired absorption, or inadequate sunlight exposure (since this vitamin is syn-thesized from the skin upon exposure to ultraviolet light)—can lead to low calcium levels and bone disease.

• Phosphorus is a mineral important for the building of bone and energy production. PTH and vitamin D regulate phosphorus levels. So, if disorders such as hyperparathyroidism or vitamin D deficiency are suspected, a blood test for phosphorus levels may be done. In chronic kidney (renal) failure, phosphorus levels are elevated because of inadequate excretion by the kidney.

Purpose of the Test

Calcium:

• To evaluate calcium metabolism and parathyroid function.

• To aid in the diagnosis of neuromuscular, skeletal, and endocrine disorders, arrhythmias,

Results

▼

➡ The blood sample is sent to a laboratory for analysis. Your doctor will review the results and consider them along with your symptoms, your physical exam, and the results of other tests. (For more on laboratory testing, see Chapter 1.)

➡ Hypercalcemia (chronically elevated blood calcium) is most commonly caused by hyperparathyroidism due to a benign parathyroid tumor.

➡ Hypocalcemia (chronically low blood calcium) may be caused by malnutrition, intestinal malabsorption, kidney failure, and acute inflammation of the pancreas (pancreatitis).

➡ Abnormal results often necessitate additional studies in order to confirm a diagnosis.

blood clotting dysfunction, and acid-base imbalance in the blood.

• To monitor people with chronic renal failure, hyperparathyroidism, and certain types of malignancies.

Parathyroid hormone:

• To aid in the evaluation of low or high blood calcium levels.

• To confirm a suspected diagnosis of hyperparathyroidism.

• To monitor patients with chronic renal failure.

Vitamin D:

• To evaluate bone diseases.

• To aid in the evaluation of abnormal calcium levels.

• To detect overdose of vitamin D or monitor therapy with vitamin D.

Phosphorus:

• To aid in the interpretation of the other tests.

Who Performs It

• A nurse or a technician.

Special Concerns

• Half of the calcium in the blood is bound to proteins (primarily albumin); the other half is known as free or ionized calcium. In most cases, the total amount of calcium (bound plus free) is measured. However, in people with low albumin levels—for example, malnourished patients—free calcium must be measured directly.

• A variety of medications may affect the test results.

• Blood levels of PTH, which vary during the day, are highest at around 2 AM and lowest at 2 PM. This pattern differs in people who work nights and sleep during the day; this fact must be taken into account when interpreting the test results.

Before the Test

• Do not eat or drink anything after midnight on the day before a PTH or phosphorus test.

• Do not eat or drink anything for 8 to 12 hours before a vitamin D test.

• No fasting is required before a blood calcium test. However, if this test is performed together with a PTH, vitamin D, or phosphorus study, you must follow the food and drink restrictions required for the other tests.

What You Experience

• A sample of your blood is drawn from a vein, usually in your arm, and sent to a laboratory for analysis. (For more on this procedure, called venipuncture, see page 32.)

Risks and Complications

• None.

After the Test

• Immediately after blood is drawn, pressure is applied (with cotton or gauze) to the puncture site.

• You may resume your normal activities and any medications that were withheld before the test.

• Blood may collect and clot under the skin (hematoma) at the puncture site; this is harmless and will resolve on its own. For a large hematoma that causes swelling and discomfort, apply ice initially; after 24 hours, use warm, moist compresses to help dissolve the clotted blood.

Estimated Cost: $

Calcium Tests continued

Cardiac Blood Tests

Cardiac Blood Tests

Description

• Analysis of a blood sample can provide important information about the heart. Some of the more significant blood components that may be measured include the following:

• **Apolipoproteins**—the protein component of lipoproteins—are not included in a standard lipid profile (see page 238), but may be tested separately. Abnormal levels may promote atherosclerosis, and may increase the risk of coronary artery disease (CAD) and stroke.

• **Homocysteine** is an amino acid. Elevated blood levels may promote atherosclerosis and CAD, as well as blood clots that can lead to a heart attack or stroke.

• **C-reactive protein (CRP)** is a substance that reflects low levels of systemic inflammation and is increased in people at risk for CAD.

• **Cardiac enzyme studies** measure certain enzymes, such as CK-MB, that are released in large amounts when the heart is diseased or damaged, as from a heart attack.

Purpose of the Test

• Apolipoproteins, homocysteine, and CRP are measured to evaluate the risk of CAD.

• Cardiac enzymes help to detect the presence of a recent or ongoing heart attack; to determine the timing of a heart attack and assess the degree of damage to the heart muscle; to determine the appropriateness of thrombolytic therapy (a treatment that is beneficial only during an ongoing heart attack); and to monitor any shortage of blood to the heart after cardiac surgery or catheterization (see page 140).

Who Performs It

• A doctor, a nurse, or a lab technician.

Special Concerns

• Pregnancy, oral contraceptives, cortisone medications, and nonsteroidal anti-inflammatory drugs (such as ibuprofen) may affect CRP in your blood and interfere with results.

• Intramuscular injections, strenuous exercise, recent surgery, and a variety of medications can raise levels of cardiac enzymes and interfere with results.

Results

➥ Abnormal apolipoprotein levels—such as an increased level of lipoprotein(a), or Lp(a)—may significantly increase your risk for CAD and heart attack. Lifestyle measures, such as diet and exercise, and lipid-lowering medications may decrease this risk.

➥ A high homocysteine level may increase your risk for CAD and heart attack. Increasing your intake of folate (as well as vitamin B_6 and vitamin B_{12}) by eating more fruits and vegetables or taking supplements may reduce homocysteine levels (however, this measure is not proven to reduce cardiovascular risk).

➥ An elevated level of CRP indicates an increased amount of systemic inflammation, which may heighten your risk of CAD. Your doctor may recommend an aspirin a day to reduce your risk of a heart attack.

➥ Elevated levels of cardiac enzymes indicate that you are experiencing or have recently suffered a heart attack. However, because these enzymes are present in many organs and levels may be increased by a number of disease states, positive test results must be correlated to your physical signs and symptoms in order to confirm a heart attack. Treatment will be administered, as needed.

Before the Test

• A 12- to 14-hour fast is required before measuring apolipoproteins (water is permitted).

• Report to your doctor any medications, herbs, or supplements you are taking. You may be advised to discontinue certain of these agents before the test. In particular, alcohol, aminocaproic acid (Amicar), and lithium should be withheld before testing for cardiac enzymes, if possible.

• No special preparations are needed before testing homocysteine or CRP.

What You Experience

• A sample of your blood is drawn from a vein, usually in your arm, and sent to a laboratory for analysis. (For more on this procedure, called venipuncture, see page 32.)

• Subsequent blood samples may be needed to measure cardiac enzymes after a heart attack (for example, 6, 12, and 24 hours after the episode and daily thereafter).

Risks and Complications

• None.

After the Test

• After blood is drawn, pressure is applied (with cotton or gauze) to the puncture site.

• Resume your normal diet and any medications withheld before the test.

• Blood may collect and clot under the skin (hematoma) at the puncture site; this is harmless and will resolve on its own. For a large hematoma that causes swelling and discomfort, apply ice initially; after 24 hours, use warm, moist compresses to help dissolve the clotted blood.

Estimated Cost: $

Cardiac Blood Tests continued

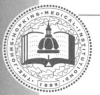

Cardiac Catheterization
(Coronary Angiography)

Cardiac Catheterization

Description

• A thin tube called a catheter is inserted into an artery in your groin or arm and is carefully threaded into your heart under the guidance of continuous x-ray imaging, or fluoroscopy (see page 205). Pressures within your heart and coronary arteries are recorded through the catheter. Next, a contrast dye is injected through the catheter to help delineate your coronary arteries and other cardiac structures on x-rays films; this portion of the test is termed coronary angiography or arteriography. (For more on angiography, see Chapter 2 and page 95.)

• In some cases, this procedure is immediately followed by treatment, such as percutaneous transluminal coronary angioplasty, which uses a catheter equipped with a small balloon to unblock coronary arteries.

Purpose of the Test

• To examine the coronary arteries, identify any blockages due to atherosclerosis, and determine the need for treatment.

• To assess the function of heart valves, coronary artery bypass grafts, and other cardiac structures.

• To evaluate pressures in the heart's chambers and the pumping function of the heart.

• To study congenital heart defects.

Who Performs It

• A cardiologist.

Special Concerns

• This procedure is performed in a hospital catheterization laboratory.

• The risks associated with this test are increased in people with bleeding disorders or poor kidney function; the test may not be possible in those with severe atherosclerosis in the arms or legs.

• People who have an allergy to shellfish or iodine may experience an allergic reaction to the contrast dye.

• Pregnant women should not undergo this test because exposure to ionizing radiation may harm the fetus.

Before the Test

• Tell your doctor if you regularly take anticoagulants or nonsteroidal anti-inflammatory drugs (such as aspirin, ibuprofen, or naproxen). You will be instructed to discontinue them for some time before the test.

• Be sure to tell your doctor if you have a known shellfish or iodine allergy or have ever had an adverse reaction to x-ray contrast dyes. You may be given a combined antihistamine-steroid preparation for several days before the test to reduce the risk of an allergic reaction.

• Do not ingest food and fluids for 6 to 8 hours before the test.

• Empty your bladder before the procedure.

• Immediately before the test, an intravenous (IV) line is inserted into a vein in your arm. You may also be given a mild sedative, but you will remain conscious throughout the procedure.

What You Experience

• You lie on your back on a padded table, and ECG leads (see page 174) are applied to mon-

---

Results
▼

➥ The doctor will examine the x-ray films and other test data for signs of significantly narrowed or blocked coronary arteries and other cardiac abnormalities.

➥ This test is usually definitive. Based on the findings, your doctor will then decide on a course of medical or surgical treatment.

itor your heart rate and rhythm.

• The area of catheter insertion (your groin or arm) is shaved, cleansed with an antiseptic to help prevent infection, and numbed with a local anesthetic. The doctor then makes a small incision and inserts a catheter into the artery; you will feel pressure during insertion, but no other discomfort.

• The doctor guides the catheter to your heart, using fluoroscopy to watch its progress on a viewing monitor.

• The contrast dye is administered through the catheter. You may feel a hot, flushing sensation for about 15 to 20 seconds after the injection; rarely, some people experience nausea and possibly vomiting.

• The doctor takes several moving and still x-ray pictures (angiograms) of your heart for later analysis.

• If you develop chest pain during the procedure, nitroglycerin may be administered.

• The test itself usually takes 1 to 2 hours.

Risks and Complications

• Possible risks include blood clot formation, bleeding, blood vessel damage, or infection at the site of catheter insertion.

• Some people may experience an allergic reaction to the iodine-based contrast dye, which can cause symptoms such as nausea, sneezing, vomiting, hives, and occasionally a life-threatening response called anaphylactic shock. Emergency medications and equipment are kept readily available.

• Rarely, the procedure may provoke a heart attack, stroke, or cardiac arrest; emergency equipment is available at the catheterization lab. Among stable patients, the risk of heart attack or death is very low (about 1 in 1,000).

After the Test

• The catheter is removed, and pressure is applied to the incision site until the bleeding stops (up to 30 minutes). A pressure bandage is then applied, and a small sandbag is typically placed over the incision site for several hours to prevent bleeding.

• You will rest in a recovery room for about 6 to 8 hours. During this time, you should not move the limb where the catheter was inserted. Nurses will check you periodically to ensure there is no bleeding at the incision site, to look for signs of delayed reaction to the contrast dye, and to monitor your blood pressure and other vital signs.

• You are encouraged to drink clear fluids during this period to avoid dehydration and help flush the contrast dye out of your system.

• Most people are able to return home after about 5 to 6 hours, though some may require overnight hospitalization.

• Before you leave, a doctor or nurse will demonstrate how to apply pressure to stop any bleeding at the incision site.

• Avoid heavy lifting and do only light activities for a few days after the test. You may develop a small lump at the insertion site, but it should disappear in a few weeks.

Estimated Cost: $$$

Cardiac Catheterization continued

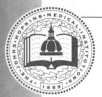

Cardiac MRI
(Magnetic Resonance Imaging of the Heart)

Cardiac MRI

Description
• Cardiac magnetic resonance imaging (MRI) uses a strong magnetic field combined with radiofrequency waves to create highly detailed, cross-sectional images of the heart and surrounding structures; these scans are examined for abnormalities. For certain cardiac studies, an MRI contrast dye such as gadolinium may be injected to provide better definition of soft tissues and blood vessels and thus enhance the images. (For more on how MRI works, see Chapter 2.)

Purpose of the Test
• To detect and evaluate heart conditions, including coronary artery disease, cardiomyopathy, pericardial disease, and masses in or around the heart.
• To identify forms of congenital heart disease, such as atrial or ventricular septal defects.
• To evaluate the extent of a heart attack and identify possible complications, such as formation of a ventricular aneurysm or thinning of the ventricular wall.
• To identify vascular disease in the chest cavity, such as an aneurysm (abnormal outpouching) or a dissection (leakage of blood between layers of the blood vessel wall) in the aorta.

Who Performs It
• A radiologist or a qualified technician.

Special Concerns
• People who experience claustrophobia may find it difficult to undergo an MRI, which takes place in a narrow, tunnel-like structure. In some cases, an open MRI—a larger unit that is open on several sides—may be used as an alternative.
• This test may not be possible for severely overweight individuals (over 300 lbs). Some open MRIs can accommodate larger patients.

• Because the MRI generates a strong magnetic field, it cannot be performed on people who have certain types of internally placed metallic devices, including pacemakers, inner ear implants, or intracranial aneurysm clips.
• The test should not be done in pregnant women because the long-term effects of MRI on the fetus are unknown.

Before the Test
• Tell your doctor if you suffer from claustrophobia. He or she may administer a sedative to help you tolerate the procedure.
• Empty your bladder before the test.
• Remove any magnetic cards or metallic objects, including watches, hair clips, belts, credit cards, and jewelry. You may be asked to disrobe and put on a hospital gown.

What You Experience
• You will lie down on a narrow padded bed that slides into a large, enclosed cylinder containing the MRI magnets.
• You must remain still throughout the scanning procedure because any motion can distort the images.

Results
▼

➡ The MRI scans are displayed on a viewing monitor and then recorded on film. The doctor will examine them for any evidence of heart disease or other abnormalities.

➡ If the doctor can make a definitive diagnosis, appropriate treatment will begin.

➡ In some cases, additional tests, such as cardiac catheterization (see page 140), may be required to establish the diagnosis and determine the extent of the problem.

• In some cases, you will receive an injection of contrast dye before or during the procedure.

• There is a microphone inside the imaging machine, and you may talk to the technician performing the scan at any time during the procedure.

• You will hear loud thumping sounds during the scanning process. To block out the noise, you can request earplugs or listen to music on earphones.

• The procedure can take up to 90 minutes.

Risks and Complications

• MRI does not involve exposure to ionizing radiation and is not associated with any risks or complications.

After the Test

• Most patients can go home right after the scan and resume their normal activities.

• Sedated patients may be monitored for a short period until the effects of the sedative have worn off.

• Blood may collect and clot under the skin (hematoma) at the dye injection site; this is harmless and will resolve on its own. For a large hematoma that causes swelling and discomfort, apply ice initially; after 24 hours, use warm, moist compresses to help dissolve the clotted blood.

Estimated Cost: $$$

Cardiac MRI continued

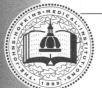

Cardiac Nuclear Scan

Cardiac Nuclear Scan

Description

• After injection of a small amount of radioactive material into the bloodstream, a special camera records the movement and uptake of the radiotracer within the heart (illustrated on page 21). The resulting images provide information about the coronary arteries and heart function. There are three common types of nuclear heart scans: the **myocardial infarction scan, myocardial perfusion scan,** and **multigated-acquisition (MUGA) scan** (also termed cardiac blood pool imaging). Each of these procedures uses a different radiotracer. The latter two scans are often done while you exercise; this is known as **stress testing.** (For more on nuclear imaging, see Chapter 2.)

Purpose of the Test

Myocardial infarction scan:

• To identify a recent heart attack, define its size and location, and determine the patient's prognosis.

Myocardial perfusion scan:

• To assess the amount of blood reaching the heart muscle and detect areas with a decreased blood supply.
• To pinpoint the location and extent of a past or recent heart attack.
• To identify blocked coronary arteries and assess the effectiveness of coronary bypass grafts or angioplasty.
• To evaluate patients who have angina (chest pain due to inadequate delivery of oxygen to the heart muscle) and inconclusive findings on an electrocardiogram, or ECG (see page 174).

MUGA scan:

• To evaluate the pumping function of the heart's left ventricle by measuring the flow of blood into the left ventricle and how much blood the heart pumps with each beat (ejection fraction).

• To assess the ability of the heart's right ventricle to pump blood into the lungs.
• To detect any abnormalities of heart wall motion.

Who Performs It

• A radiologist or a qualified technician.

Special Concerns

• This test should not be performed in pregnant women because of possible risks to the fetus.
• Other recent nuclear imaging tests, such as a thyroid or bone scan, may interfere with the results.
• A myocardial perfusion scan may yield false-positive results (see page 35) in females and in people with a heart condition called hypertrophic cardiomyopathy.
• Movement during the test, abnormalities on the ECG, or an irregular heartbeat can affect the results of a MUGA scan.

Results

▼

➡ The doctor analyzes the images obtained during the procedure for evidence of any cardiac abnormalities. If you underwent stress testing, your performance and symptoms during this phase of the test will also be evaluated.

➡ If a definitive diagnosis can be made based on the findings, your doctor will recommend that treatment be started with diet, exercise, and/or medication.

➡ In some cases, more invasive tests, such as cardiac catheterization (see page 140), may be needed to further evaluate abnormal results.

Stress testing:

• People who cannot exercise adequately because of orthopedic, arthritic, or lung disorders may instead be given dobutamine, a drug that mimics the effects of exercise by increasing the heart rate, or may be given adenosine or Persantine, which causes a relative decrease in blood flow to areas of the heart supplied by a blocked artery.

• Because this test places significant stress on the heart, it may not be appropriate for people with unstable angina, uncontrolled hypertension, severe aortic valvular heart disease, congestive heart failure, or uncontrolled heart rhythm disorders (arrhythmias).

Before the Test

• If stress testing is not being performed, no special preparation is necessary.

Stress testing:

• Antianginal drugs (such as nitroglycerin, beta-blockers, and calcium channel blockers) can affect test results by increasing your exercise tolerance. Your doctor may ask you to discontinue these medications for 1 or 2 days before the test.

• Do not eat or smoke for 4 hours before the test. Avoid caffeine and alcohol for 6 hours before the test.

• Wear comfortable shoes and loose, light-weight clothing.

• You will be asked to disrobe above the waist. (Women may wear a loose-fitting hospital gown that opens in the front.)

What You Experience

• You will lie on your back on an examination table.

• The radiotracer is injected into a vein in your arm. In some cases, an intravenous (IV) line is inserted into a vein in your arm and the radiotracer is infused through it. (Other than this injection, the procedure causes no discomfort.)

• Depending on what specific radiotracer is being used, the scanning procedure is performed from 15 minutes to 4 hours after the injection.

• A special camera is placed over the front of your chest, and you may be asked to assume various positions as the camera moves back and forth, recording multiple images of your heart. While you are being scanned, you must remain still.

• The procedure generally takes from 1 to 4 hours (sometimes there is a break of several hours between scans). Some patients may have to return 24 hours later for an additional scan.

Stress testing:

• Your blood pressure is measured, and ECG leads are attached to your chest, arm, and leg to monitor your heart activity.

• For an exercise stress test, you will begin by walking on a treadmill or pedaling a stationary bicycle.

• The pedaling tension on the cycle or the speed and grade of the incline on the treadmill are gradually increased until you reach a target heart rate (or until you are too tired to continue or have chest pain).

• For a dobutamine stress test, the doctor infuses the drug through an IV line and gradually increases the dose to mimic the effects of intensifying exercise.

• Once you achieve your target heart rate, the radiotracer is injected. You will then lie down on the examination table, and the scanning is performed.

Risks and Complications

• The trace amount of radioactive material used in this test is not associated with significant risks or complications.

• In extremely rare cases, patients may be hypersensitive to the radiotracer and may experience an adverse reaction.

Stress testing:

• Although generally safe, in rare cases stress testing may lead to complications including severe angina, heart attack, arrhythmias, a

Cardiac Nuclear Scan continued

drop in blood pressure, and fainting.

• Dobutamine may cause reactions such as flushing, palpitations, headache, and nausea, but these effects usually resolve quickly once the infusion is stopped.

After the Test

• Drink extra fluids to help your body eliminate the radioactive material.

• If you had stress testing, you will rest until your blood pressure, heart rate, and other vital signs return to normal.

• If you received an IV line, it is removed from your arm and pressure is applied to the infusion site for several minutes.

• If there are no complications, you are free to return to your normal activities and may resume any medications that were withheld before the test.

• Blood may collect and clot under the skin (hematoma) at the injection site; this is harmless and will resolve on its own. For a large hematoma that causes swelling and discomfort, apply ice initially; after 24 hours, use warm, moist compresses to help dissolve the clotted blood.

Estimated Cost: $$$

Cardiac Stress Test
(ECG Stress Test, Exercise Stress Test)

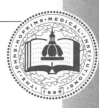

Description
• In this test, the electrical activity of the heart is monitored with ECG leads (see page 174) while you exercise on a stationary bicycle or treadmill. Abnormal ECG tracings during the test may indicate the presence of coronary artery disease or other cardiac abnormalities.

Purpose of the Test
• To detect inadequate flow of blood (ischemia) to the heart muscle and aid in the evaluation of possible coronary artery disease.
• To determine appropriate levels of exercise for people with angina (chest pain due to inadequate delivery of oxygen to the heart muscle) or other symptoms of heart disease.
• To evaluate heart function and exercise capacity after a heart attack, angioplasty, or bypass surgery.
• To identify abnormal heart rhythms (or arrhythmias) that develop during physical exercise.
• To assess the effectiveness of various drugs to treat arrhythmias or angina.
• To evaluate the heart prior to major surgery.

Who Performs It
• A doctor with a nurse or technician.

Special Concerns
• People who are unable to exercise adequately because of orthopedic, arthritic, or lung disorders may instead be given dobutamine, a drug that mimics the effects of exercise by increasing the rate and strength of the heart's contractions.
• Certain medical conditions may affect test results, including high blood pressure, valvular heart disease, left ventricular hypertrophy, severe anemia, and chronic lung disease.
• This test cannot diagnose cardiac ischemia in people with left bundle branch block (an abnormal heart rhythm); these patients may

undergo an alternative test, such as a cardiac nuclear scan with a dobutamine stress test (see page 144).
• Because this test places significant stress on the heart, it may not be appropriate for people with unstable angina, uncontrolled hypertension, severe aortic valvular heart disease, severe congestive heart failure, or uncontrolled arrhythmias.

Before the Test
• Antianginal drugs (such as nitroglycerin, beta-blockers, and calcium channel blockers) can affect test results by increasing your exercise tolerance. Your doctor may ask you to discontinue these medications for 1 or 2 days before the test.
• Do not eat, drink, or smoke for 4 hours before the test.
• Wear comfortable shoes and loose, lightweight clothing.
• At the testing facility, you will be instructed to disrobe above the waist. (Women may wear a loose-fitting hospital gown that opens in the front.)

Results
▼
➡ The doctor analyzes the ECG tracings for signs of coronary ischemia and also evaluates your performance and symptoms during the test.
➡ If a definitive diagnosis can be made based on these findings, treatment will be started with diet, exercise, and/or medication.
➡ In some cases, more invasive tests, such as cardiac catheterization (see page 140), may be needed to further evaluate abnormal results.

Cardiac Stress Test

What You Experience

• ECG leads are applied to your chest to monitor your heart rate and rhythm during the test. Pretest measurements of your heart rate and blood pressure are taken before you begin exercising.

• For an exercise stress test, you begin by walking on a treadmill or pedaling a stationary bicycle. The pedaling tension on the cycle or the speed and grade of the incline on the treadmill are gradually increased until you reach a target heart rate set by your doctor.

• For a dobutamine stress test, an intravenous (IV) line is inserted into a vein in your arm. The doctor infuses the drug and gradually increases the dose to mimic the effects of intensifying exercise. Another drug called atropine is sometimes needed to further increase your heart rate to the desired level.

• The test concludes when you achieve an adequate heart rate or develop significant symptoms, such as angina or fatigue.

• The test takes about 20 minutes.

Risks and Complications

• Although generally safe, this test carries a small amount of risk. Rare complications include severe angina, heart attack, arrhythmias, a drop in blood pressure, and fainting.

• Dobutamine may cause flushing, palpitations, headache, and nausea, but these effects usually resolve quickly once the infusion is stopped.

• Atropine can cause dry mouth and dilatation of the pupils, which may persist for an hour or so after the test.

After the Test

• You will rest until your blood pressure, heart rate, and other vital signs return to normal. The ECG leads are then removed from your chest.

• If you received dobutamine, the IV line is removed from your arm and pressure is applied to the infusion site for several minutes. Blood may collect and clot under the skin (hematoma) at the infusion site; this is harmless and will resolve on its own. For a large hematoma that causes swelling and discomfort, apply ice initially; after 24 hours, use warm, moist compresses to help dissolve the clotted blood.

• If there are no complications, you may resume your normal activities.

Estimated Cost: $$

Carotid Artery Doppler Ultrasound
(Carotid Duplex Ultrasound)

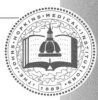

Description
• This test uses a technique called Doppler ultrasound to measure blood flow through the carotid arteries inside the neck, which supply blood to the brain. A device called a transducer is passed lightly over your neck, directing high-frequency sound waves (ultrasound) into the carotid arteries. The sound waves are reflected back at frequencies that correspond to the velocity of blood flow, and are converted into audible sounds and graphic recordings.
• **Duplex scanning** combines Doppler ultrasound with real-time ultrasound imaging of the carotid arteries, allowing calculation of the percent of narrowing in the vessels. Images are displayed on a viewing monitor and may also be recorded on film or video for later examination. (For more on Doppler and duplex ultrasound, see Chapter 2.)

Purpose of the Test
• To assess blood flow in the carotid arteries and detect any blockages, such as blood clots or atherosclerosis (narrowing due to the buildup of plaques).

Who Performs It
• A doctor or a technician who is trained in ultrasound.

Special Concerns
• None.

Before the Test
• No special preparation is necessary.

What You Experience
• You will lie on your back on an examination table, and your head will be supported to inhibit movement.
• A water-soluble gel is applied to the skin on your neck to enhance sound wave transmission.
• The examiner then moves the transducer back and forth over one side of your neck to obtain different views of the carotid artery. The other side of your neck is then checked in the same way.
• Once clear images of the carotid artery are obtained, they are recorded on film or video for later analysis.
• The test takes about 15 to 30 minutes.

Risks and Complications
• Ultrasound is painless, noninvasive, and involves no exposure to radiation. There are no associated risks.

After the Test
• The examiner removes the conductive gel from your skin.
• You may resume your normal activities.

Estimated Cost: $$

Results
▼

➡ A physician reviews the recorded images and other test data for evidence of abnormalities. High blood flow velocity indicates narrowing of the carotid arteries.

➡ If the carotid arteries are blocked, appropriate therapy will be initiated to reduce your risk of stroke.

➡ In some cases—especially if surgery to remove carotid blockages is contemplated—additional diagnostic tests, such as arteriography (see page 95), may be ordered to determine the exact location and extent of the occlusive plaques.

Carotid Artery Doppler Ultrasound

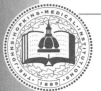

Cervical Cone Biopsy
(Cone Biopsy, Cervical Conization)

Description
• In this procedure, a cone-shaped piece of tissue is removed from the central portion of the cervix, the cylindrical area at the bottom of the uterus that opens into the vagina. This specimen is sent to a laboratory for examination. A cone biopsy is usually done to obtain a more extensive sample of cervical tissue when less invasive tests, such as colposcopy and cervical punch biopsy (see page 162), are insufficient to confirm or rule out cervical cancer. (The female reproductive system is illustrated on page 28.)

Purpose of the Test
• To detect cervical cancer and determine whether it is invasive when the results of colposcopy and cervical punch biopsy are insufficient for a definitive diagnosis.
• To evaluate the extent and severity of cervical cancer and guide treatment decisions after cancer is detected with a Pap smear (see page 279), colposcopy, and cervical punch biopsy.
• Used therapeutically to remove abnormal cervical tissue.

Who Performs It
• A gynecological surgeon assisted by a nurse.

Special Concerns
• Cone biopsy is usually performed under general anesthesia. However, in some cases only local anesthesia is required.

Before the Test
• Tell your doctor if you regularly take anticoagulants or nonsteroidal anti-inflammatory drugs (such as aspirin, ibuprofen, or naproxen). You will be instructed to discontinue them for some period before the test. Also mention any other medications, herbs, or supplements that you take.
• You will go to the hospital for certain routine blood and urine tests 1 or 2 days before the procedure.
• If general anesthesia is to be used, do not eat or drink anything for at least 8 hours before the test.
• You will be asked to disrobe and put on a hospital gown.
• Empty your bladder before the test.
• If local anesthesia is being used, you will be given a sedative about 30 minutes before the procedure.
• If general anesthesia is being used, the medication is administered through an intravenous (IV) needle or catheter inserted into a vein in your arm. A tube may be inserted through your windpipe to ensure you breathe properly during the procedure.

What You Experience
• You will be positioned on your back with your knees bent and your feet raised and resting in stirrups.
• A speculum—a metal or plastic instrument that pushes apart the walls of the vagina—is

---

Results
▼

➡ A pathologist examines the tissue sample under a microscope for the presence of unusual cells. (For more on microscopic examination, see Chapter 1.) Cone biopsy usually results in a definitive diagnosis.

➡ If no cancer is found, no further tests are necessary.

➡ If cervical cancer or a precancerous condition is found, further surgery may be scheduled. Additional tests, such as a bone scan (see page 329), may also be performed to determine if cancer has spread.

inserted to expose the cervix. If local anesthesia is being used, the medication is injected into the cervix.

• The doctor uses a scalpel or laser to remove a cone-shaped portion of tissue from the center of the cervix. (The widest part of the cone is taken from the opening of the cervix, while the middle and tip of the cone are taken from the cervical canal leading to the uterus.)

• The edges of the cervix are then sutured, or a cautery device is used to seal the blood vessels with an electric current.

• The instruments and speculum are then withdrawn.

• Cone biopsy takes up to 30 minutes.

Risks and Complications

• Possible complications include heavy bleeding and, rarely, infection, inadvertent perforation of the uterus (which requires surgical repair), or impaired menstrual flow.

• Cone biopsy may lead to increased risk of miscarriages and possible infertility because the cervix may be weakened by the surgery.

Scar tissue may also interfere with dilatation of the cervix during labor and thus reduce the chances for vaginal childbirth.

After the Test

• You will remain in a recovery room until you recover from the effects of sedation or anesthesia. During this time, your vital signs will be monitored and you will be observed for any evidence of complications.

• Arrange for someone to drive you home.

• You may experience mild to moderate cramping. Pain-relieving medication may be prescribed to allay any discomfort.

• You may experience slight bleeding. Use sanitary napkins rather than tampons.

• After 2 or 3 days, you may return to your normal activities. However, you should avoid sexual intercourse, tampons, and douching for 6 weeks to allow the cervix to heal adequately.

• Call your doctor immediately if you develop heavy bleeding or discharge or a fever.

Estimated Cost: $$

Cervical Cone Biopsy continued

Chest CT Scan
(Computed Tomography Scan of the Chest)

Description
• In this test, a body scanner delivers x-rays to the chest region at many different angles. A computer then compiles this information to construct highly detailed, cross-sectional images of the chest cavity. In some cases, a contrast dye may be injected to better define tissues and organs on the images. This procedure is very useful for detecting abnormalities in the chest region that cannot be found with conventional x-rays. (For more on how CT scans work, see Chapter 2.)

Purpose of the Test
• To obtain an image of the lungs and other chest structures that is more accurate than a routine chest x-ray.
• To determine the precise anatomy of chest structures prior to surgery.
• To identify bleeding or fluid collections in the lungs or other regions of the chest.
• To evaluate a chest injury.

Who Performs It
• A radiologist or a qualified technician.

Special Concerns
• CT scans are not usually done during pregnancy because exposure to ionizing radiation may harm the fetus.
• People who experience claustrophobia may find it difficult to undergo a CT scan, which takes place in a narrow, tunnel-like structure.
• This test may not be possible for severely overweight individuals (over 300 lbs).
• People with allergies to iodine or shellfish may experience an allergic reaction to the iodine-based contrast material.

Before the Test
• Inform your doctor if you have an allergy to iodine or shellfish. You may be given a combined antihistamine-steroid preparation to reduce the risk of an allergic reaction.
• Tell your doctor if you suffer from claustrophobia. He or she may prescribe a sedative that can help you tolerate the procedure.
• You may be asked to fast for 4 to 6 hours before the procedure if a contrast dye is to be used or if sedation is likely to be necessary.
• Remove any metal objects, including watches, hair clips, and jewelry.
• If a contrast dye is to be administered, an intravenous (IV) needle or catheter is inserted into a vein in your arm immediately before the test begins.

What You Experience
• You are asked to lie on your back on a narrow table that is then advanced into the CT scanner.
• The scanner, which encircles you, takes pictures at different intervals and varying levels over your chest area, so you will feel the table move during the test. The resulting images are displayed on a viewing monitor and recorded on x-ray film.
• You must remain still because any movement can distort the image on the scan.

Results
▼
➡ The doctor will examine the CT scans for evidence of any abnormality.
➡ If a definitive diagnosis can be made, appropriate treatment will be initiated, depending on the specific problem.
➡ In some cases, additional tests, such as a chest MRI (see page 154) or bronchoscopy (see page 134), may be needed to establish a diagnosis and determine the extent of the problem.

• The examiner may advise you on how to control your breathing at several points during the procedure.

• A contrast dye may be administered through the IV line in your arm to help define blood vessels and various tissues.

• The test may take 30 to 45 minutes. However, if a contrast dye is used, the procedure time may be doubled.

Risks and Complications

• CT scans involve exposure to low levels of radiation.

• Some people may experience an allergic reaction to the iodine-based contrast dye, which can cause symptoms such as nausea, sneezing, vomiting, hives, and occasionally a life-threatening response called anaphylactic shock. Emergency medications and equipment are kept readily available.

After the Test

• If contrast dye was used, blood may collect and clot under the skin (hematoma) at the injection site; this is harmless and will resolve on its own. For a large hematoma that causes swelling and discomfort, apply ice initially; after 24 hours, use warm, moist compresses to help dissolve the clotted blood.

• You are encouraged to drink clear fluids to avoid dehydration and help flush the contrast dye out of your system.

• Delayed allergic reactions to the contrast dye, such as hives, rash, or itching, may appear 2 to 6 hours after the procedure. If this occurs, your doctor will prescribe antihistamines or steroids to ease your discomfort.

Estimated Cost: $$$

Chest CT Scan continued

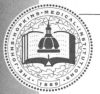
Chest MRI
(Magnetic Resonance Imaging of the Chest)

Chest MRI

Description
• Magnetic resonance imaging (MRI) uses a strong magnetic field combined with radiofrequency waves to create highly detailed, cross-sectional images of internal structures; these scans are examined for abnormalities. MRI of the chest is particularly valuable for providing detailed images of blood vessels and soft tissues in the chest cavity, such as the lungs and their surrounding membrane, or pleura (illustrated on page 23) the lymph nodes (illustrated on page 19). (For more on how MRI works, see Chapter 2.)

Purpose of the Test
• To detect and evaluate abnormalities, such as tumors or other growths, in chest organs and tissues.
• To detect and evaluate blood vessels problems in the chest cavity, such as an aneurysm (abnormal outpouching) or stenosis (narrowing) of the aorta; blood vessel malformations in the lungs; and certain abnormalities of the cardiac blood vessels.
• To clarify findings from previous x-rays or CT scans of the chest.

Who Performs It
• A radiologist or a qualified technician.

Special Concerns
• People with claustrophobia may find it difficult to undergo this procedure, which takes place in a narrow, tunnel-like structure. In some cases, an open MRI—a larger unit that is open on several sides—may be used as an alternative.
• This test may not be possible for severely overweight individuals (over 300 lbs). Some open MRI scanners can accommodate larger patients.
• Because the MRI generates a strong magnetic field, it cannot be performed on people who have certain types of internally placed metallic devices, including pacemakers, inner ear implants, or intracranial aneurysm clips.
• The test is not commonly done in pregnant women because the long-term effects of MRI on the fetus are unknown.

Before the Test
• Tell your doctor if you suffer from claustrophobia. He or she may prescribe a sedative that can help you tolerate the procedure.
• For your comfort, you will be instructed to empty your bladder before the test.
• Remove any magnetic cards or metallic objects, including watches, hair clips, belts, credit cards, and jewelry.
• You may be asked to disrobe and put on a hospital gown.

What You Experience
• You will lie down on a narrow padded bed that slides into a large, enclosed cylinder containing the MRI magnets.

Results
▼
➥ The MRI scans are displayed on a viewing monitor and then recorded on film. The doctor will examine them for evidence of any abnormality.

➥ If a definitive diagnosis can be made based on these images, your doctor will recommend an appropriate course of treatment, depending on the specific problem.

➥ In some cases, additional tests, such as a chest CT scan (see page 152) or bronchoscopy (see page 134), may be required to establish a diagnosis or determine the extent of a problem.

- You must remain still throughout the scanning procedure because any motion can distort the images.
- There is a microphone inside the imaging machine, and you may talk to the technician performing the scan at any time during the procedure.
- You will hear loud thumping sounds as the scanning is performed. To block out the noise, you can request earplugs or listen to music on earphones.
- The entire procedure may require up to 90 minutes.
- No discomfort is associated with this test.

Risks and Complications

- MRI does not involve exposure to ionizing radiation. The test is not associated with any risks or complications.

After the Test

- Most patients can go home promptly after the scan is completed and resume their usual activities.
- Sedated patients may be monitored for a short period until the effects of the sedative have worn off.

Estimated Cost: $$$

Chest MRI continued

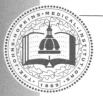

Chest X-ray
(Chest Radiography)

Description

• X-ray beams are passed through the chest, producing images of the internal structures on a special type of film. This basic imaging test is often part of the initial evaluation in people being assessed for lung or heart disorders. (For more on how x-rays work, see Chapter 2.)

Purpose of the Test

• To detect and evaluate abnormalities in the lungs, including pneumonia; pneumothorax (leakage of air outside the lungs and into the pleural cavity, resulting in a collapsed lung); and tumors.

• To provide an initial assessment of the size of the heart.

• To locate fluid accumulation in the lung or pleural space (the space between the lung and chest wall).

• To detect fractures of bones in the chest.

• To locate foreign bodies (such as coins or small objects) that may have been swallowed.

• To screen for lung diseases in apparently healthy individuals who have been exposed to environmental toxins such as asbestos. (For more on screening tests, see Chapter 3.)

• To aid in the placement of devices for other tests, such as a pulmonary artery catheter.

Who Performs It

• An x-ray technician.

Special Concerns

• In general, pregnant women should not undergo this test because exposure to ionizing radiation may harm the fetus. If the test is deemed necessary, a lead apron should be placed over the woman's abdomen to shield the fetus.

• Obesity and scarring from previous lung diseases or chest surgery may make interpretation of x-ray films difficult.

• To prevent radiation-related problems, a lead shield may be placed over the ovaries in women or testicles in men.

Before the Test

• Remove any metal objects, including watches, hair clips, and jewelry.

What You Experience

• You will be positioned, either sitting, standing, or lying down, in front of an x-ray machine.

• You are asked to take a deep breath and hold it while the x-ray is being taken, in order to provide a clear view of the chest. It is important to remain still throughout the procedure because any motion can distort the image. Several views may be taken.

• The test generally takes 10 to 15 minutes.

Risks and Complications

• This test involves minimal radiation exposure.

After the Test

• No special aftercare is needed.

Estimated Cost: $

Results
▼

➥ The doctor will examine the x-ray films for any evidence of heart or lung disease or other abnormalities.

➥ If a definitive diagnosis can be made based on the images, appropriate treatment will be initiated.

➥ In many cases, additional tests, such as a chest MRI (see page 154), a chest CT scan (see page 152), or a lung biopsy (see page 245), may be required for further evaluation.

Coagulation Studies
(Blood Clotting Tests)

Description

• When a break occurs in a blood vessel wall—due to a skin cut or abrasion, for example—a process called coagulation occurs that leads to the formation of a blood clot, which stops the bleeding. First, blood cells called platelets aggregate, or clump, at the injury site; at the same time, the injured cells and platelets both trigger the release of special substances, called clotting factors, into the bloodstream. The clotting factors activate a complex series of events that results in the production of a long-stranded protein called fibrin. At the injury site, strands of fibrin interlock to form a meshwork that traps platelets and red blood cells, completing the blood clot. Blood coagulation studies—the most common ones are covered here—assess whether your blood clots normally and help to identify the origin of any clotting problems.

• **Prothrombin time (PT)** and **activated partial thromboplastin time (APTT)** are tests that evaluate the release of specific clotting factors by measuring the time it takes for a clot to form after certain reagents are added to a blood sample. The PT test is often performed periodically to monitor patients who regularly take the anticoagulant drug warfarin (Coumadin, Panwarfin), while APTT is used to evaluate therapy with the anticoagulant heparin (which is usually used to treat patients after an acute episode such as a blood clot or heart attack).

• **Platelet count**—one of the most essential tests of platelet function—estimates the number of platelets in your blood using an automated system. The results are confirmed with a visual estimate by a pathologist who examines a blood sample under a microscope.

• **Bleeding time** measures the time required for a clot to form and stop bleeding after a standardized skin incision. It is used to evaluate platelet function and is typically performed, along with a platelet count, in people with a personal or family history of bleeding disorders, or as a preoperative safety measure before a scheduled surgery.

Purpose of the Test
PT and APTT:
• To evaluate blood coagulation.
• To screen patients for bleeding tendencies before a scheduled surgery.
• To monitor the response of people taking anticoagulant drugs.

Platelet count:
• To evaluate platelet production; assess the effects of chemotherapy or radiation treatment

---

Results
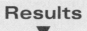

➡ The blood sample is sent to a laboratory for analysis. Your doctor will review the results for evidence of a blood clotting abnormality.

➡ A wide variety of conditions may cause abnormal results on coagulation studies. For example, people with liver disease often have a prolonged PT, since this test screens for clotting factors that are produced by the liver. An abnormal platelet count and prolonged bleeding time may be caused by bone marrow disease, chemotherapy or radiation therapy for cancer, and liver disease. Additional tests—such as further blood clotting studies, a complete blood count (see page 164), or a bone marrow biopsy—may be necessary to pinpoint the cause of the problem.

➡ Prolonged PT or APTT results—meaning the blood takes too long to clot—in people taking anticoagulants may indicate the need for a dosage adjustment.

Coagulation Studies

on platelet production; and aid in the diagnosis of decreased (thrombocytopenia) or increased (thrombocytosis) number of platelets.

Bleeding time:
• To evaluate platelet function.
• To screen patients for bleeding tendencies before a scheduled surgery.

Who Performs It
• A nurse or a technician draws the blood sample.

Special Concerns
• A variety of medications may affect the results of coagulation studies in people who take anticoagulant medication. In addition, a diet rich in green, leafy vegetables may cause a shortened PT time in those receiving treatment with anticoagulants.
• The bleeding time test should not be performed in people with extremely low platelet counts, those who are taking anticoagulant medication, and those who have had lymph nodes dissected (for example, breast cancer patients) on the test side (the other arm should be used, if possible).
• The bleeding time test will leave two small, hairline scars that will be nearly invisible after they have healed. More severe scarring may occur in people who tend to form large scars, or keloids.

Before the Test
• Report to your doctor any medications, herbs, or supplements you are taking. You may be advised to discontinue certain of these agents before the test.

What You Experience
PT, APTT, and platelet count:
• A sample of your blood is drawn from a vein in your arm and sent to a laboratory for analysis. (For more on venipuncture, see page 32.)

Bleeding time:
• A blood pressure cuff will be wrapped around your upper arm and then inflated so that it feels tight.
• An area high on your forearm will be cleansed with an antiseptic solution. After it has dried, 1 or 2 small incisions are made in the skin. (Alternatively, 3 small punctures are made with a lancet, or a puncture is made in the earlobe.)
• The examiner will start a stopwatch, and then blot the drops of blood with filter paper every 30 seconds until bleeding stops.
• The incisions and tightness of the blood pressure cuff may cause some discomfort.
• The test takes about 10 minutes.

Risks and Complications
• The bleeding time test carries a small risk of excessive bleeding or skin infection. In addition, scars may occur in people who are prone to keloid formation.

After the Test
• Immediately after blood is drawn, pressure is applied (with cotton or gauze) to the puncture or incision site. (For people on anticoagulant therapy, additional pressure may be needed to control the bleeding.)
• After a bleeding time test, the incisions are covered with a small piece of gauze and an adhesive bandage. (However, in people with bleeding disorders such as hemophilia, a pressure bandage is kept over the incisions for 24 to 48 hours to prevent further bleeding.)
• After bleeding has stopped, you may leave the testing facility.
• Resume taking any medications that were withheld before the test, according to your doctor's instructions.
• Blood may collect and clot under the skin (hematoma) at the puncture site; this is harmless and will resolve on its own. For a large hematoma that causes swelling and discomfort, apply ice initially; after 24 hours, use warm, moist compresses to help dissolve the clotted blood.

Estimated Cost: $

Colonoscopy

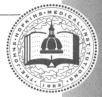

Description

• In this test, a flexible, lighted viewing tube (colonoscope) is passed through the anus, rectum, the full length of the large intestine (or colon), and sometimes into the lower part of the small intestine. (These structures are illustrated on page 25 of the body atlas.) The colonoscope is equipped with fiberoptic cables that enable a physician to visually inspect the lining of these organs for any evidence of disease or abnormality. In addition, instruments may be passed through the scope to obtain tissue biopsies or stool samples for microscopic examination.

• Colonoscopy is primarily performed in people with symptoms of a bowel abnormality (for example, blood in the stool, recent changes in bowel habits, or abdominal pain) when the cause is unclear or when the results of less invasive tests, such as sigmoidoscopy (see page 323) or barium enema (see page 104), are negative or inconclusive. It may also be done therapeutically to perform procedures such as polyp removal.

Purpose of the Test

• To detect and evaluate inflammatory or ulcerative bowel disease, polyps, tumors, bleeding, and other bowel abnormalities.

• To further evaluate tumors, ulcers, and narrowed passages (strictures) detected by a barium enema.

• To screen for colon cancer or precancerous polyps in people with a high risk of developing the disease, such as those with a strong family history of colorectal cancer or familial polyposis.

• To monitor patients who have been treated for colorectal cancer for recurrence.

• To monitor patients with inflammatory bowel disease for the development of colorectal cancer.

• Used therapeutically to remove polyps, stop active bleeding, dilate narrowed passages, or remove an obstruction.

Who Performs It

• A gastroenterologist.

Special Concerns

• Although colonoscopy may provoke some anxiety, the procedure usually causes only minor discomfort. You will receive a sedative medication before the test.

• You must wait at least a week after having a barium x-ray procedure before undergoing colonoscopy, since the presence of barium in the abdomen interferes with visual inspection of the colon.

• Colonoscopy should not be performed in people with a suspected colon perforation or

Results

▼

➡ During the visual inspection of the bowel, the doctor will note any abnormalities such as bleeding, inflammation, abnormal growths, or ulcers.

➡ Various laboratory tests may be necessary to pinpoint a diagnosis. For example, biopsied tumors and excised polyps are examined under a microscope by a pathologist for evidence of cancer or another abnormality. (For more on laboratory testing, see Chapter 1.)

➡ If no abnormality is found, your doctor will recommend a schedule of periodic follow-up exams to monitor your health.

➡ If a problem is diagnosed based on the findings of this test, appropriate medical or surgical treatment will be recommended.

Colonoscopy

an extremely dilated colon (megacolon), in women who are about to give birth, or in those who have had a recent heart attack or abdominal surgery.

• The procedure may not be possible in people with painful anorectal conditions such as fissures or hemorrhoids; diverticulitis (inflammation in the sacs of the colon); active bleeding in the bowel or rectum; or acute colon inflammation.

• Colonoscopy may be performed in a hospital or an outpatient setting.

Before the Test

• Inform your doctor if you regularly take non-steroidal anti-inflammatory drugs (such as aspirin, ibuprofen, or naproxen) or anticoagulants such as warfarin (Coumadin, Panwarfin). These medications must be discontinued for several days before the test to reduce the risk of bleeding.

• Cleansing your intestine before colonoscopy is essential to provide clear visibility during the procedure. Your doctor will give you specific instructions.

• Typically, you should consume only clear liquids (such as water, bouillon, or gelatin) for 24 to 48 hours before the scheduled procedure, and drink large amounts of water on the day before. Do not eat or drink anything after midnight on the day before the test.

• In addition, your doctor will prescribe an oral laxative agent to take on the day before the procedure. (Sometimes, instead of a laxative, the bowel cleansing is accomplished by drinking a gallon of nonabsorbable salty liquid—for example, GoLYTELY, Colyte, or NuLYTELY.)

• On the morning of the procedure, a cleansing enema may be administered at the testing facility.

• Immediately before the test, an intravenous (IV) needle or catheter is inserted into a vein in your arm. A mild sedative medication is usually administered, but you will remain conscious throughout the procedure (so-called conscious sedation).

What You Experience

• You lie on your side on a table, with your knees drawn to your chest, and you are draped to minimize any embarrassment.

• The doctor begins by inserting a gloved, lubricated finger into your rectum to perform a manual examination.

• Next, the lubricated scope is gently inserted through the anus and rectum and then into the colon.

• You may experience some abdominal cramping or feel the urge to defecate as the instrument is inserted and advanced. Breathe deeply and slowly through your mouth to relax your abdominal muscles and reduce this discomfort.

• In order to advance the scope through the deepest portion of the colon, the doctor or a nurse may help you to lie on your back. The doctor may palpate your abdomen or use fluoroscopy (see page 205) to help guide the passage of the scope.

• As the scope is slowly withdrawn, the doctor carefully inspects the lining of your colon, rectum, and anus, looking for any abnormalities.

• Small amounts of air will be instilled through the scope to dilate the intestinal passage for better viewing. This may cause you to feel bloated and to pass gas.

• Depending on the circumstances, a biopsy forceps or other instruments may be inserted through the scope to obtain tissue or stool specimens. Polyps may be entirely removed using an electrocautery device. (These procedures are painless, since the lining of the colon contains no pain receptors.) Tissue and fluid samples will be sent to a laboratory for analysis.

• The procedure time typically ranges from 30 to 60 minutes.

Risks and Complications

• Possible complications include bleeding, impaired respiration due to oversedation, and, rarely, perforation of the rectum or colon. Perforation requires surgery to repair the hole in the colon.

After the Test

• You will rest in a recovery room until the sedative wears off (usually about an hour). During this time, your vital signs will be checked periodically, and you will be observed for signs of complications.

• Arrange for someone to drive you home.

• You may experience flatulence or gas pains for several hours after the procedure.

• If a biopsy was performed, you may have a small amount of rectal bleeding for several hours.

• Rest in bed for the remainder of the day and drink only clear liquids and no alcohol for 24 hours.

• After 24 hours, you may resume your normal activities and any medications withheld before the test.

• Blood may collect and clot under the skin (hematoma) at the IV insertion site; this is harmless and will resolve on its own. For a large hematoma that causes swelling and discomfort, apply ice initially; after 24 hours, use warm, moist compresses to help dissolve the clotted blood.

• Contact your doctor immediately if you develop fever, chills, excessive rectal bleeding, or abdominal pain or distention.

Estimated Cost: $$$ to $$$$

Colonoscopy continued

Colposcopy and Cervical Punch Biopsy

Colposcopy and Cervical Punch Biopsy

Description

• In this test, a doctor uses a colposcope—a long, thin tube equipped with a magnifying lens and a light—to visually inspect the vagina and cervix (the bottom of the uterus that opens into the vagina) for abnormalities. (The female reproductive system is illustrated on page 28.) Photographs may be taken of any suspicious lesions. In some cases, the cervix may be biopsied to obtain tissue samples for microscopic examination; this procedure is called cervical punch biopsy. Colposcopy is most commonly performed to evaluate women who have had an abnormal Pap smear (see page 279).

Purpose of the Test

• To confirm the presence of precancerous conditions (such as cervical intraepithelial neoplasia, or CIN) or cervical cancer detected by a Pap smear.
• To evaluate suspicious vaginal or cervical lesions identified during a pelvic exam.
• To monitor women receiving conservative treatment for precancerous CIN.
• To monitor women at high risk for developing reproductive cancers, such as those whose mothers took diethylstilbestrol (DES) during pregnancy.

Who Performs It

• A gynecologist.

Special Concerns

• Punch biopsy should ideally be performed one week after your last menstrual period has ended, since menstrual blood can obscure the view of the cervix.
• In some cases, cervical punch biopsy may be performed without the aid of a colposcope. Instead, an applicator stick is used to apply iodine and stain the normal cervical tissue (but not abnormal tissue) to identify sites for biopsy.

Before the Test

• Do not apply any vaginal creams or medications for 24 hours prior to the procedure.
• Empty your bladder just before the test.
• You will be asked to undress from the waist down and put on a drape or hospital gown.

What You Experience

• You will lie on your back on an examining table with your knees bent and feet resting in stirrups.
• The doctor gently inserts a speculum—a metal or plastic instrument that pushes apart the walls of the vagina to provide a view of the cervix—into your vagina. The device may feel cold and uncomfortable, but causes no pain. Relax and breathe through your mouth to ease the insertion.
• A cotton swab, small brush, or wooden spatula may be inserted through the speculum to perform a Pap smear.

Results

▼

➥ During visual inspection of your vagina and cervix, the doctor will note any abnormalities.
➥ If a biopsy was obtained, a pathologist examines the tissues sample under a microscope for the presence of unusual cells. (For more on microscopic examination, see Chapter 1.)
➥ If a definitive diagnosis can be made, your doctor will recommend an appropriate course of medical or surgical treatment, depending on the specific problem.
➥ If results are unclear, more invasive tests, such as a cone biopsy of the cervix (see page 150), may be needed to confirm a diagnosis and determine the extent of the problem.

• The cervix is cleansed with a solution of acetic acid that removes excess mucus and helps highlight any abnormal areas.

• The colposcope is passed through the speculum and focused on the cervix. The doctor will note abnormal areas (with, for example, an unusual tissue color or blood vessel pattern). Photographs or sketches may be made of any abnormalities.

• If a biopsy is performed, a special scissors-like instrument (biopsy forceps) is inserted through the speculum or colposcope and used to snip tiny specimens from selected sites on the cervix. You may feel a brief pinching sensation as each sample is taken.

• Following a biopsy, the doctor may apply pressure or use special solutions or a cautery device to control any bleeding. If bleeding continues, the doctor may insert a tampon (you should leave it in place for 8 to 24 hours, according to your doctor's instructions).

• The procedure takes 10 to 15 minutes.

Risks and Complications

• Colposcopy alone is not associated with any risks or complications.

• Rare complications associated with cervical punch biopsy include excessive bleeding and infection.

After the Test

• You may return home (someone should accompany you home after a biopsy).

• If you had a biopsy, avoid strenuous activity for 8 to 24 hours. Your doctor will also instruct you to avoid sexual intercourse, douching, and tampons for several days to 1 week until the biopsy sites have healed.

• You may experience mild cramping after a biopsy. An over-the-counter pain reliever, such as ibuprofen, should provide some relief.

• Slight bleeding may also follow a biopsy. Use sanitary napkins rather than tampons. You may also develop a foul-smelling, gray-green vaginal discharge for several days.

• Inform your doctor if you experience heavy bleeding (more than during menstruation) or vaginal discharge that persists for more than 21 days.

Estimated Cost: $$

Colposcopy and Cervical Punch Biopsy continued

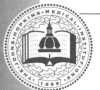

Complete Blood Count
(CBC)

Complete Blood Count *(sidebar)*

Description

• As blood continuously circulates through the body, it performs many vital functions—including carrying oxygen to and waste products from body tissues, helping to fight infection, and maintaining blood vessel integrity. Whole blood is made up of 2 major components: plasma (which is essentially water that contains hundreds of dissolved substances) and blood cells (which include red and white blood cells and platelets). A complete blood count (CBC) assesses the number and size of these different types of cells. The following tests are commonly included in a CBC, or in some cases may be performed alone:

• **Red blood cell (RBC) count** estimates the number of RBCs in the blood. The primary function of RBCs is to carry oxygen from the lungs to the body's tissues and to carry carbon dioxide (a waste product) from the tissues back to the lungs for elimination. A low RBC count indicates anemia, while a high count carries a risk that the RBCs will clump together and block capillaries.

• **Hemoglobin**—the iron-containing pigment that gives RBCs their red color—is a protein that enables the RBCs to transport oxygen and carbon dioxide. The total hemoglobin test estimates the amount of hemoglobin in the blood, and gives an idea of the blood's ability to carry oxygen. (Though not part of a CBC, a laboratory technique called electrophoresis [see page 31] may be used to detect the presence of abnormal hemoglobins, which often do not work as well as normal ones.)

• **Hematocrit**—which assesses the amount of space (volume) RBCs take up in the blood—is determined by measuring the volume of RBCs after a blood sample is spun in a centrifuge. (Values are given as a percentage of the blood that is red cells.)

• **Red blood cell indices** incorporate the results of the RBC count, hemoglobin, and hematocrit tests to provide further information about the size, hemoglobin concentration, and hemoglobin content of an average RBC. These values help to categorize different types of anemia.

• **Reticulocyte count** measures the number of newly formed RBCs, or reticulocytes, in the blood and gives an idea of RBC production by the bone marrow. (This value is expressed as a percentage of the total RBC count.) This test helps to distinguish between different types of anemias, or to monitor treatment for anemia.

• **White blood cell (WBC) count** estimates the number of WBCs in the blood. These cells—which fight infection and promote wound healing—are drawn to sites of infection and inflammation, where they engulf and digest invaders such as bacteria and other microorganisms or foreign bodies. This test may be done alone to detect the presence of an infec-

Results
▼

➡ Your blood sample is sent to a laboratory for analysis. The doctor will review the results—and consider them along with your symptoms, your physical exam, and the results of other tests—for evidence of a blood disorder or another problem. (For more on blood tests, see Chapter 1.)

➡ A CBC is often used as an initial test to indicate potential health problems. Abnormal results may necessitate additional tests, such as a bone marrow aspiration and biopsy (see page 117), to establish a definitive diagnosis.

➡ If an abnormality is found and the doctor can make a definitive diagnosis, appropriate treatment will begin.

tion (values may rise dramatically) or to monitor response to cancer treatment.

• **White blood cell differential** measures the proportion of the various types of WBCs in the blood as well as their structure. (There are five different kinds of WBCs that respond in varying degrees to the presence of infection or inflammation.) This test helps to determine the severity of an infection, suggests the type of organism responsible, and also provides important information about the immune system.

• **Platelet count** is an estimate of the number of platelets in the blood. Platelets, or thrombocytes, are blood cells that clump together, or aggregate, at sites of blood vessel injury and work together with various clotting factors to promote the formation of blood clots. This process, called coagulation, is essential to stop bleeding and repair tissue injuries. (For more information, see page 157.)

• **Blood smear** is a test that involves spreading blood on a slide which is then stained with a special dye and examined under a microscope. This test can provide additional diagnostic information to a CBC by identifying changes in cell color, size, and shape and the type of cells in circulation, as well as the presence of cell inclusions. For example, sickle cell anemia can be detected by the presence of characteristic unusually shaped red cells, and leukemia by the presence of very immature white cells (blast cells) in the blood.

Purpose of the Test

• Used as a general screening test to provide information about the state of a person's health, for example, before a scheduled surgery.

• To detect or evaluate blood cell disorders, such as anemia (an abnormal decrease in RBCs), polycythemia (an excess of RBCs), leukopenia (an abnormal decrease in WBCs), leukemia (a type of cancer that affects the WBCs), and thrombocytopenia (a decrease in blood platelets).

• To monitor drug therapy and drug toxicity.

Who Performs It

• A nurse or a technician will draw the blood sample.

Special Concerns

• None.

Before the Test

• Certain medications may alter CBC test values. Inform your doctor of any medications you regularly take. You may be asked to discontinue certain of these agents before the test.

What You Experience

• A sample of your blood is drawn from a vein in your arm and sent to a laboratory for analysis. (For more on this procedure, called venipuncture, see page 32.)

Risks and Complications

• None.

After the Test

• Immediately after blood is drawn, pressure is applied (with cotton or gauze) to the puncture site.

• Resume your normal activities and any medications withheld before the test.

• Blood may collect and clot under the skin (hematoma) at the puncture site; this is harmless and will resolve on its own. For a large hematoma that causes swelling and discomfort, apply ice initially; after 24 hours, use warm, moist compresses to help dissolve the clotted blood.

Estimated Cost: $

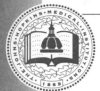
Cultures and Microscopic Exams for Infectious Disease

Description

• Infectious diseases are caused by tiny microorganisms such as bacteria, viruses, fungi, and parasites. To help identify the organism responsible for infection, doctors usually obtain samples of body fluid or tissue for laboratory analysis. Depending on the suspected infection, any fluid in the body—including blood, urine, sputum, cerebrospinal fluid, and genital secretions—may be examined, as well as stool or tissue biopsies. Microscopic examination and cultures are two of the primary methods used to help diagnose infectious diseases; the other, antigen/antibody testing, is discussed on page 91.

• **Microscopic examination** can provide a preliminary, tentative identification of certain infectious agents by revealing their size, shape, and cellular structure. The Gram stain test—in which a sample is smeared on a microscopic slide and stained with a special dye—is used to classify all bacteria as either gram positive (blue staining) or gram negative (red staining). The presence of specific inflammatory cells may also provide clues about the type of infection. The acid-fast smear involves spreading a sample on a slide, dyeing it, and treating it with an acid-alcohol solution to identify acid-fast bacteria (which will not be decolorized by the acid-alcohol). This test is often used to examine sputum and support a diagnosis of tuberculosis, or TB (since cultures for TB may take up to 2 months to grow). In addition, microscopic exams are necessary to identify parasites and their eggs.

• **Cultures** generally take longer to perform than microscopic exams—from a day to several weeks—but are necessary to identify the organism with certainty and provide a definitive diagnosis. This technique involves placing a specimen in an environment, or medium, that is designed to promote the growth of specific organisms. (The medium is typically a jelly-like substance that contain nutrients to encourage the organisms to reproduce.) Cultures can be used to screen for a wide variety of bacteria, or can be focused to look for specific agents. In some cases, various antimicrobial drugs (such as antibiotics) are then added to a culture to determine which treatment is most effective for killing the offending organism; this is known as drug sensitivity testing.

Purpose of the Test

• To identify the microorganism causing an infection and, in some cases, to help determine the best course of treatment.

• The acid-fast bacilli test may be done to monitor treatment for tuberculosis.

Who Performs It

• Varies according to what type of tissue or fluid sample is required.

Special Concerns

• Several rapid diagnostic tests have recently been developed to detect the influenza virus, or "the flu," within 30 minutes (viral culture for the flu usually takes days). These tests are

Results

▼

➡ The sample is sent to a microbiology or bacteriology laboratory for microscopic examination and/or culturing. (For more on laboratory tests, see Chapter 1.)

➡ In many cases, your doctor will issue a preliminary diagnosis and prescribe a treatment based on your history, symptoms, physical exam, and the results of any initial microscopic studies. Once the final results of a culture and/or drug sensitivity test are in, treatment may be refined accordingly.

increasingly being used to identify the flu early, and thus reduce unnecessary use of antibiotics (which are only effective for bacterial infections) and help to determine if antiviral treatment should be prescribed.

• Many sexually transmitted diseases, such as Chlamydia and gonorrhea, are now diagnosed by DNA probe—a test that is positive if DNA from the particular bacterium is present—which requires only a urine sample.

• Recent antimicrobial therapy, for example, with antibiotic drugs, can interfere with the accuracy of this test.

Before the Test

• Preparation varies according to what type of tissue or fluid sample is required. Your doctor will provide specific instructions.

What You Experience

• A sample of body fluid, tissue, cells, or stool is obtained and sent to a laboratory for analysis. A variety of procedures may be used, depending on what type of sample is needed. These techniques vary from noninvasive—such as collecting fluid with a swab (as with a throat culture)—to more invasive means involving significant risks, such as tissue biopsy (see page 38), bronchoscopy (see page 134), bone marrow aspiration (see page 117), or lumbar puncture (see page 243).

Risks and Complications

• Possible risks vary according to what type of tissue or fluid sample is required.

After the Test

• Post-test care varies according to what type of tissue or fluid sample is required.

Estimated Cost: $

Cultures and Microscopic Exams for Infectious Disease continued

Cystography

(Voiding Cystourethrography)

Description

• In this imaging test, the bladder is filled with a contrast dye to highlight this organ on x-rays or fluoroscopic films. In some cases, additional films are obtained as you urinate to reveal any abnormalities of the urethra or urinary dysfunction (a procedure called voiding cystourethrography, or VCUG). The recorded images are then examined for abnormalities. (For more on contrast x-rays and fluoroscopy, see Chapter 2.)

• A similar procedure, called urethrography, involves instilling contrast dye into the urethra but not as far as the bladder. Used almost exclusively in males, this test helps to diagnose structural problems in the urethra, such as obstructions.

Purpose of the Test

• Cystography is used to detect structural abnormalities of the bladder such as tumors; traumatic injury; or abnormal pouches or protrusions (diverticula).

• VCUG can identify abnormalities of the bladder and urethra, as well as urinary dysfunction, such as backward flow (reflux) of urine from the bladder to the kidneys.

Who Performs It

• A radiologist and a technician.

Special Concerns

• Pregnant women should not undergo this test because exposure to ionizing radiation may harm the fetus.

• This test is not appropriate in people with acute bladder or urethral infection.

• During this test, men will wear a lead shield over the testes to shield against excess radiation. However, in women it is not possible to shield the ovaries without blocking the view of the bladder.

• People with allergies to iodine or shellfish may experience an allergic reaction to iodine-based contrast dyes, but this is rare.

• Results may not be accurate if you have had other recent x-rays using a contrast dye or if there is feces or gas in the bowels.

• Embarrassment may prevent some individuals from urinating during VCUG.

Before the Test

• Inform your doctor if you have a known allergy to iodine or shellfish.

• The morning of the test, you should drink only clear liquids for breakfast.

• At the testing facility, you will be asked to disrobe and put on a hospital gown.

What You Experience

• You will lie on your back on an x-ray table. You may be given a sedative, if necessary.

• A thin, soft tube, called a Foley catheter, is inserted through the urethra and into the bladder. You may feel some discomfort during catheter insertion.

• The examiner instills a contrast dye solution through the catheter until your bladder feels full, and then clamps the catheter closed. You

Results

➥ A radiologist (and possibly a urologist) will examine the images for evidence of any abnormality.

➥ If a definitive diagnosis can be made, appropriate treatment will be initiated.

➥ In some cases, additional urologic tests, such as cystoscopy (see page 170) or ultrasound of the kidneys (see page 80), may be needed to establish a diagnosis and determine the extent of the problem.

may experience a sensation of fullness and the urge to urinate.

• A series of x-rays or fluoroscopic films is obtained. You will be asked to assume a variety of positions as they are taken.

• If a VCUG is being done, the catheter is removed and you are asked to urinate (if you cannot do so while lying down, you may stand up). During urination, additional films are taken of the bladder and urethra.

• In rare cases, a small amount of air may be insufflated through the catheter into the bladder after the dye is eliminated, and more images are obtained (this is called the double-contrast technique).

• This test takes 30 to 45 minutes.

Risks and Complications

• X-ray exams involve minimal exposure to radiation. Although radiation exposure is still small with fluoroscopy, you receive a higher dose than during standard x-ray procedures.

• Some patients may develop a bladder infection after this procedure.

• Rarely, some people may experience an allergic reaction to the iodine-based contrast dye, which can cause symptoms such as nausea, sneezing, vomiting, hives, and occasionally a life-threatening response called anaphylactic shock. Emergency medications and equipment are kept readily available.

After the Test

• You may experience some burning as you urinate the first few times after the test. Drink plenty of fluids to help flush the dye from your bladder and reduce this sensation, and to prevent any accumulation of bacteria.

• You may return home and resume your usual activities.

• Contact your doctor if you develop lower abdominal pain or a fever.

Estimated Cost: $$

Cystography continued

Cystoscopy

Description

• In this test, a flexible or rigid viewing tube (cystoscope) is passed through the urethra and into the bladder (illustrated on page 26). Fiberoptic cables permit a physician to visually inspect these structures. In addition, various instruments may be passed through the scope to obtain fluid or tissue samples for laboratory examination, and to perform diagnostic or therapeutic procedures. This test is often performed on people with urinary symptoms such as bloody urine, frequency, urgency, incontinence, or urinary retention.

Purpose of the Test

• To detect abnormalities of the urethra and bladder, including inflammation, tumors, stones, or narrowed passages.
• To help determine the cause of urinary dysfunction or recurrent urinary tract infections.
• To obtain fluid or tissue samples from the lower urinary tract.
• To perform therapeutic measures, such as removal of stones; placement of a catheter or stents to drain the ureters; or transurethral resection of the prostate (TURP), a treatment that removes excess tissue from the inner portion of the prostate in men with prostate enlargement (known as benign prostatic hyperplasia or BPH).

Who Performs It

• A physician, usually a urinary tract specialist (urologist).

Special Concerns

• If cystoscopy is being performed for diagnostic purposes, it can usually be done under local anesthesia. However, general or spinal anesthesia will be administered if a bladder or tissue biopsy is required or if therapeutic measures (such as TURP or the removal of stones) are planned.

• The procedure should be postponed if you currently have a urinary tract infection.

Before the Test

• If general or spinal anesthesia is required, do not eat or drink anything after midnight on the day before the procedure. No fasting is required before local anesthesia.
• Drink plenty of fluids on the night before the procedure.
• At the testing facility, you will be asked to disrobe and put on a hospital gown.
• An intravenous (IV) needle or catheter may be inserted into a vein in your arm immediately before the procedure begins and any medications, such as a sedative or general anesthesia, are administered.
• If spinal anesthesia is used, the medication is injected into your lower spinal column to numb the lower half of your body. You will remain conscious throughout the procedure.

Results

▼

➥ During the visual inspection of your urinary tract, the doctor will note any abnormalities.

➥ If tissue or fluid samples were taken, specimen containers may be sent to several different laboratories for analysis. For example, biopsied tissue may be inspected under a microscope for the presence of unusual cells, or urine may be cultured (see page 166) for infectious organisms. (For more on laboratory tests, see Chapter 1.)

➥ This test usually results in a definitive diagnosis. Your doctor will recommend appropriate medical or surgical treatment, depending on the specific problem.

• If general anesthesia is being used, a thin tube attached to a breathing machine will be inserted through your mouth and into your windpipe to help you breathe.

What You Experience

• You will lie on your back with your knees bent, legs spread apart, and feet resting in stirrups. Lie very still throughout the procedure to prevent trauma to the urinary tract.

• If applicable, a local anesthetic jelly is instilled into your urethra to numb it.

• The cystoscope is gently inserted into the urethra and passed into the bladder. Fluid is infused through the scope to fill the bladder. This will create an urge to urinate, but this step is necessary to stretch the bladder walls and provide the doctor with a better view of the area.

• If appropriate, a biopsy sample or urine specimen is taken and sent to a laboratory for analysis, or therapeutic procedures are performed.

• The cystoscope is slowly withdrawn.

• The procedure usually takes about 25 to 30 minutes.

Risks and Complications

• If general anesthesia is necessary, the procedure carries the associated risks.

• Rare complications include infection, urinary retention (inability to void due to swelling), and inadvertent perforation of the bladder.

After the Test

• Do not attempt to walk or stand alone directly after the procedure. Dizziness or fainting may occur.

• If a local anesthesia was used, you are free to leave after the test. After general or spinal anesthesia, you will remain in the hospital until you recover from the effects of the anesthetic. During this time, your vital signs will be monitored, and you will be observed for any signs of complications.

• Drink plenty of fluids (but no alcohol) to prevent accumulation of bacteria in your bladder and to reduce the slight burning sensation that may occur during urination (which may persist for 1 or 2 days).

• You may be given an antibiotic to reduce the risk of infection.

• It is common to have a temporary pink tinge to your urine at first. However, if bright red blood or blood clots are present, notify your doctor.

• Call your doctor immediately if you experience pain in your back, stomach, or side, urinary difficulties, chills, or fever.

Estimated Cost: $$

Cystoscopy continued

Doppler Studies of the Extremities
(Segmental Limb Pressures)

Description

• This test uses a technique called Doppler ultrasound to evaluate blood circulation in the major arteries in the arms or legs. A device called a transducer is passed lightly over different areas of your limbs, directing high-frequency sound waves (ultrasound) at particular arteries. The sound waves are reflected back at frequencies that correspond to the velocity of blood flow, and are converted into audible sounds and graphic recordings.

• **Duplex scanning** combines Doppler ultrasound with real-time ultrasound imaging of the arteries, allowing calculation of the percent of narrowing in the vessels. Images are displayed on a viewing monitor and may also be recorded on film or video for later examination. (For more on Doppler and duplex ultrasound, see Chapter 2.)

• **Segmental limb pressures** are measured by combining Doppler ultrasound with blood pressure measurements at various locations in the arms and legs. By detecting differences in blood pressure at specific locations in different limbs, this test helps to diagnose arterial blockages and other circulation problems. It is most commonly performed in people suspected of having peripheral arterial disease (PAD)—narrowing of arteries in the legs due to the accumulation of plaques (atherosclerosis) that is characterized by leg pain upon exercise.

• **The ankle-brachial index (ABI),** which is determined by recording segmental limb pressures, is the most useful initial test to identify PAD. The ABI is calculated by dividing the systolic blood pressure (that is, the pressure as the heart contracts) in the ankle by the systolic pressure in the brachial artery in the arm. Normally, the ankle pressure should be slightly higher, resulting in an ABI of 1.0 or greater. PAD is indicated if the ABI is less than 1.0; the lower the ABI, the more severe the disease. ABI measurements are usually taken at rest and after a designated amount of exercise on a treadmill.

Purpose of the Test

• To evaluate arterial blood flow in the arms or legs and detect blockages, trauma, or other circulation problems.

• To aid in the diagnosis of PAD, determine the location and extent of any arterial blockages, and (with the treadmill test) determine the severity of functional impairment due to PAD.

• To monitor the progression of known PAD and evaluate the effectiveness of treatments such as arterial bypass grafts in the legs.

• To detect and evaluate possible arterial trauma.

Who Performs It

• A nurse or a technician who is trained in ultrasound.

Results

➡ A physician reviews the ultrasound images, ABI and exercise ABI, and other test data for evidence of any abnormality. If an arterial blockage is indicated, comparing blood pressures at various locations in the leg can help to determine where it is located.

➡ In some cases, additional tests, such as arteriography (see page 95) or magnetic resonance angiography (see page 253), are required to further evaluate abnormal findings and determine an appropriate course of treatment.

➡ If no further tests are warranted, your doctor will recommend an appropriate schedule of follow-up exams and/or treatment.

Special Concerns

• Blood pressure readings in the thigh may not be possible in obese patients, since a standard cuff may not be large enough to fit.

• Individuals who have extremely rigid (or calcified) arteries may show falsely elevated ankle pressures. This is most common in people with diabetes, but may also be found in people on long-term corticosteroid therapy, kidney dialysis patients, and kidney transplant recipients. To obtain more accurate results, the ABI should be calculated using pressures from the foot or toes instead of the ankle in these patients.

• Arterial plethysmography (see page 296) is sometimes performed concurrently with this test.

Before the Test

• Avoid cigarette smoking for at least 30 minutes before the test, since smoking constricts the peripheral arteries and can interfere with the accuracy of the results.

• You will be asked to remove any clothes covering your legs and arms. You may wear shorts and a short-sleeved shirt or a hospital gown during the test.

• You may be asked to rest for about 20 minutes prior to the test.

What You Experience
Duplex scanning:

• You will lie down on a table or bed.

• A small amount of water-soluble gel is applied to the skin on the areas being examined to enhance sound wave transmission.

• The examiner movers the transducer back and forth over the selected limbs to obtain different views of the artery or arteries being examined.

• Once clear images are obtained, they are recorded on film or video for later analysis.

• The test usually takes 20 to 30 minutes.

Segmental limb pressures with ABI index:

• You will lie on either a bed or table with your arms at your sides.

• Blood pressure cuffs are wrapped above the elbow on both arms. The cuffs are inflated, and blood pressure is measured in the brachial artery on both sides. (The higher of the 2 pressures is used to calculate your ABI.)

• To examine segmental pressures in the legs, cuffs are then placed at various points—typically, at the thigh, calf, ankle, foot, and toe level. If the arms are being tested, cuffs are placed on the upper arms, forearm, and sometimes the hand or fingers.

• A small amount of water-soluble gel is applied to various areas of skin on the limb being examined to enhance sound wave transmission.

• Each cuff is inflated in turn and blood pressures are measured at each site on the limb. This is done with the aid of a ultrasound transducer that is held against the skin.

• This procedure is repeated in the other leg or arm.

• To determine your exercise ABI, you will be asked to walk on a treadmill for a few minutes (your doctor will specify the treadmill setting and time period). Your ankle pressure is measured before and after the exercise.

• The test usually takes 30 to 45 minutes.

Risks and Complications

• Ultrasound is painless, noninvasive, and involves no exposure to radiation. There are no associated risks.

After the Test

• The examiner removes the conductive gel from your skin.

• You are free to leave the testing facility and resume your normal activities.

Estimated Cost: $$

Doppler Studies of the Extremities continued

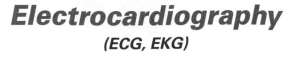

Electrocardiography
(ECG, EKG)

Electrocardiography

Description
• Small metal sensors (electrodes or leads) are applied to the skin to record the electrical current generated by the heart with every contraction. The leads transmit this information to a machine that provides a graphic representation of the heart's electrical activity.

Purpose of the Test
• To detect heart problems, including a recent or ongoing heart attack, abnormal heart rhythms (arrhythmias), coronary artery blockage, areas of damaged heart muscle (as from a prior heart attack), enlargement of the heart muscle, and inflammation of the sac surrounding the heart (pericarditis).
• To detect noncardiac conditions such as electrolyte imbalances and lung diseases.
• To monitor recovery from a heart attack, progression of heart disease, or the effectiveness of certain heart medications or a pacemaker.
• To rule out hidden heart disease in patients about to undergo surgery.

Who Performs It
• A doctor, a nurse, or a technician.

Special Concerns
• Patients at high risk for dangerous arrhythmias may undergo a special ECG procedure called signal-averaged electrocardiography, in which the ECG is performed for 15 to 20 minutes and results over this period are averaged.

Before the Test
• Tell your doctor if you take any heart medications, which may affect the results.

What You Experience
• You will disrobe and lie down on a table.
• ECG leads are attached to your chest, arms, and legs. A special gel may be applied to these areas to allow for better electrical conduction.

• The electrical impulses generated by your heart are transmitted through the leads to the ECG machine, which prints them as a series of waves (tracings) on a strip of paper. For the most accurate results, remain still, relaxed, and silent.
• The test usually takes 5 to 10 minutes.

Risks and Complications
• None.

After the Test
• The leads are removed and any electrode gel is wiped away with a damp cloth.

Estimated Cost: $

Results
▼

➡ Results are determined by a doctor who examines the ECG tracings for abnormalities; sometimes a computer is used to help interpret the findings. (In some cases, ECG results may be transmitted over telephone lines to be evaluated at a diagnostic center or clinic.)
➡ If the ECG indicates an abnormality, additional tests—such as Holter monitoring (see page 221), echocardiography (see page 367), or electrophysiology studies (see page 182)—may be needed to establish a diagnosis.
➡ If the ECG reveals an ongoing heart attack, treatment to stabilize your condition is begun immediately.
➡ If results are normal, no further testing is usually needed. However, a normal resting ECG does not eliminate the possibility of heart disease. Further tests may still be needed.

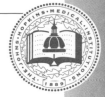

Electroencephalography
(EEG, Electroencephalogram)

Description

• Small metal sensors (electrodes) are applied to your scalp to record the electrical signals produced by nerve cells in the brain. The electrodes transmit this information to a machine that magnifies the electrical activity and provides a graphic representation of brain waves. This test is usually done while you are awake, but in one variation (called a sleep EEG), you must stay awake the night beforehand, and brain activity is then recorded after you are given a sedative to help you sleep. Another test, called polysomnography (see page 337), measures EEG activity and other body functions, such as breathing and heart rate, during one full night of sleep.

Purpose of the Test

• To identify and evaluate the cause of seizures.
• To aid in the diagnosis of intracranial (within the skull) lesions, such as an abscess or tumor.
• To evaluate brain wave activity in people with brain or spinal cord infections (such as meningitis or encephalitis); head injury; and psychiatric conditions.
• To diagnose a stroke and determine the extent of damage that has occurred.
• To monitor brain wave activity during surgery.
• To help evaluate sleep disorders.
• To diagnose a coma.
• To confirm brain death.

Who Performs It

• A doctor, a nurse, or a technician who is trained in EEG.

Special Concerns

• This test is usually conducted in a special room designed to eliminate electrical interference and minimize distractions.
• A variety of medications (including sedatives, anticonvulsants, tranquilizers, and barbiturates), caffeinated beverages, failure to eat before the test, or the presence of bright or flashing lights may alter the results of the test.
• You must remain still during the test. Any excess movement can interfere with the accuracy of results.

Before the Test

• Inform your doctor of any medications you regularly take. Certain of these agents may need to be discontinued for 1 or 2 days before the test.
• Wash your hair the night before the test, and do not use hair spray, gel, or other hair care products after shampooing.
• Be sure to eat a normal meal before the test, since low blood sugar (hypoglycemia) may interfere with test results. However, you should avoid caffeine-containing beverages, such as coffee, tea, or cola, on the morning of the test day.

Results

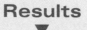

➥ A neurologist will evaluate your brain wave patterns for evidence of any abnormality. For example, seizure activity is indicated by rapid, spiking waves, while cerebral lesions such as tumors or blood clots will result in abnormally slow EEG waves. The presence of an inflammatory brain disease, such as meningitis or encephalitis, may cause diffuse and slow brain waves.

➥ If a definitive diagnosis can be made, appropriate therapy will be initiated.

➥ In most cases, additional imaging tests of the brain—such as a CT scan (see page 121), an MRI (see page 119), or a nuclear scan (see page 123)—are necessary to pinpoint the location of any abnormality.

Electroencephalography

Electroencephalography continued

• You are asked to stay up as late as possible on the night before a sleep EEG.

What You Experience

• You will either sit in a reclining chair or lie down on a bed.

• For most studies, 18 electrodes are attached to your scalp with a special adhesive paste or gel in a specified pattern, plus 1 on each earlobe and 1 on the forehead. (Less commonly, electrodes with tiny needles are placed in the skin of the scalp. These may cause a pricking sensation during insertion.)

• You are asked to relax, close your eyes, and lie still as the EEG recording is being taken. The examiner will note any movements, such as blinking, swallowing, or talking, that may affect the test results.

• Periodically, the examiner will stop the procedure to allow you to reposition yourself and get comfortable. Fatigue and restlessness can alter brain wave patterns.

• You may be asked to breathe deeply and rapidly (hyperventilate) for 3 minutes to stimulate hidden brain wave abnormalities not evident during the resting EEG.

• "Photostimulation" may also be conducted by flashing a light at variable speeds over your face when your eyes are open or closed. This is intended to produce abnormal activity present in seizures that are stimulated by light.

• If you are undergoing a sleep EEG, you are given a sedative medication and brain wave activity is measured as you fall asleep, while you are asleep, and as you wake.

• The procedure typically takes 45 minutes to 2 hours.

Risks and Complications

• EEG is a safe procedure. However, people who are susceptible to seizures may have one during the test.

After the Test

• The electrodes are removed and the adhesive paste is washed away with acetone. You may need to use acetone and wash your hair at home to remove any residue.

• Unless you are actively having seizures or you underwent a sleep EEG, you may drive home immediately. If you've had a sleep EEG, you will be observed until the sedative wears off, and someone should drive you home.

• Resume taking any medications withheld before the test, according to your doctor's instructions.

Estimated Cost: $$$

Electromyography
(EMG)

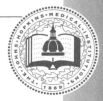

Description
• Small needle sensors (electrodes) are used to record the electrical activity in selected muscles during rest and as they contract during movement. The electrodes transmit this information to a machine that provides a graphic representation of the muscles' electrical discharge; the resulting data show how well the muscles work. Electroneurography (see page 180), which evaluates the function of nerves in a similar manner, is often performed at the same time as EMG in order to fully evaluate people experiencing weakness or paralysis.

Purpose of the Test
• To aid in the diagnosis of primary muscle disorders, such as muscular dystrophy; degenerative nerve diseases such as amyotrophic lateral sclerosis (Lou Gehrig's disease); and neuromuscular diseases (which affect both nerves and muscles), such as myasthenia gravis.

Who Performs It
• A doctor, a physical therapist, or a trained technician.

Special Concerns
• People with a widespread skin infection should not take this test because the infection may pass into the muscle via the needle electrodes.
• Because the needles may cause intramuscular bleeding, people with bleeding disorders or those who take anticoagulants should not undergo this procedure.
• Obesity or edema (swelling) may make it difficult to insert the electrodes into the muscle.
• A variety of medications may interfere with the results of this test.

Before the Test
• Tell your doctor if you regularly take any medications, herbs, or supplements—particularly anticoagulants, nonsteroidal anti-inflammatory drugs (such as aspirin, ibuprofen, or naproxen), muscle relaxants, and anticholinergic medications. You will be instructed to discontinue certain agents before the test.
• Fasting is not usually required. However, your doctor may ask you to refrain from smoking or drinking caffeinated beverages for 2 to 3 hours prior to the test.
• Wear loose clothing that permits access to the muscle being studied. In some cases, you may be instructed to undress and put on a hospital gown.

What You Experience
• You will either lie down on a bed or sit in a chair, depending on which muscles are being tested. A metal plate is placed underneath you to serve as a reference electrode.
• The skin over the selected muscle is cleansed with an antiseptic and a small needle electrode—which is very thin and resembles a stick pin—is inserted into the muscle. A refer-

Results
▼
➡ The function of your muscles is indicated by the strength and pattern of their electrical activity. Normally, there is no electrical activity in a muscle at rest. If a muscle disease is present, there may be electrical activity in the rested state and abnormal activity when the muscle contracts.
➡ Your doctor will consider the test results—as well as your symptoms, your physical exam, and the results of other tests—in order to diagnose any muscle disease and identify the muscles affected.
➡ If a definitive diagnosis can be made, appropriate therapy will be initiated.

Electromyography

ence electrode is inserted under the skin nearby. You may experience some discomfort due to the needles.

• The electrodes record the electrical activity while the muscle is relaxed. You will then be asked to contract the muscle gradually, with increasing forcefulness. The impulses are transmitted to a machine that amplifies the signals and displays them. Sometimes the signals are converted into audio and played through a speaker.

• The procedure may be repeated at other locations.

• EMG generally takes about 30 to 60 minutes.

Risks and Complications

• Rarely, blood may collect and clot under the skin (hematoma) at the needle insertion sites, causing swelling and discoloration. This is harmless but may cause some discomfort.

After the Test

• You may be given pain-relieving medication to allay any soreness around the electrode insertion sites.

• Resume your normal activities and any medications withheld before the test.

• If a large hematoma develops at the needle insertion sites, apply ice initially; after 24 hours, use warm, moist compresses to help dissolve the clotted blood.

Estimated Cost: $$

Electron-Beam CT Scan

(Ultrafast Computed Tomography)

Description

• A focused beam of electrons is used to generate x-rays of the heart. This relatively new imaging technique works so quickly that it captures images of the heart between beats, avoiding the distortion associated with conventional CT scanning, and can detect calcium deposits associated with atherosclerosis (the buildup of plaques) in the coronary arteries. (For more on CT scans, see Chapter 2.)

Purpose of the Test

• To detect coronary artery disease (CAD) in its early stages in people at moderate risk.
• To help determine whether lipid-lowering drugs are necessary in patients with a high cholesterol level but no other risk factors for heart disease.
• To assess the effectiveness of treatment with lipid-lowering medications.
• To help determine the cause of chest pain in emergency room patients with no history of CAD and normal initial test results.

Who Performs It

• A radiologist or a qualified technician.

Special Concerns

• People who experience claustrophobia may have difficulty undergoing a CT scan, which takes place in a narrow, tunnel-like structure.
• This test may not be possible for severely overweight individuals (over 300 lbs).
• Pregnant women should not undergo this test because exposure to ionizing radiation may harm the fetus.

Before the Test

• Tell your doctor if you suffer from claustrophobia. He or she may prescribe a sedative that can help you tolerate the procedure.
• Remove any jewelry or other metallic objects that may interfere with clear x-ray images.

What You Experience

• You are asked to lie on your back with your arms above your head on a narrow examining table that slides into the center of the CT scanner.
• Remain as motionless as possible while the scanner takes multiple x-ray images of your heart. You will be asked to hold your breath during a portion of the scan.
• The procedure takes about 5 to 8 minutes.

Risks and Complications

• There are no risks associated with the low levels of radiation from a CT scan.

After the Test

• Most patients can go home promptly after the scan.
• Sedated patients may be monitored for a short period until the effects of the sedative have worn off.

Estimated Cost: $$$

Results

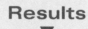

➡ A physician examines the scans for evidence of calcium deposits in the coronary arteries (seen as white specks on the x-rays). Detection of calcium indicates a high probability of CAD.

➡ If CAD is diagnosed, treatment will begin with diet, exercise, and/or medication.

➡ In some cases, additional tests, such as a cardiac stress test (see page 147), may be required to establish a diagnosis and determine the extent of the problem.

Electron-Beam CT Scan

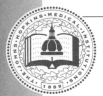

Electroneurography

(ENG, Nerve Conduction Studies)

Description

• Electroneurography (ENG) measures the conduction of electrical signals along nerve pathways in the body. (For more on the nervous system, see page 16 of the body atlas.) To perform the test, small, patch-like sensors (electrodes) are applied to the skin at specific locations to measure the electrical activity of particular peripheral nerves—that is, nerves outside of the brain and spinal cord. By stimulating a nerve at one site and then recording the time it takes for the nerve impulse to travel to a second point, this test is able to measure the velocity of nerve conduction. The detection of slowed conduction velocity with ENG indicates possible nerve disease or trauma.

• This test is typically performed in conjunction with electromyography, or EMG (see page 177)—which measures the electrical activity of muscles—in order to fully evaluate people who are experiencing weakness or paralysis. This combined procedure may be called electromyoneurography.

Purpose of the Test

• To identify peripheral nerve damage or destruction and establish the precise location of the problem.

• To differentiate peripheral nerve disease from muscular injury.

Who Performs It

• A doctor or a technician.

Special Concerns

• Because this test reflects the condition of the best surviving nerve fibers, normal values for ENG may be obtained if only a few fibers remain intact. For this reason, the test results may sometimes be normal despite the presence of extensive nerve damage.

Before the Test

• Be sure to wear loose-fitting clothes on the day of the procedure so that it will be easy to expose the relevant nerves and muscles during the test.

• Do not use any hand cream or lotion to ensure that the test electrodes will adhere properly to your skin.

What You Experience

• A special electrical paste is applied to the skin overlying the particular muscle or muscle group that is served by the nerve being evaluated.

Results

▼

➥ The nerve conduction velocity is calculated based on the distance between the stimulating and recording electrodes and the time elapsed between the nerve impulse and the resulting muscle contraction. The strength, or amplitude, of the nerve signal is also measured.

➥ Your doctor will evaluate the results for evidence of peripheral nerve disease. Since normal values vary in different nerves and from person to person, your symptoms and physical exam and the results of other tests will also be considered in order to make an accurate diagnosis.

➥ If a definitive diagnosis can be made, appropriate therapy will be initiated.

➥ Additional laboratory tests may be needed to identify the underlying cause of any nerve damage—for example, diabetes or hypothyroidism.

• Several electrodes are then placed on your skin—one that will stimulate a particular nerve with an electrical impulse, and the others to record the muscle response to this stimulus.

• A very mild electrical shock is delivered to the stimulating electrode, causing the muscles under the recording electrodes to contract. The shock is so small that most people cannot perceive it.

• The response of the muscle to this stimulus is recorded by the other electrodes.

• This process is repeated at other locations to test different nerves.

• This test takes approximately 15 minutes to perform.

Risks and Complications

• There are no significant risks or complications associated with this procedure.

After the Test

• The examiner will remove the electrode gel from your skin.

• You are free to leave the testing facility and resume your normal activities.

Estimated Cost: $$$ to $$$$

Electroneurography continued

Electrophysiology Studies
(EPS)

Description

• This test evaluates the electrical conduction system of the heart, which controls the rate and timing of the heart's contractions. A catheter with an electrode tip is inserted into a vein in the groin and threaded to the heart. The electrode records the heart's electrical activity, and is then used to send pacing signals to the heart in an attempt to produce abnormal heart rhythms (arrhythmias) and thus pinpoint their origin. EPS is sometimes combined with a treatment called radiofrequency ablation, in which radiofrequency energy is used to obliterate small areas of the heart that induce arrhythmias.

Purpose of the Test

• To localize the source of cardiac arrhythmias and other defects in the heart's electrical system.
• To assess the effectiveness of various antiarrhythmic drugs or monitor antiarrhythmic drug therapy.
• To evaluate the potential effectiveness of a pacemaker or automatic implantable cardioverter-defibrillator (another type of implanted pacing device).

Who Performs It

• A cardiologist specializing in EPS, assisted by specially trained nurses and technicians.

Special Concerns

• Because EPS may induce arrhythmias, this test must take place under carefully controlled conditions in a cardiac catheterization laboratory.
• People with severe bleeding disorders or a recent blood clot in the lungs or extremities are not candidates for this procedure.
• Certain medications, including painkillers, sedatives, and tranquilizers, may interfere with test results. Inform your doctor of any medications you are taking.

Before the Test

• Do not eat or drink anything for 6 to 8 hours before the test.
• Empty your bladder right before the test.

What You Experience

• An intravenous (IV) line is inserted into a vein in your arm to allow administration of medications during the test.
• You lie on your back on a table, and ECG leads (see page 174) are applied to monitor your heart rate and rhythm.
• The skin at the site of catheter insertion (usually the groin, but occasionally the arm or neck) is shaved and then swabbed with an antiseptic, and a local anesthetic is administered to numb the area. The doctor then makes a small incision and inserts a catheter into the vein; you will feel pressure during insertion, but no other discomfort.
• The doctor threads the catheter to your heart using continuous x-ray imaging, or fluoroscopy (see page 205), to watch its progress on a viewing monitor.
• Once the catheter has been guided to your heart, recordings are made of your heart's electrical activity, and various parts of the electrical conduction system are stimulated with pacing signals. This process may induce

---

Results

▼

➡ Depending on the results of this test, your doctor will recommend an appropriate treatment, such as antiarrhythmic medication, a pacemaker, or an automatic implantable cardioverter-defibrillator.

➡ If radiofrequency ablation was performed, it may be a definitive treatment for your cardiac arrhythmia.

arrhythmias, causing you to experience light-headedness, dizziness, or palpitations.

• Your vital signs are monitored throughout the procedure, and the medical staff may continually engage you in light conversation to ensure you are stable and conscious. Report to them any symptoms you experience due to arrhythmias.

• Different antiarrhythmic drugs may be injected into your IV line to evaluate how well they stop the abnormal rhythms, and to select the best medication for you.

• If the doctor decides that radiofrequency ablation is appropriate, it will be performed directly after EPS is completed.

• The procedure may take from 1 to 4 hours.

Risks and Complications

• Serious complications of EPS include induced arrhythmias leading to ventricular tachycardia or fibrillation (life-threatening arrhythmias that can cause cardiac arrest and death); perforation of the heart muscle; stroke or heart attack due to a catheter-induced blood clot; peripheral vascular problems; hemorrhage; and inflammation of the vein (phlebitis) at the site of catheter insertion.

• When performed by experts, the risk associated with EPS is very low, but emergency equipment is available if serious complications arise.

After the Test

• After the procedure is completed, you must remain in a hospital bed for a few hours, with pressure placed on the site of catheter insertion to prevent bleeding.

• Your blood pressure and other vital signs will be monitored periodically during this time, and the catheter insertion site will be checked for signs of bleeding.

• If radiofrequency ablation was performed during this procedure, you must remain in the hospital overnight.

• You may resume your normal diet and any medications withheld before the test.

Estimated Cost: $$$

Electrophysiology Studies continued

Electroretinography
(ERG)

Electroretinography

Description
• This test evaluates the functioning of the retina—the light-sensitive layer of tissues that lines the back of the eye. Normally, retinal photoreceptor cells (called cones and rods) receive light and transform it into electrical impulses that are sent to the brain. In ERG, small sensors (electrodes) embedded in contact lenses are applied to the eyes to record the electrical responses of the retina to light stimuli.

Purpose of the Test
• To assess functioning of photoreceptors and relay cells in the retina.
• To help diagnose or evaluate certain retinal disorders, including hereditary conditions such as retinitis pigmentosa; toxic retinopathies resulting from medications, chemicals, or metallic foreign bodies; circulatory problems in retinal blood vessels; degenerative diseases such as diabetic retinopathy; and remote ocular effects of some cancers.

Who Performs It
• An ophthalmologist or a trained technician.

Special Concerns
• None.

Before the Test
• The examiner administers eye drops to dilate your pupils.
• You will wait in a dark room or a room lit only with a soft red light.
• When your pupils are dilated, anesthetic eye drops are given to numb the eyes.

What You Experience
• Contact lenses (containing electrodes) are placed on each eye. A background patch electrode is applied to the forehead or earlobe.
• Electrical activity of the retina, induced by a flash of light, is first recorded in the dark and then after your eyes have adapted to the light. Different light stimuli, such as a reversing checkerboard light pattern, may be used. The intensity, color, and frequency of the light may be varied.
• The procedure usually takes about 30 to 45 minutes.

Risks and Complications
• None.

After the Test
• Do not rub your eyes for at least 30 minutes (until the anesthesia wears off) to avoid injuring the cornea.
• Your pupils may stay dilated for 3 to 4 hours. You may find it more comfortable to wear dark glasses until your vision has returned to normal.
• Arrange for someone else to drive you home.

Estimated Cost: $$

Results
▼

➡ The electrical responses of the retina are displayed as waves on a viewing monitor and recorded on paper or photographic film. The patterns of waveforms are examined for abnormalities.

➡ A doctor will review the test results. These findings will be considered along with your symptoms, your eye exam, and the results of other tests—such as fluorescein angiography (see page 203) and visual field testing (see page 389)—in order to diagnose any retinal disease or condition.

Endometrial Biopsy

(Uterine Biopsy)

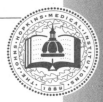

Description

• In this test, a thin, flexible tube (catheter) is passed through the vagina and cervix and into the uterus (illustrated on page 28). A suction device attached to the catheter is used to obtain tissue samples from the lining of the uterus (endometrium); these specimens are sent to a laboratory for analysis.

• Alternatively, the cervix may be dilated and surgical instruments may be used to scrape tissue samples from the endometrium while you are under local or general anesthesia. This procedure, called dilatation and curettage (D&C), is more painful and entails more risk than suction biopsy; thus, it is generally reserved for cases where suction biopsy cannot be done. (It may also be used as a treatment to stop heavy bleeding or remove residual tissue after miscarriage or abortion.)

Purpose of the Test

• To evaluate abnormal uterine bleeding, such as heavy or prolonged periods of bleeding after the menopause, especially in women over age 35 with a family history of endometrial cancer.

• To diagnose endometrial cancer, polyps, or inflammatory conditions.

• To document ovulation and help evaluate the cause of infertility.

• To monitor endometrial health in women taking estrogen replacement therapy (ERT) without progesterone (since this regimen increases the risk of developing endometrial cancer).

Who Performs It

• A gynecologist, an infertility specialist, or a specially trained physician's assistant performs suction biopsy.

• D&C is performed by a gynecologist in a hospital operating room or surgery clinic.

Special Concerns

• Endometrial biopsy is not appropriate in women with an active infection of the vagina or cervix (such as gonorrhea or a yeast infection) or those in whom the cervix cannot be visualized (due to irregular position or prior surgery, for example).

• The time of the menstrual cycle can affect the accuracy of results. If you are being evaluated for fertility, the test should be done approximately 2 days before you expect your period to begin.

• Suction biopsy may be performed using local anesthesia, but anesthesia is not usually required.

Before the Test

• You may be given a pregnancy test before the procedure to ensure you are not pregnant; if the test is positive, the procedure will be canceled.

• Empty your bladder just before the test.

• You will be asked to undress from the waist down and put on a drape or hospital gown.

• Your doctor may give you an over-the-counter pain reliever, such as ibuprofen, and/or a mild sedative about 30 minutes before the procedure.

• If you are undergoing a D&C under general anesthesia, do not eat or drink anything for at least 8 hours before the procedure.

Results

▼

➥ A pathologist examines the tissue samples under a microscope. (For more on microscopic examination, see Chapter 1.)

➥ This test usually results in a definitive diagnosis. If tissue abnormalities are detected, your doctor will recommend a course of medical or surgical treatment, depending on the specific problem.

Endometrial Biopsy continued

What You Experience
Suction biopsy:
• You will lie on your back on an examining table with your knees bent and your feet placed in stirrups.
• The examiner will conduct a manual pelvic exam—which involves inserting a gloved, lubricated finger into the vagina—to determine the size, shape, and location of the uterus.
• Next, a lubricated speculum—a metal or plastic instrument that pushes apart the walls of the vagina to provide a view of the cervix—is gently inserted. The device may feel cold and uncomfortable, but causes no pain. Relax and breathe through your mouth to ease the insertion.
• The cervix is cleansed.
• A narrow, flexible catheter attached to a vacuum device is inserted through the vagina and cervix into the uterus. Suction is initiated to obtain samples from the endometrium. You may feel some cramping as this is done.
• The tissue samples and instruments are withdrawn.
• The procedure takes only about 5 minutes to perform.

D&C:
• A general anesthetic medication is administered through an intravenous (IV) needle or catheter inserted into a vein in your arm.
• The doctor inserts a speculum into your vagina and uses a special clamp to grip the cervix.
• Your cervix is slowly opened, or dilated, using blunt metal instruments of increasing diameter.
• A spoon-shaped instrument called a curette is inserted into the uterus to scrape tissue from the endometrium.
• The tissue samples and instruments are removed.
• This procedure takes about 30 minutes.

Risks and Complications
• Rare but serious complications include infection, severe bleeding, and inadvertent perforation of the uterine wall (which requires surgical repair).
• Rarely, D&C may result in damage to the bladder or bowel. If general anesthesia is used, it entails all of the associated risks.

After the Test
• You will remain in a recovery room until the effects of sedation or anesthesia wear off. You may return home and should rest for about 24 hours. (If you received general anesthesia, be sure to arrange for a ride home.)
• You may experience mild cramping for several days. Over-the-counter pain relievers, such as ibuprofen, may help. (A prescription painkiller may be given after D&C.)
• You may experience slight vaginal bleeding for 1 or 2 days after suction biopsy, and for up to several weeks after D&C. Use sanitary napkins rather than tampons.
• Avoid sexual intercourse and do not douche for 72 hours after a suction biopsy, and for at least 2 weeks after D&C.
• Call your doctor if you experience severe pain, excessive vaginal bleeding, abnormal vaginal discharge, or fever.

Estimated Cost: $$

Endoscopic Retrograde Cholangiopancreatography (ERCP)

Description

- ERCP combines the use of a thin, flexible, lighted viewing tube (endoscope) with x-rays to visualize the pancreatic ducts and the bile ducts in and near the liver (biliary tract). The doctor inserts the scope into your mouth and guides it through the digestive tract until the point where the bile and pancreatic ducts open into the first part of the small intestine, or duodenum (illustrated on page 25 of the body atlas). A contrast dye is then injected through the scope to delineate the ducts on x-ray films and uncover any abnormalities. In addition, instruments may be passed through the scope to obtain tissue or fluid samples for laboratory analysis or to perform therapeutic procedures.
- This procedure is usually ordered after less invasive tests, such as abdominal CT scanning or ultrasound, fail to provide a definitive diagnosis. (For more on contrast x-rays, see Chapter 2.)

Purpose of the Test

- To detect bile duct obstructions in and near the liver and gallbladder—such as tumors, stones, and abnormal narrowings (strictures)—that may be causing pain and jaundice (yellowing of the skin).
- To diagnose or to rule out cancer of the pancreas.
- To determine the cause of recurrent pancreatic inflammation.
- To evaluate the pancreas prior to surgery.
- Used therapeutically to remove bile duct stones, dilate narrow ducts, unblock obstructions caused by tumors, and open the muscular ring at the point where the common bile duct enters the duodenum.

Who Performs It

- A doctor who is specially trained in endoscopic procedures.

Special Concerns

- This procedure is associated with fewer complications than percutaneous transhepatic cholangiography (see page 287).
- ERCP may not be appropriate for people with an infectious disease; acute inflammation of the pancreas; an abnormal narrowing or obstruction of the esophagus or duodenum; pancreatic pseudocysts (a condition in which pancreatic fluids break through the ducts and collect in spaces in the pancreas); inflammation of the bile ducts (cholangitis); or severe heart or lung disease.
- People with allergies to iodine or shellfish may experience an allergic reaction to the iodine-based contrast dye.
- Pregnant women should not undergo this test because exposure to ionizing radiation may harm the fetus.

Results

▼

➡ The doctor examines the x-rays for evidence of stones, tumors, strictures, or other abnormalities in the biliary and pancreatic ducts. In some instances, this review will prompt immediate interventions during ERCP, such as placement of a stent to widen a narrowed duct.

➡ If any tissue, cell, or fluid samples were obtained, the specimen containers may be sent to several different laboratories for examination. The samples will be analyzed for evidence of infection, inflammation, or cancer. (For more on laboratory testing, see Chapter 1.)

➡ If a definitive diagnosis cannot be made, additional tests may be ordered.

Endoscopic Retrograde Cholangiopancreatography

• Residual barium in the abdomen following recent contrast x-rays of the digestive tract may interfere with visualization of the biliary and pancreatic ducts on the x-rays.

Before the Test

• Inform your doctor if you regularly take anticoagulants or nonsteroidal anti-inflammatory drugs (such as aspirin, ibuprofen, or naproxen). You will be instructed to discontinue these medications for some time before the test.

• Tell your doctor if you've ever had an allergic reaction to iodine or shellfish or to an anesthetic medication.

• Do not eat or drink anything after midnight on the day before the test.

• At the testing facility, you will be asked to disrobe from the waist up and put on a hospital gown.

• You will be advised to empty your bladder before the test.

• Immediately before the test, an intravenous (IV) needle or catheter is inserted into a vein in your arm. You will receive a mild sedative medication, but will remain conscious throughout the procedure.

What You Experience

• You are positioned on your side on an x-ray table.

• A local anesthetic (lidocaine) is sprayed on the back of your throat to suppress the gag reflex. (You may still experience mild gagging as the scope passes through your throat.) A plastic mouthpiece is inserted into your mouth to hold it open.

• The doctor inserts the endoscope into your mouth and carefully passes it down the throat, through the esophagus and stomach, and into the duodenum. Continuous x-ray imaging, or fluoroscopy (see page 205), may be used to guide the progress of the scope on a viewing monitor.

• The doctor closely inspects the internal structures through the scope, looking for any abnormalities.

• Several medications may be administered through the IV line or through the scope to relax the opening from the duodenum into the common bile duct, to remove air bubbles, and to otherwise improve the view through the scope.

• A thin tube, or catheter, is then advanced through the scope until it reaches the point at which the common bile duct opens into the duodenum.

• A contrast dye is infused through the catheter into the bile and pancreatic ducts, and a series of x-ray films is obtained. You may feel a brief flushing sensation as the dye is infused.

• You may need to wait as the initial films are developed, so that additional x-rays can be taken if necessary.

• If appropriate, the physician may insert instruments through the scope to remove tissue samples for analysis; to remove stones; to dilate any narrow segments; or to perform other procedures.

• Throughout the procedure, excess saliva is suctioned from your mouth, your blood pressure and oxygen levels are monitored, and fluids are administered through the IV line.

• The procedure usually takes 1 to 2 hours.

Risks and Complications

• Some people may experience an allergic reaction to the iodine-based contrast dye, which can cause symptoms such as nausea, sneezing, vomiting, hives, and occasionally a life-threatening response called anaphylactic shock. Emergency medications and equipment are kept readily available.

• Rare complications after ERCP include inflammation of the pancreas (pancreatitis); infection; perforation of the esophagus, stomach, or duodenum; bleeding; and respiratory arrest due to oversedation.

• Severe complications develop in fewer than 1% of procedures.

• Certain medications administered during the test may cause side effects such as dry mouth, nausea, or urine retention.

After the Test

• You are taken to a recovery room, where your vital signs are monitored and you are observed for any adverse reaction to the anesthetic or other complications.

• Once the sedation wears off, you may usually return home. Arrange for someone to drive you.

• If therapeutic procedures were performed, you may need to stay in the hospital overnight for observation.

• You may experience a feeling of fullness, cramping, or flatulence for several hours after the test.

• Do not eat or drink until your gag reflex returns, usually in a few hours. (Touching the back of the throat with a tongue depressor tests for this reflex.) You may then drink fluids and have a light meal, according to your doctor's instructions.

• You may have a sore throat for several days. Lozenges or a warm saline gargle may provide some relief.

• Contact your doctor immediately if you develop abdominal or back pain or blood in the stool after this test.

Estimated Cost: $$$ to $$$$

Endoscopic Retrograde Cholangiopancreatography continued

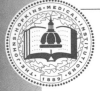

Enteroclysis
(Small Bowel Enema)

Enteroclysis

Description

• In this procedure, a thin tube, or catheter, is inserted through your nose or mouth and passed through your stomach into the small intestine, or small bowel (illustrated on page 25). Barium sulfate is infused directly into the small bowel; this contrast agent is opaque to x-rays and thus reveals any structural or tissue abnormalities on the x-ray images. Because the barium bypasses your stomach—avoiding dilution by its digestive juices—this test can provide a more accurate picture of the small bowel than a small bowel series (see page 373). (For more on contrast x-rays, see Chapter 2.)

Purpose of the Test

• To detect and evaluate Crohn's disease, an inflammatory condition affecting the last portion of the small intestine (ileum).
• To diagnose Meckel's diverticulum, a sac that pushes through the wall of the small bowel.
• To help identify the site of small bowel obstructions.
• To aid in the diagnosis of tumors.

Who Performs It

• A radiologist.

Special Concerns

• When perforation of the upper gastrointestinal tract is suspected, barium is not used because leakage of the dye could worsen any existing infection. A water-soluble contrast agent, diatrizoate (Gastrografin), is usually substituted.
• Pregnant women should not undergo this test because exposure to ionizing radiation may harm the fetus.
• Barium in the intestine from previous contrast x-rays, such as a barium swallow (see page 106), may interfere with the results.
• Patients with unstable vital signs must be closely monitored during this test.

Before the Test

• Be sure to inform your doctor of all drugs you regularly take. Some medications may need to be discontinued for 24 hours before the test.
• Do not eat, drink, or smoke after midnight on the day before the test.
• You may be instructed to take a mild laxative or perform a mild cleansing enema on the day before the test.
• Remove any metallic objects, such as jewelry, watches, dentures, or hairpins, before the test begins.
• An intravenous (IV) catheter is inserted in a vein in your arm so that medications can be administered as needed during the procedure.

What You Experience

• You are asked to lie on your back on an x-ray table. Before the test begins, you may receive an IV sedative to relax you.
• A catheter is then passed through your nose or mouth. (A local anesthetic is usually sprayed inside your nose or throat to make the catheter insertion more comfortable.)
• With the aid of fluoroscopy (see page 205), which transmits continuous, moving x-ray images onto a viewing screen, the radiologist guides the catheter through your stomach and into the initial portion of the small bowel.
• A small balloon at the tip of the catheter is

Results

➥ The doctor will examine the recorded x-ray images for evidence of any abnormality.
➥ If a definitive diagnosis can be made, appropriate treatment will be initiated.
➥ In some cases, additional tests, such as a small bowel biopsy (see page 338), may be needed to further evaluate abnormal results.

inflated to prevent barium from flowing back into your stomach.

• Barium is administered through the catheter. (In some cases, the bulking agent methylcellulose is also given to distend the walls of the small bowel further and provide a clearer picture of the area.) You may feel a sensation of fullness in your abdomen.

• The radiologist observes the flow of barium through the small bowel via fluoroscopy.

• At various points during the exam, you will be instructed to move into different positions as spot x-ray films are taken of any abnormalities. As each x-ray is taken, you should hold your breath and remain as still as possible.

• Once the exam is completed, the doctor deflates the balloon and removes the catheter.

• The procedure takes about 1 hour.

Risks and Complications

• Although radiation exposure is minimal, you receive a higher dose of radiation than during standard x-ray procedures.

• The barium may accumulate and block the intestines if it is not excreted within a few days.

After the Test

• Your vital signs are monitored in a recovery area until you are alert.

• If you received a sedative, someone should drive you home.

• If a local anesthetic was administered inside your throat, do not eat or drink until your gag reflex returns, usually in a few hours. (Touching the back of the throat with a tongue depressor tests for this reflex.)

• Drink plenty of fluids to help eliminate the barium. Your doctor may also give you a mild laxative to purge your body of the contrast agent.

• Your stool will be chalky and light-colored initially, but should return to normal color after 1 to 3 days.

Estimated Cost: $$

Enteroclysis continued

Esophageal Function Studies

Description

• In this series of tests, special probes are passed into the esophagus—the muscular passage that contracts and relaxes to carry food from the throat to the stomach—to evaluate its swallowing function. These tests also measure the efficiency of the lower esophageal sphincter (LES), the circular muscle that acts as a valve to prevent backflow of stomach contents and acid into the esophagus (a disorder known as gastroesophageal reflux). One or more of the following tests are typically included:

• **Esophageal manometry** records the muscular contractions (swallowing waves) of the esophagus and measures the pressure of the LES (when pressure is too low, reflux of stomach acid occurs; when it is too high, it is difficult for food to pass from the esophagus to the stomach).

• **The acid reflux test** uses a pH probe to measure acid-base levels in the esophagus. Reflux of gastric acid from the stomach causes a noticeable drop in pH levels.

• **The acid perfusion test** (also known as the Bernstein test) attempts to reproduce the symptoms of gastroesophageal reflux by instilling hydrochloric acid into the esophagus. If the acid causes discomfort, then gastroesophageal reflux is indicated; if not, a cause other than reflux is responsible for your symptoms.

• **The acid clearing test** measures the ability of the esophagus to clear itself of hydrochloric acid. People with normal esophageal function are able to clear the acid in less than 10 swallows.

Purpose of the Test

• To identify and evaluate esophageal disorders—such as gastroesophageal reflux, diffuse esophageal spasm, and esophagitis (inflammation of the esophagus)—in people with symptoms such as heartburn, chest pain, or difficulty swallowing.

• To distinguish the pain caused by heartburn from similar pain caused by cardiac disorders.

Who Performs It

• An esophageal technician in an endoscopy laboratory.

Special Concerns

• If gastroesophageal reflux is suspected, a barium swallow (see page 106) or esophagogastroduodenoscopy (see page 194) may first be used to establish a diagnosis. Esophageal function studies are typically done only if the initial treatment fails to relieve symptoms.

• A number of medications can interfere with the results of these tests by either decreasing or increasing gastric acid secretion or relaxing the LES and promoting reflux.

• Eating before this test may interfere with results.

• The acid perfusion test should not be done in people with esophageal varices (abnormally dilated blood vessels), congestive heart failure, and certain other cardiac disorders.

Before the Test

• Be sure to inform your doctor of any heartburn medications or other drugs you regularly take. You may be advised to discontinue certain drugs before the test.

Results
▼

➡ Your doctor will review the test results and consider them along with your symptoms to reach a diagnosis.

➡ If results indicate gastroesophageal reflux, certain lifestyle and dietary changes will be prescribed, as well as medications to reduce stomach acid secretion.

Esophageal Function Studies

• Avoid tobacco and alcohol for 24 hours before the test.

• Do not eat or drink anything for at least 8 hours before the test.

What You Experience

• Immediately before the test, your blood pressure and pulse are taken. A local anesthetic may be sprayed into your throat.

• Very thin, soft tubes are passed into your nose or mouth, down through your esophagus, and into your stomach. (You may feel a gagging sensation initially, but it will pass.)

• One of the tubes, called a manometry probe, is attached to a pressure transducer that records pressures in the LES and esophagus as the probe is slowly withdrawn from the stomach.

• Next, you are asked to swallow water, and the probe records the swallowing waves of the esophagus. The probe is withdrawn.

• For the acid reflux test, another thin tube with a pH meter at the tip is used, and you will be asked to perform several maneuvers (such as drawing your knees to your chest). The movements may be repeated after hydrochloric acid is instilled through the probe into your stomach. If the probe registers a drop in pH, gastroesophageal reflux is indicated.

• For the acid perfusion test, hydrochloric acid and salt water are alternately instilled through the pH probe into the esophagus. Tell the examiner if and when you experience any discomfort or chest pain; if symptoms occur with the acid, but not the salt water, you may have an inflamed esophagus due to chronic reflux.

• For the acid clearing test, hydrochloric acid is instilled through the pH probe into the esophagus and you will be asked to swallow about every 30 seconds. If it takes more than 10 swallows to clear the acid, reflux is indicated.

• These tests usually take from 30 minutes to 1 hour. In some cases, you will remain in the hospital for 12 to 24 hours while a probe continuously measures acidity in your esophagus.

Risks and Complications

• There is a possibility of inadvertent aspiration of stomach contents into the lungs.

After the Test

• You may experience a sore throat, which can be eased with soothing lozenges.

• Resume your usual diet and any medications withheld before the test.

Estimated Cost: $$$

Esophageal Function Studies continued

Esophagogastroduodenoscopy
(EGD, Upper Gastrointestinal Endoscopy)

Description

• In this test, a flexible, lighted viewing tube (endoscope) is passed into the throat and through the esophagus, the stomach, and the uppermost portion of the small intestine, or duodenum (illustrated on pages 24 and 25). Fiberoptic cables permit a physician to visually inspect the lining of these digestive organs for any signs of disease or abnormality; in some cases, instruments are passed through the scope to obtain tissue biopsies for microscopic examination. EGD may also be done therapeutically, for example, to remove polyps, control bleeding, or remove a swallowed object.

Purpose of the Test

• To detect abnormalities of the esophagus, stomach, and duodenum, particularly in people with gastrointestinal (GI) symptoms—such as heartburn, difficulty swallowing, weight loss, abdominal pain, and diarrhea—that have not been explained by contrast x-rays such as a barium swallow (see page 106) or upper GI series (see page 373).
• To confirm a diagnosis of esophageal or stomach cancer or some other abnormality found on a contrast x-ray.
• To evaluate the stomach or duodenum after surgery.
• Used therapeutically to remove polyps, widen narrowed passages, stop active bleeding, or remove obstructions.

Who Performs It

• A physician who is trained in endoscopic procedures.

Special Concerns

• EGD should not be done in people with uncontrolled bleeding in the GI tract (until they are stable); those with esophageal diverticula (abnormal outpouchings); if there is a suspected perforation of the GI tract; or in people who have had recent upper GI surgery.
• The procedure may not be possible if food or blood is present in the stomach.
• You must wait at least 2 days after having a barium test before undergoing this procedure; the presence of barium interferes with visual inspection.
• This test may provoke some anxiety, but it is not painful. You will not be able to speak when the scope is in your throat, but your breathing will not be affected.
• In some cases, an extra long endoscope may be used to visualize or perform biopsies of the small intestine beyond the duodenum; this procedure is known as enteroscopy.

Before the Test

• You will be instructed to fast for 6 to 12 hours before the test.
• Inform your doctor if you regularly take nonsteroidal anti-inflammatory drugs (such as aspirin, ibuprofen, or naproxen). These med-

Results

▼

➡ The doctor will note any abnormalities such as bleeding, inflammation, abnormal growths, or ulcers that were discovered during the visual inspection.

➡ Various laboratory tests may be necessary to pinpoint a diagnosis. For example, tissue samples may be cultured (see page 166) to identify the presence of infectious organisms, such as *Helicobacter pylori* (a bacterium believed to be responsible for some stomach ulcers). Biopsied tumors and excised polyps are examined under a microscope for signs of cancer or another abnormality. (For more on laboratory testing, see Chapter 1.)

ications must be discontinued for 7 days before the test to reduce the risk of bleeding.
• If you wear dentures, contacts, or glasses, remove them prior to the test.
• A sedative medication will likely be administered through an intravenous (IV) catheter inserted in a vein in your arm. You may drift into a light sleep during the procedure.

What You Experience
• You lie on your left side on a table.
• A local anesthetic (such as lidocaine) is sprayed into your mouth and throat to suppress the gag reflex when the scope is inserted. A plastic mouthpiece may be inserted to hold your mouth open and prevent you from biting down on the scope.
• Next, you will bend your head forward and open your mouth. The doctor will guide the scope into your throat with his finger. When the scope reaches a certain point, the doctor will straighten your head to aid the advancement of the scope down through your esophagus.
• If needed, the doctor may instill a small amount of air through the scope to dilate the esophagus and stomach for better viewing. This may cause you to belch or pass gas.
• The doctor carefully inspects the lining of your esophagus, stomach, and duodenum, looking for any abnormalities.
• If appropriate, a biopsy forceps or other instruments may be inserted through the scope to obtain tissue samples or cells for laboratory analysis. If necessary, surgical treatments may be performed through the scope, such as obliteration of polyps with heat.
• Upon completion of the visual inspection, excess air and gastric secretions are removed through the scope, and the scope is withdrawn.
• The procedure usually takes from 20 to 30 minutes.

Risks and Complications
• Possible complications include bleeding from a biopsy site; aspiration of stomach contents into the lungs; low blood pressure or breathing difficulties due to oversedation; and inadvertent perforation of the esophagus, stomach, or duodenum.

After the Test
• You will rest in a recovery room until the sedative medication wears off. Your vital signs will be checked periodically, and you will be observed for signs of complications. Arrange for someone to drive you home.
• Do not eat or drink until your gag reflex returns, usually in a few hours. (Touching the back of the throat with a tongue depressor tests for this reflex.)
• You may experience belching, flatulence, or gas pains after the procedure.
• You may feel hoarse or have a sore throat for several days. Lozenges or a warm saline gargle may provide some relief.
• If a biopsy was performed, you may have black, tarry stools due to bleeding for a short period of time.
• Contact your doctor immediately if you develop a fever, or if you experience persistent difficulty swallowing; black, tarry stools; or bloody vomit.

Estimated Cost: $$$

Esophagogastroduodenoscopy continued

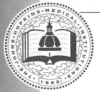

Evoked Potential Studies
(Evoked Brain Potentials, Evoked Responses)

Description
• These tests measure the brain's response to stimuli that are delivered through sight, hearing, or touch. These sensory stimuli evoke minute electrical potentials that travel along nerves to the brain, and can be recorded with patch-like sensors (electrodes) that are attached to the scalp. These signals are transmitted to a computer, where they are amplified, averaged, and displayed. The 3 major types of evoked potential studies are described here.
• **Visual evoked potentials,** which are produced by exposing the eye to a reversible checkerboard pattern or strobe light flash, help to detect vision impairment caused by optic nerve damage, particularly from multiple sclerosis.
• **Auditory evoked potentials,** generated by delivering clicks to the ear, are used to identify the source of hearing loss. They help to differentiate between damage to the acoustic nerve and damage to auditory pathways within the brainstem.
• **Somatosensory evoked potentials,** produced by electrically stimulating a peripheral sensory nerve—that is, a nerve responsible for sensation in an area of the body—can be used to diagnose peripheral nerve damage and locate brain and spinal cord lesions.

Purpose of the Test
• To assess the function of the nervous system.
• To aid in the diagnosis of nervous system lesions and abnormalities.
• To monitor the progression or treatment of degenerative nerve diseases such as multiple sclerosis.
• To monitor brain activity and nerve signals during brain or spine surgery, or in patients who are under general anesthesia.

Who Performs It
• A neurologist, a nurse, or a lab technician.

Special Concerns
• It may be difficult to determine visual evoked potentials accurately in people with extremely impaired vision.
• Earwax, severe inflammation of the middle ear, or severe hearing impairment may interfere with the results of auditory evoked potential studies.
• Severe sensory loss (neuropathy) may interfere with the results of somatosensory evoked potential studies.
• Muscle spasms in the head or neck may also interfere with test results.

Before the Test
• Wash your hair the night before the test, and do not use hair spray, gel, or other hair care products after shampooing.
• Your hair should be free of any braids, pins, or jewelry.
• Avoid taking sedative drugs, such as benzodiazepines and barbiturates, before the test.
• Remove all jewelry and metal objects before the procedure.

Results
▼

➡ A neurologist will evaluate the electrical tracings, or wave forms, for any abnormalities that indicate damage to the nerve pathways leading to the brain from your eyes, ears, or limbs.

➡ In most cases, further testing will be needed to provide more specific information or further evaluate abnormal findings. Additional tests may include a brain CT scan (see page 121), magnetic resonance angiography (see page 119), or electroneurography (see page 180).

What You Experience
Visual evoked potentials:
• You sit in a chair, about 3 feet away from a TV screen.
• A special adhesive paste is used to attach electrodes to your scalp.
• The eye that is not being tested is usually covered with a patch.
• You are asked to focus your gaze on a dot at the center of the TV screen as it displays a visual stimulus, usually a rapidly moving checkerboard pattern.
• Electrical activity in the optic nerve and brain is recorded by the electrodes.
• The procedure is repeated for the other eye.
• Each eye is usually tested twice. The entire procedure takes about 30 to 45 minutes.

Auditory evoked potentials:
• You will sit in a soundproof room and put on headphones.
• Electrodes are attached to the top of your head and to the earlobe of the ear being tested.
• A series of clicking sounds is delivered through the headphones to one ear, then the other. Signals produced by the brain in response to the clicks are recorded.
• Each ear is usually tested twice. The entire procedure takes about 30 to 45 minutes.

Somatosensory evoked potentials:
• Recording electrodes are attached to your scalp and neck. Stimulating electrodes may be placed over your wrist, lower back, knee, or ankle.
• Mild, painless electrical shocks are delivered to the stimulating electrodes. The stimulus lasts for about 2 minutes at a time and may cause some twitching and tingling in the target area.
• The brain's response to the shocks is measured by the recording electrodes.
• The procedure takes about 30 minutes.

Risks and Complications
• Evoked potential studies are painless and carry no significant risk. The mild electrical shocks delivered in the somatosensory tests are usually perceived as a tingling sensation.

After the Test
• The electrodes are removed and the adhesive paste is washed away.
• You may resume taking any medications that were withheld before the test, according to your doctor's instructions.

Estimated Cost: $$

Evoked Potential Studies continued

Fecal Fat

(Fecal Lipids)

Fecal Fat

Description
• In this test, stool samples are collected for 3 days and then analyzed for their fat (lipid) content. Normally, most dietary fat is absorbed by the small intestine (small bowel). Excessive amounts of lipids in the stool indicate improper absorption of fat due to an abnormality in the lining of the small bowel, or improper digestion of fat caused by a problem with the bile acids or digestive enzymes secreted by the pancreas or liver.

Purpose of the Test
• To confirm the diagnosis of steatorrhea (excessive excretion of fecal lipids) in people with large, greasy, foul-smelling stools or diarrhea.

Who Performs It
• A laboratory technician.

Special Concerns
• Don't use a container with a waxy coating to collect the stool samples. The wax may mix with the sample and interfere with the test results.
• Don't take laxatives or mineral oil or use enemas during the test period.

Before the Test
• Inform your doctor if you regularly take any medications. Certain drugs may affect fecal fat levels and must be discontinued briefly before the test.
• For 3 days before the test—and throughout the testing period—you should ingest at least 100 grams of fat per day.
• Avoid alcohol and any products with the fat substitute olestra.

What You Experience
• Collect all of your stool in a dry, clean container over the testing period of 3 days. You will either be given one large container or several smaller containers for each sample.
• Be careful not to contaminate the samples with urine or toilet paper.
• Keep the containers refrigerated and tightly closed between samples.

Risks and Complications
• There are no risks or complications associated with this test.

After the Test
• You will be instructed to take the stool specimens to a laboratory.
• Resume your normal diet and any medications withheld before the test.

Estimated Cost: $$

Results

▼

➥ The fat content of your stool is calculated. If the test is positive for steatorrhea, a wide variety of conditions may be responsible, including bile duct obstructions, pancreatic disease, and inflammatory intestinal disorders such as Crohn's disease.

➥ Further tests, such as an upper GI series (see page 373), will be necessary to determine the cause of steatorrhea.

Fecal Occult Blood Test

Description

• In this test, three separate stool specimens are analyzed for trace amounts of blood that cannot be detected with the naked eye (occult blood). Normally, extremely small quantities of blood are excreted in the feces; by using microscopic and chemical analysis, this test can detect larger amounts that indicate bleeding in the gastrointestinal tract. Doctors currently recommend that all adults over age 50 have an annual fecal occult blood test to screen for colorectal cancer. (For more on screening tests, see Chapter 3.)

Purpose of the Test

• To detect bleeding in the gastrointestinal tract, which may be caused by many different disorders, including ulcers, inflammatory bowel disease, ulcerative colitis, cancer, and hemorrhoids.
• To screen for premalignant growths in the colon or rectum and for colorectal cancer in asymptomatic individuals.

Who Performs It

• A laboratory technician.

Special Concerns

• False-negative results may be caused by taking vitamin C supplements or antacids or by delaying transport of the stool samples for analysis.
• False-positive results may result from failure to follow dietary or medication restrictions, or the presence of bleeding gums, hemorrhoids, menstrual blood, or watery stools. (For more on false-positives and false-negatives, see page 35.)

Before the Test

• All of the following instructions should be carried out for three days before the test to maximize the accuracy of results.
• Avoid eating any red meat, poultry, fish, or peroxidase-rich fruits and vegetables, especially turnips, radishes, melons, and horseradish.
• Do not take vitamin C supplements or eat large quantities of foods, such as citrus fruits, that contain this vitamin.
• Eat a high-fiber diet, containing whole grains, beans, and vegetables that do not contain peroxidase, to increase the bulk of the stools.
• Do not take any antacids, iron supplements, steroids, and nonsteroidal anti-inflammatory drugs such as aspirin, ibuprofen, or naproxen. (Your doctor may also instruct you to avoid certain other medications that you regularly take).
• Do not drink alcohol and avoid any other substances that may irritate the digestive tract.

Results

▼

➥ Your stool samples are analyzed using various methods. They may be examined under a microscope, and may also be treated with special chemicals that can identify hemoglobin, a red blood cell pigment. (For more on laboratory testing, see Chapter 1.)

➥ If occult blood is detected, your doctor will first attempt to rule out any unrelated factors, such as bleeding gums, that might account for this finding.

➥ Because occult blood may result from bleeding at almost any point along the digestive tract, this test is generally used as an initial evaluation in people who show symptoms of gastrointestinal bleeding. Additional tests—such as contrast x-rays (see pages 104, 106, and 373) or endoscopy (see pages 194 and 323) of the digestive tract—are required to identify the site and extent of the bleeding.

Fecal Occult Blood Test continued

• If your gums tend to bleed, avoid brushing your teeth.

• Women should not begin testing during their menstrual period or during the first three days after the end of their period.

What You Experience

• Your doctor will give you the kit to use for the test.

• You will collect stool samples in a clean plastic container for three consecutive days.

• Use the wooden applicator supplied with the kit to smear a portion of each sample onto a specimen card.

• When you have completed the stool sampling, bring the specimens to your doctor or to a testing laboratory so they can be analyzed for occult blood.

Risks and Complications

• There are no risks or complications associated with this test.

After the Test

• After you have completed the stool sampling process, you may resume your normal diet and any medications that were discontinued before the test.

Estimated Cost: $

Fine Needle Aspiration of a Neck Mass

Description

• In this procedure, a long, thin needle is inserted through the skin to withdraw (aspirate) a column of cells from a growth in the neck. This specimen is sent to a laboratory for microscopic examination. Fine needle aspiration is typically performed to evaluate a neck mass that was detected on an imaging test, such as a CT scan (see page 212) or an MRI scan (see page 214). Common sites include the thyroid gland (see page 18), parotid salivary gland (see page 24), or lymph nodes (see page 19).

Purpose of the Test

• To determine whether a neck mass is benign or malignant (cancerous).

Who Performs It

• The procedure is conducted by a surgeon, a pathologist, or another physician trained in fine needle aspiration.
• In some cases, a radiology technician may assist.

Special Concerns

• Fine needle aspiration may be performed in a doctor's office, an outpatient surgery facility, or a hospital, depending on the exact procedure.

Before the Test

• If you are anxious about undergoing this procedure, your doctor may administer a sedative to relax you.
• You will be instructed to empty your bladder just before the test.
• You will be asked to disrobe above the waist and put on a hospital gown.

What You Experience

• In most cases, a local anesthetic is injected to numb the site of needle insertion, but it is not always necessary. This injection may cause mild discomfort.
• The doctor inserts a thin needle through the skin into the neck mass and withdraws cells from the mass. Sometimes several samples are obtained.
• If you did not receive a local anesthetic, you may experience mild discomfort during needle insertion. However, it is important that you remain very still during the procedure.
• For a mass that is located deep in the neck, ultrasound imaging or CT scanning may be used to guide the placement of the needle. (These imaging techniques are described in Chapter 2.)
• Pressure is placed on the needle insertion site until bleeding has stopped, and small bandage is applied.
• The procedure usually takes only about 5 minutes.

Results

➡ The specimen is sent to a pathology laboratory and examined under a microscope for the presence of abnormal cells. Possible findings include inflammation due to bacterial or viral infection, benign tumors, and cancer. (For more information about microscopic examination, see Chapter 1.)

➡ If a definitive diagnosis can be made, your doctor will recommend an appropriate course of medical or surgical treatment.

➡ On rare occasions, the cells obtained by fine needle aspiration are insufficient to make a diagnosis. In this case, the procedure may need to be repeated, or a surgical biopsy under general anesthesia may be necessary.

Fine Needle Aspiration of a Neck Mass continued

Risks and Complications

• The most common complication is swelling or bruising due to collection of blood under the skin (hematoma) at the needle insertion site. This is harmless and will resolve on its own, but may cause some discomfort and slight, temporary difficulty swallowing.

• Serious complications—such as bleeding (hemorrhage), infection, or inadvertent puncture of other structures in the neck—are extremely rare.

After the Test

• You may be instructed to place pressure on the aspiration site for some minutes to minimize the chance of a hematoma. Otherwise, you are free to leave the testing facility.

• Your doctor may recommend that you avoid strenuous physical activity for 24 hours.

• For a large hematoma at the needle insertion site, you should apply ice initially. After 24 hours, use warm, moist compresses to help dissolve the clotted blood and relieve discomfort.

• Your doctor may recommend taking an over-the-counter pain reliever, such as aspirin, acetaminophen, or ibuprofen, to allay any postprocedure discomfort.

• Call your doctor if you develop excessive pain or bleeding or if you develop a fever.

Estimated Cost: $$$

Fluorescein Angiography

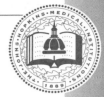

Description

• Fluorescein dye is injected into a vein in the arm. As it circulates through blood vessels in the eye, a rapid series of photographs is taken with a special camera. The camera uses a cobalt blue light to intensify the yellow-green color produced by the dye in the blood vessels of the retina (the light-sensitive layer of tissues that lines the back of the eye) and choroid (the layer of tissue behind the retina).

Purpose of the Test

• To reveal fine details of retinal circulation that are not visible with a routine eye exam.
• To diagnose and evaluate a variety of eye diseases, including age-related macular degeneration, or AMD (a degenerative condition of the most sensitive area of the retina, or macula); diabetic retinopathy (deterioration of the retina resulting from diabetes); circulatory or inflammatory disorders; and tumors.
• To assist in the planning of laser treatments for neovascular AMD, diabetic retinopathy, and other disorders.

Who Performs It

• An ophthalmological photographer.

Special Concerns

• The presence of cataracts or blood in the vitreous (the jelly-like mass that fills the cavity of the eyeball) may limit or preclude use of fluorescein angiography because clear pictures cannot be obtained. The procedure may be performed after cataracts are removed.
• This test should not be done in people with a known allergy or sensitivity to fluorescein dye or dilating eye drops.

Before the Test

• Inform your doctor if you have any allergies, use any medications, or have another eye disorder such as glaucoma.

• If you have glaucoma, do not use any eye drop medication on the day of the test.
• The examiner will administer eye drops to dilate your pupils. It may take 15 to 40 minutes to achieve maximum dilation.

What You Experience

• You are asked to place your head in a brace with a padded chin rest and forehead bar. Keep your teeth together, focus your eyes straight ahead, and breathe and blink normally.
• Several preliminary photographs may be taken.
• Fluorescein dye is injected into a vein in your arm. You may feel mild discomfort and a feeling of warmth or nausea soon after the dye is injected.
• As the dye passes through the blood vessels in the back of your eye over the next 30 to 60 seconds, a series of photographs is taken using a special camera.
• In some cases, additional photographs may

Results
▼

➡ An ophthalmologist will examine the photographs for abnormalities, such as blood vessel leakage or blockage, bleeding (hemorrhage), or new vessel growth.

➡ Depending on the results, the doctor will recommend appropriate course of treatment, if possible. You may be referred to a low vision center for advice on measures to help you manage daily activities with vision loss.

➡ If fluorescein angiography cannot produce an adequate image of any abnormal blood vessels, a similar procedure that uses a different dye, called indocyanine green angiography, is sometimes performed.

be taken as much as 30 minutes later.
• The test usually takes about 30 minutes.

Risks and Complications
• Transient nausea or vomiting occurs in 2% to 4% of patients.
• Minor allergic reactions to the fluorescein dye may produce hives or asthmatic symptoms.
• In rare cases, a severe, potentially fatal allergic reaction may occur. Emergency medications and equipment and trained personnel are present in most facilities performing this test.

After the Test
• Since your pupils will remain dilated for 3 to 4 hours, arrange for someone to drive you home. Your vision may remain blurred for up to 12 hours.
• The fluorescein dye may result in a harmless yellow discoloration of the skin and urine for 24 to 48 hours.
• Blood (hematoma) or fluorescein may collect under the skin at the injection site; this is harmless and resolves on its own. For a large hematoma that causes swelling and discomfort, apply ice initially; after 24 hours, use warm, moist compresses to help dissolve the clotted blood.

Estimated Cost: $$

Fluoroscopy

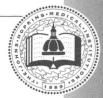

Description

• A continuous stream of x-rays is passed through the body and projected onto a fluorescent viewing screen to provide real-time images of internal structures in motion. (The images can be recorded on film or video for later viewing.) Fluoroscopy is performed on its own to evaluate the movement of the diaphragm and lungs, but it is most often used in conjunction with other tests—for example, to guide catheter placement during cardiac catheterization. (For more on fluoroscopy, see Chapter 2.)

Purpose of the Test

• To evaluate the motion of the diaphragm, lungs, and other structures in the chest during breathing.
• To detect obstructions of the airways or blood vessels.
• To guide the placement of catheters, endoscopes (thin tubes used for viewing internal structures), and other instruments in various medical procedures.

Who Performs It

• A radiologist or a qualified technician.

Special Concerns

• Pregnant women should not undergo this test because exposure to ionizing radiation may harm the fetus.
• During the test, any movements other than those requested by the examiner may affect the results.

Before the Test

• Remove any clothing or jewelry covering the area being examined.
• Additional preparation may be needed if a contrast dye is being administered, or if the test is being done in conjunction with another exam.

What You Experience

• An x-ray tube is suspended or held over your body; it transmits continuous images to a viewing monitor.
• Depending on the nature of the examination, the examiner may ask you to assume different positions, cough, breathe in and out, and perform other movements while you are exposed to the x-rays.
• When performed alone, fluoroscopy usually takes about 5 minutes.

Risks and Complications

• Although radiation exposure is minimal, you receive a higher dose than during standard x-ray procedures.

After the Test

• You are free to resume your normal activities unless you need to observe restrictions associated with other tests performed in conjunction with fluoroscopy.

Estimated Cost: $$

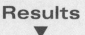

Results

➡ A physician will examine the test images and video for evidence of any abnormality.
➡ If a definitive diagnosis can be made, appropriate treatment will be initiated.
➡ In some cases, additional tests may be needed to further evaluate abnormal results.

Fluoroscopy

Gallium Scan

Gallium Scan

Description

• In this nuclear imaging test, you are given an intravenous injection of a radioactive form of gallium (gallium-67), and a special camera records the movement and uptake of this radioactive material throughout your body. The camera data are then translated by computer into two-dimensional images that are recorded on film. Gallium-67 tends to concentrate in areas of inflammation and infection, abscesses, and benign and malignant tumors. The recorded images will show any areas of unusual gallium concentration that may require further investigation. (For more on nuclear imaging, see Chapter 2.)

Purpose of the Test

• To detect primary and metastatic cancers and inflammatory lesions.
• To evaluate malignant lymphoma and identify tumors that recur after chemotherapy or radiation therapy.
• To determine the stage of lymphomas and lung cancer.
• To monitor the response to treatment for infection, inflammation, or tumor.
• To clarify focal defects (areas that appear altered due to disease) in the liver.

Who Performs It

• A radiologist or a technician trained in nuclear medicine.

Special Concerns

• Nuclear imaging tests should not be performed in pregnant or breastfeeding women because of possible risks to the fetus or infant.
• This procedure should be performed before any barium contrast x-rays of the digestive tract because the presence of residual barium may impair visualization of gallium activity in the bowel.

• Uptake of the radioactive gallium by the liver and spleen may prevent the detection of abnormal lymph nodes near the aorta (illustrated on page 20) in patients with Hodgkin's disease, leading to false-negative results (see page 35).

Before the Test

• A laxative or a cleansing enema is usually administered prior to the scan to minimize increased gallium uptake within the bowel.
• You will be asked to disrobe above the waist and put on a hospital gown. Remove any jewelry, dentures, or other metal objects that could affect the scan.

What You Experience

• A technologist will inject the radioactive gallium into a vein in your hand or arm.
• About 4 to 6 hours later, a total-body scan may be performed.
• You will lie on a table and a large scanning camera, which detects the gamma rays being emitted by the radioactive gallium, is slowly passed over your body.

Results

▼

➡ A physician will analyze the recorded images for evidence of a suspected disorder.
➡ If a definitive diagnosis can be made based on these images, appropriate therapy will be initiated, depending on the specific problem.
➡ In some cases, additional diagnostic imaging tests, such as a CT scan, ultrasound, or a PET scan, may be necessary to clarify the results. (These imaging procedures are also described in Chapter 2.)

• The images provided by the camera are recorded on film.

• Additional scans are taken periodically, usually 24, 48, and 72 hours after the injection of gallium.

• During the scanning process, you will be asked to assume different positions, including lying on your back, stomach, and side.

• Each scan usually takes about 30 to 60 minutes to perform.

Risks and Complications

• The trace amount of radioactive material used in this test is not associated with any risks or complications.

After the Test

• You are free to leave and resume your normal activities.

• Drink extra fluids to help your body eliminate the radioactive gallium.

• Blood may collect and clot under the skin (hematoma) at the injection site; this is harmless and will resolve on its own. For a large hematoma that causes swelling and discomfort, apply ice initially; after 24 hours, use warm, moist compresses to help dissolve the clotted blood.

Estimated Cost: $$$

Gallium Scan continued

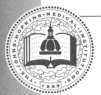

Gastrointestinal Nuclear Scans
(GI Nuclear Scans)

Description

• In this test, a small amount of radioactive material is introduced into your body, and a special camera records the movement and uptake of the radiotracer within different organs of the gastrointestinal (GI) tract. The resulting images provide information about these organs and the function of your digestive system. There are five common types of GI nuclear scans. In the **gallbladder nuclear scan, GI bleeding scan,** and **liver-spleen scan,** a radiotracer is injected into one of your veins. The **gastroesophageal reflux scan** and **gastric emptying scan** require ingesting a radiotracer orally. (For more on nuclear imaging, see Chapter 2.)

Purpose of the Test
Gallbladder nuclear scan:
• To detect an acute infection of the gallbladder (cholecystitis), blockage of a bile duct, or signs of rejection of a transplanted liver.

GI bleeding scan:
• To identify the locations of bleeding in the GI tract.

Liver-spleen scan:
• To assess liver function; screen for liver metastases (cancer spread into surrounding tissues); detect tumors, cysts, and abscesses in the liver and spleen; or demonstrate enlargement of the liver or spleen.

Gastroesophageal reflux scan:
• To measure the emptying rate of the esophagus and detect gastroesophageal reflux (backflow of stomach acid into the esophagus) in people with persistent symptoms such as heartburn, regurgitation, or difficulty swallowing.

Gastric emptying scan:
• To aid in the diagnosis of digestive disorders in people with symptoms that suggest delayed stomach emptying, such as unexplained nausea, vomiting, bloating, or early sensation of fullness. Possible causes include an obstruction (such as a peptic ulcer) and gastroparesis (a condition caused by nerve damage that primarily occurs in people with diabetes).

Who Performs It
• A radiologist or a technician.

Special Concerns
• This test should not be performed in pregnant or breastfeeding women because of possible risks to the fetus or infant.
• Residual radioactive material from other recent nuclear imaging tests, such as a thyroid or bone scan, may interfere with the results.
• Movement during the test can interfere with the results.
• In the gastric emptying scan, eggs are usually used to hold the radiotracer. If you are allergic to eggs, notify your doctor. Another food can be substituted.

Before the Test
• Do not eat or drink anything for at least 2 hours before a gallbladder scan.

Results

▼

➡ A physician analyzes the recorded images for any abnormalities in the structure or function of the organ being examined.

➡ If a definitive diagnosis can be made, appropriate treatment will be initiated, depending on the specific problem.

➡ In some cases, additional tests may be needed for further evaluation of abnormal results.

• Do not eat or drink anything after midnight on the day before a gastric emptying scan.

• No fasting is required for a liver-spleen scan or a GI bleeding scan.

• For a gastroesophageal reflux scan, you should eat a full meal just before the test.

• Remove any jewelry or metal objects before the test begins.

What You Experience

• For the gallbladder, GI bleeding, and liver-spleen scans, a radiotracer is injected into a vein in your arm. (Other than the minor discomfort of this injection, the procedure is painless.)

• The gastric emptying scan requires eating a meal of scrambled eggs that has been mixed with a radiotracer, while for the gastroesophageal reflux scan, the radioactive material is ingested in a liquid mixture.

• You are placed in various positions under a large scanning camera, which detects the gamma rays being emitted by the radiotracer. You will be asked to remain still while the pictures are taken.

• The initial scans may take up to an hour. Scanning may then be repeated periodically to assess organ function. For example, to evaluate gastric emptying, sequential images of the stomach are obtained at 15- to 30-minute intervals over several hours. To detect GI bleeding, which is often intermittent, delayed films may be taken up to 24 hours after the initial scans.

Risks and Complications

• The trace amount of radioactive material used in these tests is not associated with significant risks or complications.

• In extremely rare cases, patients may be hypersensitive to the radiotracer and may experience an adverse reaction.

After the Test

• You may resume your normal activities.

• Drink extra fluids to help your body eliminate the radioactive material.

• If the radiotracer was administered by injection, blood may collect and clot under the skin (hematoma) at the injection site; this is harmless and will resolve on its own. For a large hematoma that causes swelling and discomfort, apply ice initially; after 24 hours, use warm, moist compresses to help dissolve the clotted blood.

Estimated Cost: $$$

Gastrointestinal Nuclear Scans continued

Glucose Tests

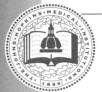

Glucose Tests

Description

• Diabetes mellitus is a disorder characterized by abnormally high blood glucose levels (hyperglycemia). Glucose, a type of sugar, is the body's primary source of energy. In type 1 diabetes, blood glucose is elevated because the pancreas produces little or no insulin—the hormone that permits cells to remove glucose from the blood; in type 2 diabetes, high blood glucose develops because the body's cells are resistant to insulin. The following glucose tests are performed to diagnose or monitor diabetes.

• A single blood sample taken anytime after eating that day may be sufficient for a diagnosis; a blood glucose level above 200 milligrams per deciliter (mg/dL) associated with the classic symptoms of hyperglycemia—thirst, frequent urination, and weight loss—indicates that diabetes is present.

• **Fasting blood glucose** measures blood glucose levels after a 12- to 14-hour fast. While levels normally decrease during fasting, they remain persistently high in people with diabetes. A fasting glucose value above 125 mg/dL on at least 2 tests indicates diabetes.

• **Postprandial blood glucose** measures blood glucose levels 2 hours after eating a meal. This test is usually done in people who have symptoms of hyperglycemia, or when the results of a fasting glucose test suggest possible diabetes, but are inconclusive. Values of 200 mg/dL or more indicate diabetes.

• **The oral glucose tolerance test** is not necessary in most cases, but is the method of choice to detect diabetes when results from the fasting and postprandial tests are borderline or inconclusive. In this test, glucose levels in the blood and urine are measured periodically for several hours following the ingestion of a beverage containing a specified dose (usually 75 grams) of glucose.

• **Hemoglobin A1c (HbA1c),** also known as the glycosylated hemoglobin or glycohemo-globin test, is used to monitor the effectiveness of therapy in people already diagnosed with diabetes. This test measures the amount of glucose attached to hemoglobin (the oxygen-carrying protein in red blood cells), which increases as blood glucose levels rise. Since hemoglobin circulates in the blood until the red blood cells die (half the red blood cells are replaced every 12 to 16 weeks), the HbA1c test is a useful tool for measuring average blood glucose values over the previous 2 to 3 months.

Purpose of the Test

• The fasting, postprandial, and oral glucose tolerance tests are used to diagnose type 1 or type 2 diabetes mellitus.

• HbA1c is used to monitor the effectiveness of dietary or drug therapy in the management of diabetes mellitus.

Who Performs It

• A lab technician or nurse.

Special Concerns

• A wide variety of factors—including medica-

Results

▼

➡ Chemical tests are performed on the blood and urine samples to measure the level of glucose. These results and the presence of risk factors for diabetes will help your doctor in making a diagnosis. (For more on laboratory testing, see Chapter 1.)

➡ If you test positive for diabetes, the condition can be treated with dietary measures, exercise, and, if necessary, oral glucose-lowering medications or insulin injections.

tions, some herbs and supplements, diet, recent illness, pregnancy, infection, stress, smoking, caffeine, and strenuous exercise—may affect blood glucose levels and interfere with the accuracy of results.

Before the Test
• Report to your doctor any medications, herbs, or supplements you are taking. You may be advised to discontinue certain of these agents before all of these tests, except HbA1c.

Fasting glucose test:
• Fast for 12 to 14 hours before the test (but no longer than 16 hours). Water is permitted.

Postprandial glucose test:
• A fasting blood glucose test is performed to establish the pre-test blood glucose level.
• You will be instructed to eat a balanced meal containing at least 75 grams of carbohydrates, and then fast for 2 hours.
• Do not smoke or perform any strenuous activities after the meal.

Oral glucose tolerance test:
• Your doctor will advise you to maintain a high-carbohydrate diet for 3 days before the test.
• You should fast for 12 to 14 hours before the test. Water is permitted.
• Do not smoke, exercise strenuously, or drink coffee or alcohol for 8 hours before the test.
• Your doctor may weigh you to determine the appropriate amount of glucose to include in the test beverage.
• You may want to bring something to read during the test.

HbA1c test:
• No advance preparation is necessary.

What You Experience
Fasting, postprandial, and HbA1c tests:
• A sample of your blood is drawn from a vein, usually in your arm, and sent to a laboratory for analysis. (For more on this procedure, called venipuncture, see page 32.)

Oral glucose tolerance test:
• Blood will be drawn using venipuncture and a urine specimen will be obtained to determine fasting glucose levels.
• You will be given a glucose-laden beverage. It will be very sweet. (It may be diluted with a small amount of lemon juice and water.)
• You won't be allowed to eat anything until the test is complete, but you may drink water.
• Additional blood samples are taken at 30 minutes, 60 minutes, and hourly intervals after you drink the glucose beverage.
• Urine specimens are taken at hourly intervals.
• The total test time is usually 3 hours, but may last up to 6 hours.

Risks and Complications
• The fasting, postprandial, and HbA1c tests are associated with no risks.
• You may experience symptoms of hypo-glycemia (weakness, restlessness, hunger, sweating, nervousness) during the oral glucose tolerance test. Tell your doctor immediately if this happens. If these symptoms persist, you will be given orange juice, and the test will be discontinued.

After the Test
• After blood is drawn, pressure is applied (with cotton or gauze) to the puncture site.
• You may be given a snack or some orange juice after the oral glucose tolerance test.
• You may resume your normal diet, activities, and any medications withheld before the test.
• Blood may collect and clot under the skin (hematoma) at the puncture site; this is harmless and will resolve on its own. For a large hematoma that causes swelling and discomfort, apply ice initially; after 24 hours, use warm, moist compresses.

Estimated Cost: $$

Glucose Tests continued

Head and Neck CT Scan
(Computed Tomography Scan of the Head and Neck, Cranial CT Scan)

Description

• A body scanner delivers x-rays to the head and neck area at many different angles. A computer then compiles this information to construct highly detailed, cross-sectional images of internal structures. In some cases, a contrast dye may be injected to better define tissues and blood vessels on the images. This procedure is used to detect abnormalities outside of the skull; for a description of a brain CT scan, see page 121. (For more on CT scanning, see Chapter 2.)

Purpose of the Test

• To detect inflammation, tumors and other masses, and other abnormalities in the head and neck region, including the mouth, tongue, salivary glands, throat (pharynx), sinuses, nasal cavities, vocal cords (larynx), and ear.
• To investigate the cause of hearing loss, detect bone or soft tissue damage in the ear, confirm abnormalities of the cochlea (a cone-shaped tube in the inner ear), and identify candidates for a cochlear implant.
• To determine the extent of head or neck tumors before treatment for cancer, and to monitor the area for recurrence after cancer therapy.

Who Performs It

• A radiologist and/or a trained technician.

Special Concerns

• CT scans are not usually done during pregnancy because exposure to ionizing radiation may harm the fetus.
• People who experience claustrophobia may find it difficult to undergo a CT scan, which takes place in a narrow, tunnel-like structure.
• People with allergies to iodine or shellfish may experience an allergic reaction to the iodine-based contrast material.

Before the Test

• Inform your doctor if you have an allergy to iodine or shellfish. You may be given a combined antihistamine-steroid preparation to reduce the risk of an allergic reaction.
• Tell your doctor if you suffer from claustrophobia. He or she may prescribe a sedative that can help you tolerate the procedure.
• If a contrast dye is to be used, drink large amounts of fluids on the day before the test to prevent dehydration. Do not eat or drink anything for 1 to 2 hours before the test. (Fasting is unnecessary before noncontrast CT scans.)
• Remove any hair clips, jewelry, dentures, glasses, and other metal objects from your head and neck.
• If a contrast dye is to be administered, an intravenous (IV) needle or catheter is inserted into a vein in your arm immediately before the test begins.

What You Experience

• You will lie on your back on a narrow table, and your head and neck are advanced into the CT scanner. Your head is immobilized

Results

▼

➡ A radiologist will examine the CT images for evidence of any abnormality.

➡ If a definitive diagnosis can be made, appropriate treatment will be initiated, depending on the specific problem.

➡ In some cases, additional tests, such as fine needle aspiration of a head or neck mass (see page 201), laryngoscopy (see page 236), or thyroid ultrasound (see page 360), may be needed to establish a diagnosis and determine the extent of the problem.

but your face is left uncovered.

• The scanner takes pictures at different intervals and varying levels over your head and neck area, so you will feel the table move during the test. The resulting images are displayed on a viewing monitor and recorded on x-ray film.

• You must remain still because any movement can distort the image on the scan.

• A contrast dye may be administered through the IV line in your arm to help define blood vessels and various tissues. (Upon injection of the dye, you may experience a brief flushing sensation and a metallic taste in the mouth.)

• The test usually takes 30 minutes to 1 hour. However, if a contrast dye is used, the procedure time may be longer because scans are taken before and after the dye is administered.

Risks and Complications

• Although radiation exposure is minimal, you will receive a higher dose of radiation than during standard x-ray procedures.

• Some people may experience an allergic reaction to the iodine-based contrast dye, which can cause symptoms such as nausea, sneezing, vomiting, hives, and occasionally a life-threatening response called anaphylactic shock. Emergency medications and equipment are kept readily available.

After the Test

• If contrast dye was used, you are encouraged to drink clear fluids to avoid dehydration and help flush the dye out of your system.

• You may leave the testing facility and resume your normal diet and activities.

• Blood may collect and clot under the skin (hematoma) at the dye injection site; this is harmless and will resolve on its own. For a large hematoma that causes swelling and discomfort, apply ice initially; after 24 hours, use warm, moist compresses to help dissolve the clotted blood.

• Delayed allergic reactions to the contrast dye, such as hives, rash, or itching, may appear 2 to 6 hours after the procedure. If this occurs, your doctor will prescribe antihistamines or steroids to ease your discomfort.

Estimated Cost: $$$

Head and Neck CT Scan continued

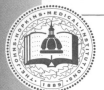

Head and Neck MRI
(Magnetic Resonance Imaging of the Head and Neck)

Head and Neck MRI

Description
• This test uses a strong magnetic field combined with radiofrequency waves to create highly detailed, cross-sectional images of internal structures in the head and neck area; these scans are examined for abnormalities. For certain studies, an MRI contrast dye such as gadolinium may be injected to provide better definition of soft tissues and blood vessels and thus enhance the images. This procedure is used to detect abnormalities outside of the skull; for a description of a brain MRI, see page 119. (For more on how MRI works, see Chapter 2.)

Purpose of the Test
• To detect inflammation, tumors and other masses, and other abnormalities in the head and neck region, including the mouth, tongue, salivary glands, throat (pharynx), sinuses, nasal cavities, vocal cords (larynx), and ear.
• To investigate the cause of hearing loss and detect soft tissue damage in the inner ear.
• To determine the extent of head or neck tumors before treatment for cancer, and to monitor the area for recurrence after cancer therapy.

Who Performs It
• A radiologist and/or a trained technician.

Special Concerns
• People who experience claustrophobia may find it difficult to undergo an MRI, which takes place in a narrow, tunnel-like structure. In some cases, an open MRI—a larger unit that is open on several sides—may be used as an alternative.
• Because the MRI generates a strong magnetic field, it cannot be performed on people who have certain types of internally placed metallic devices, including pacemakers, inner ear implants, or intracranial aneurysm clips.

• The test should not be done in pregnant women because the long-term effects of MRI on the fetus are unknown.

Before the Test
• Tell your doctor if you suffer from claustrophobia. He or she may administer a sedative to help you tolerate the procedure.
• Remove any magnetic cards or metallic objects, including watches, hair clips, belts, credit cards, and jewelry.

What You Experience
• You will lie down on a narrow padded bed.
• Your head and neck are advanced into the large, enclosed cylinder containing the MRI magnets.
• You must remain still throughout the procedure because any motion can distort the scan. Your head will likely be placed in a cradle to restrict movement.
• You may receive an injection of contrast dye before or during the procedure.

Results
▼

➡ The MRI scans are displayed on a video monitor and then recorded on film. The doctor will examine the images for evidence of any abnormality.

➡ If a definitive diagnosis can be made based on the images, appropriate treatment will be initiated, depending on the specific problem.

➡ In some cases, additional tests, such as fine needle aspiration of a head or neck mass (see page 201), laryngoscopy (see page 236), or thyroid ultrasound (see page 360), may be needed to establish a diagnosis and determine the extent of the problem.

• There is a microphone inside the imaging machine, and you may talk to the technician performing the scan at any time during the procedure.

• You will hear loud thumping sounds as the scanning is performed. To block out the noise, you can request earplugs or listen to music on earphones.

• The procedure lasts about 15 minutes but can take longer if a contrast dye is used.

Risks and Complications

• MRI does not involve exposure to ionizing radiation and is not associated with any risks or complications.

After the Test

• Most patients can go home right after the scan and resume their usual activities.

• Sedated patients may be monitored for a short period until the effects of the sedative have worn off.

• If a contrast dye was used, blood may collect and clot under the skin (hematoma) at the injection site; this is harmless and will resolve on its own. For a large hematoma that causes swelling and discomfort, apply ice initially; after 24 hours, use warm, moist compresses to help dissolve the clotted blood.

Estimated Cost: $$$

Head and Neck MRI continued

Hearing Tests

Description

• In order to hear normally, the three parts of the ear—the outer, middle, and inner ear—must work together. The outer ear canal directs sound waves toward the tympanic membrane (eardrum), which conducts them to the three connected bones in the middle ear. These bones then vibrate to conduct sound into the inner ear, where a coiled tube called the cochlea converts sound vibrations into nerve impulses and passes them to the 8th cranial nerve (acoustic nerve) leading to the brain. Hearing tests are designed not only to detect the presence of hearing loss, but also to determine where in this process a hearing problem originates. Impaired sound transmission through the outer and middle ear is known as conductive hearing loss; dysfunction of the cochlea, acoustic nerve, or higher nerve pathways is termed sensorineural hearing loss; both conditions together are known as mixed hearing loss. A thorough hearing evaluation usually involves several of the following tests:

• **Pure tone audiometry,** the standard test of hearing level, measures the ability to hear tones at different pitches and volumes—first as the sound is transmitted through air, and then as it travels through vibrations of the bone. By comparing these two types of sound conduction, this test can help to differentiate between conductive, sensorineural, and mixed hearing loss.

• **The speech recognition test** assesses your ability to hear conversational speech by measuring the lowest volume at which you can recognize a series of two-syllable words at least 50% of the time.

• **The word recognition test** evaluates how well you understand single-syllable words that are more difficult to hear (sometimes in the presence of background noise). Poor word recognition results from the sound distortion caused by hearing loss and may be improved by a hearing aid.

• **Acoustic immittance tests** measure the flow of sound energy into the ear and the resistance to that flow, and are valuable for evaluating the eardrum and middle ear for possible conductive hearing loss. In tympanometry, a special probe is used to alter air pressure in the middle ear and measure how sound conduction responds to this change. The acoustic reflex test measures the involuntary contraction of muscles in the middle ear in response to a loud sound (acoustic reflex); this reaction serves to protect the ear from potentially damaging noise levels. This test not only helps to confirm conductive hearing loss, but also may help to diagnose problems affecting the acoustic nerve (which initiates the acoustic reflex).

Results
▼

➡ Your doctor will review the test results, and consider them along with your symptoms, the visual inspection of your ear, and findings from other tests to reach a diagnosis. In addition to disease or injury affecting ear structures, possible causes for hearing loss include degenerative changes in the ear associated with aging, certain drugs, or repetitive exposure to loud noises. The extent of hearing loss, its treatment, and your prognosis depend on the nature of the problem.

➡ If your hearing tests, symptoms, and physical exam suggest the presence of a lesion along the hearing pathway, your doctor may recommend an imaging test of the head and neck, such as an MRI (see page 214) or a CT scan (see page 212), to determine the precise type and location of the lesion.

• **Otoacoustic emissions (OAEs)** are measurable sounds generated by a healthy cochlea in response to sound stimulation; they are produced by the movement of tiny cells, called hair cells, on the cochlear surface. In this test, a thin probe simultaneously emits a series of clicking noises into the ear and, with a tiny microphone, records the resulting OAEs produced by the cochlea. The absence of OAEs indicates cochlear damage. OAEs are typically measured to determine whether sensorineural hearing loss is due to cochlear dysfunction, or to problems beyond the cochlea affecting the acoustic nerve or brain (known as the retrocochlear area).

• **The auditory brainstem response (ABR)** is the involuntary electrical response that starts in the cochlea, travels through the acoustic nerve and the brainstem, and finally arrives in the hearing centers of the higher brain every time a sound is heard. In this test, clicking sounds or tones are used to stimulate the ABR thousands of times; these responses are measured by electrodes and transmitted to a computer that records and analyzes them. The resulting data help to evaluate the function of your sensorineural hearing tissue and identify the location of any cochlear or retrocochlear lesions.

Purpose of the Test

• To reveal the presence, type, and extent of hearing loss.

• The acoustic immittance, otoacoustic emissions, and ABR tests may also help to determine the cause of a hearing problem by identifying lesions or dysfunction in particular regions of the ear.

Who Performs It

• These tests are usually done by a doctor who specializes in hearing disorders (audiologist).

• The ABR test may also be performed by a neurologist or neurology technician.

Special Concerns

• Pure tone audiometry should be performed at least 16 hours after exposure to loud noises, such as loud music or heavy workplace noise.

In addition, the presence of tinnitus (ringing in the ear) may interfere with the results of this test.

• Because disorders of the middle or inner ear may disturb equilibrium as well as hearing, balance tests are sometimes performed in conjunction with hearing tests (see page 101).

Before the Test

• Wash your hair on the night before ABR testing, and do not consume coffee, tea, or caffeinated soft drinks for at least 4 hours before the test.

• Before pure tone audiometry, your ears may be checked for excess wax blockage. If necessary, you may be sent to a physician for wax removal.

What You Experience
Pure tone audiometry:

• You will enter a soundproof room and put on earphones.

• A series of tones is played into one ear. You are instructed to give a signal, such as raising a finger or pressing a button, to indicate that you heard the sound. The volume of the tones is lowered progressively until you can no longer hear them, and will then be intensified and lowered several more times. This process is then repeated in the other ear.

• Next, you will remove the earphones and put on a special headband with a small plastic piece that sits behind your ear and conducts sound vibrations through the bone. The series of tones is repeated, and you are again asked to signal when you hear them. This is done in one ear, then in the other.

• In some cases, background noise will be played into one ear to ensure it is not helping the other to hear the tones.

• The test takes about 20 minutes.

Speech and word recognition tests:

• You will wear earphones in a soundproof booth. (Speech recognition testing often follows pure tone audiometry.)

• For speech recognition, you will hear a series

Hearing Tests continued

of common, two-syllable words in one ear. You will be asked to repeat every word as you hear it. The volume of the words is lowered progressively until you can no longer hear them, and will then be intensified and lowered several more times. This procedure is repeated in the other ear.

• Word recognition testing follows a similar procedure, but uses one-syllable words. In some cases, the words will be presented first in quiet and then in the presence of background noise.

• Each of these tests takes about 10 minutes.

Acoustic immittance tests:

• A special probe is inserted into one ear so that no air can pass in or out of the ear; it feels like an earplug and may cause minor discomfort. (In some cases, silicone putty may be applied around the ear opening to ensure an airtight seal.)

• During tympanometry, the probe will change the pressure in your middle ear. (In rare cases, this may induce transient vertigo; tell the examiner if this happens.)

• For the acoustic reflex test, you will hear a loud tone emitted by the probe, but you do not need to respond. A loud noise may then be presented continuously for 5 to 10 seconds.

• Do not move, speak, or swallow as these tests are being performed. The examiner will warn you when to expect loud tones so you will not be startled.

• These tests take about 2 to 3 minutes each.

Otoacoustic emissions:

• A soft rubber probe is inserted into your outer ear canal and you will hear a series of clicking noises.

• You should sit quietly during the test.

• The test takes about 5 minutes.

Auditory brainstem response:

• You will lie on a bed or reclining chair. The skin on your forehead may be rubbed with a mild abrasive pad or gel to remove excess dry skin, and a special electrode gel is applied to improve electrical conductivity.

• Electrodes are placed on your forehead and on each earlobe, and then the lights are usually dimmed.

• Earphones are placed over your ears, and you will hear a long series of tones and clicking noises in one ear, and then the other.

• The electrodes and paste are removed with warm water and a washcloth.

• Testing usually takes less than 1 hour.

Risks and Complications

• None.

After the Test

• You may return home and resume your normal activities.

• Any electrode paste residue after ABR testing can be removed easily by washing your hair.

Estimated Cost: $$

HIV and AIDS-related Blood Tests

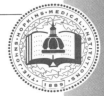

Description

• The human immunodeficiency virus (HIV) is an infectious viral organism that attacks immune cells and gradually destroys the ability of your immune system to fight against infection and disease. The last stage of HIV infection is known as acquired immunodeficiency syndrome, or AIDS. People with AIDS will eventually die from infection, cancer, or another ailment because their failing immune system is unable to combat the disease. The following are the major blood tests used to diagnose HIV infections and monitor the progression of the condition.

• **Enzyme-linked immunosorbent assay (ELISA)** tests for the presence of antibodies to HIV in the blood. If such antibodies are present, they will adhere to a plate coated with fragments of the HIV virus. The ELISA reagent will detect the bound antibodies and change color, indicating a positive result. ELISA, which is faster and less expensive than other HIV blood tests, is commonly used as the initial screening test for HIV infection. Positive results are confirmed by a repeat ELISA and a Western blot test.

• **Western blot** also tests for the presence of antibodies to HIV in the blood. In this test, a blood sample is exposed to a special paper that is impregnated with selected fragments of the HIV virus. Any anti-HIV antibodies that are present in the blood will bind to the viral fragments, producing a characteristic pattern. The Western blot very rarely produces false-positive results and is used to confirm the presence of HIV infection in people who test positive with ELISA.

• **CD4 count,** or T-cell assay, is a test to measure the level of the immune system's CD4 cells, which are part of the body's defense against infection. As HIV targets and destroys CD4 cells in the initial stages of infection, CD4 levels fall sharply. Later, as the body starts to cope with the infection, CD4 cell counts rise again. Eventually, however, the rate of CD4 destruction exceeds that of CD4 cell creation, and the CD4 count declines. Measuring the CD4 cell count is thus an effective way of assessing the condition of the immune system and monitoring the effects of treatment for HIV infection.

• **Viral load** is a test that provides a direct measurement of the quantity of HIV virus in your blood. The genetic material of the virus (RNA) is usually measured by the polymerase chain reaction (PCR), which can amplify and detect small amounts of specific RNA sequences in a blood sample. This test is valuable for the management of HIV infection because the viral load can aid in determining your prognosis and evaluating your response to treatment. People with high levels of HIV RNA in their blood, for example, are more likely to progress to AIDS than those with low viral levels.

Purpose of the Test
ELISA and Western blot:

• To screen for HIV infection in individuals at high risk for the disease.
• To screen donated blood for HIV.

Results
▼

➡ Your blood sample is sent to a laboratory for analysis.

➡ If you test positive for the HIV antibody with the ELISA or Western blot test, you will undergo a thorough health evaluation—including CD4 count, viral load, a skin test for tuberculosis, and various other blood tests.

➡ Depending on the stage of HIV infection—as determined by the CD4 count and viral load—your doctor may prescribe medications to reduce the amount of virus in your body and delay the progression of the condition.

HIV and AIDS-related Blood Tests continued

CD4 count and viral load:
- To determine the stage of HIV infection.
- To aid in deciding when to start anti-HIV medications.
- To monitor the response to therapy.

Who Performs It
- A doctor, a nurse, or a technician draws a blood sample.

Special Concerns
- The ELISA and Western blot assays cannot detect HIV infection until antibodies develop, which may take from 6 to 24 weeks after exposure. Thus, false-negative results can occur in the early incubation stage of HIV infection.
- False-positive results occur in about 2 out of every 1,000 people tested with ELISA. The Western blot assay produces very few false-positives, although it may rarely give ambiguous results. In such cases, the test is repeated. (For more on false-positives and false-negatives, see page 35.)
- A recent viral illness and certain medications can alter the CD4 count.
- CD4 counts vary from hour to hour throughout the day and must be evaluated in the context of your symptoms.
- Certain illnesses and some vaccinations may temporarily increase your viral load.
- Because the viral load test does not measure the extent of existing damage to your immune system, it must be used in conjunction with the CD4 cell count.

Before the Test
- You will receive counseling about the test and the implications of the results.

What You Experience
- A sample of your blood is drawn from a vein, usually in your arm, and sent to a laboratory for analysis. (For more on this procedure, called venipuncture, see page 32.)

Risks and Complications
- None.

After the Test
- Immediately after blood is drawn, pressure is applied (with cotton or gauze) to the puncture site.
- You are free to resume your usual activities.
- Blood may collect and clot under the skin (hematoma) at the puncture site; this is harmless and will resolve on its own. For a large hematoma that causes swelling and discomfort, apply ice initially; after 24 hours, use warm, moist compresses to help dissolve the clotted blood.

Estimated Cost: $$

Holter Monitoring
(Ambulatory ECG Monitoring)

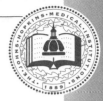

Description
• ECG leads (see page 174) are attached to a small, portable device that continuously records heart rate and rhythm over a 24-hour period or longer. Results are then analyzed with the assistance of a computer to identify heart rhythm disturbances (arrhythmias) or other cardiac problems.

Purpose of the Test
• To detect and classify arrhythmias, especially in people with symptoms such as fainting, dizziness, palpitations, shortness of breath, or atypical chest pain.
• To evaluate the status of patients recuperating from a heart attack.
• To test the effectiveness of antiarrhythmic drugs or a pacemaker.
• To detect silent ischemia (deficient blood flow to the heart without symptoms such as angina) in patients with suspected heart disease but normal results on a resting ECG.

Who Performs It
• A doctor, a nurse, or a technician.

Special Concerns
• None.

Before the Test
• No special preparation is needed.

What You Experience
• ECG leads are applied to your chest or abdomen and taped securely in place. The leads are hooked up to a portable device that records your ECG on a small cassette tape or digital recorder. The device weighs about 2 lbs and is strapped or belted to your body.
• The most common type of monitor records continuously for 24 hours. Another device can be worn for 5 to 7 days; you must activate it yourself whenever symptoms arise.

• Go about your normal daily schedule and keep a careful diary of your activities (including walking, climbing stairs, sleeping, and sexual activity), any physical symptoms (such as dizziness), and medication doses—along with the time of day. (Most recording devices also have an "event" button that you press whenever you experience symptoms.)
• Bathing or showering is usually prohibited, but sponge baths are permitted. Try to avoid external magnetic or electrical sources, such as metal detectors, electric blankets or toothbrushes, or high voltage areas, though they will probably not affect your results.
• Be careful not to dislodge the leads; wearing a loose-fitting top that buttons in the front can help. If a lead loosens, the monitor light will flash and you should notify your doctor.

Risks and Complications
• None.

After the Test
• Return to the doctor's office or laboratory so the monitor and leads can be removed.

Estimated Cost: $$

Results
▼

➤ The ECG recording is interpreted by a computer and a report is printed. A cardiologist reviews the results along with your diary.
➤ If a cardiac arrhythmia or another problem is detected, treatment will be initiated.
➤ This test may fail to detect an arrhythmia if symptoms do not occur during the monitoring period. If your results are normal, it is up to your doctor to decide if further testing is needed.

Holter Monitoring

Hysteroscopy

Hysteroscopy

Description

• A thin, rigid viewing tube, called a hysteroscope, is inserted through the vagina and cervix and into the uterus. Fiberoptic cables permit the examiner to directly inspect the uterine cavity and endometrium (the tissue that lines the uterus) for any signs of disease or abnormality. If necessary, instruments (such as a tiny scissors or small electrical loop used to cut tissue) may be passed through the scope to perform therapeutic procedures. (The female reproductive system is illustrated on page 28.)

Purpose of the Test

• To help evaluate women with abnormal uterine bleeding, postmenopausal bleeding, infertility problems (when a deformity within the uterine cavity is suspected), or repeated miscarriages.
• To detect or evaluate uterine abnormalities, such as polyps, fibroids, and intrauterine adhesions (scar tissue inside the uterine cavity).
• Used therapeutically to remove polyps, small fibroids, and displaced intrauterine devices (IUDs).

Who Performs It

• A gynecologist trained in hysteroscopy.

Special Concerns

• Hysteroscopy is not appropriate in women who have pelvic inflammatory disease (PID) or vaginal discharge.
• Hysteroscopy is sometimes performed in conjunction with other procedures, such as laparoscopy (see page 234) or endometrial biopsy (see page 185).
• Depending on the extent of the procedure, hysteroscopy can be performed under general, regional, or local anesthesia, or with just a mild pain reliever and no anesthetic medication.
• If you still have menstrual periods, schedule the procedure for the week after the end of your menstrual cycle (before ovulation), to allow for better viewing conditions and to avoid interfering with a newly formed pregnancy.

Before the Test

• If general anesthesia is required, do not eat or drink anything after midnight on the day before the procedure.
• If the procedure will be performed under local anesthesia, you may be given a sedative before the test to relax you.
• You will be asked to disrobe and put on a hospital gown.
• Empty your bladder just before the test.
• Before the procedure begins, the doctor may perform a complete pelvic exam and may take cultures (see page 166) of the vagina and cervix.
• For general anesthesia, an intravenous (IV) needle or catheter is inserted into a vein in your arm and the medication is administered. In some cases, a thin tube attached to a breathing machine will be inserted through

Results

▼

➥ During the visual inspection of your uterus, the doctor will note any abnormality.

➥ If tissue samples or cultures are taken, specimen containers may be sent to several different laboratories for examination. (For more on laboratory tests, see Chapter 1.) Your doctor will review the results for any evidence of any abnormality.

➥ This test usually results in a definitive diagnosis. Your doctor will recommend an appropriate course of medical or surgical treatment, depending on the specific problem.

your mouth and into your windpipe to ensure you breathe properly during the procedure.

What You Experience

• You will lie on your back with your knees bent and your feet placed in stirrups.

• The vaginal area will be cleansed with an antiseptic, and the doctor will gently insert a lubricated speculum—a metal or plastic instrument that pushes apart the walls of the vagina to provide the examiner with a view of the cervix. This device may feel uncomfortable, but causes no pain. Relax and breathe through your mouth to ease the insertion.

• A local anesthetic is injected to numb the cervix. Alternatively, you will be under general anesthesia or a spinal (epidural) anesthetic will be injected into the spinal column to numb the pelvic region.

• The hysteroscope is carefully passed through the vagina and cervix and into the uterus. (If necessary, the cervix may be opened, or dilated, using blunt metal instruments of increasing diameter to ease insertion of the scope.) Magnifying devices provide the doctor with a direct view inside the cavity. An image of the area may also be transmitted onto a TV screen and photographs may be taken for later examination.

• The doctor may instill liquid or gas (such as carbon dioxide) through the hysteroscope to distend the uterine walls so that the tissue is easier to see.

• If appropriate, small instruments may be inserted through the scope to perform therapeutic procedures. If more detailed or complicated surgical procedures are necessary, the outside of the uterus may be viewed concurrently with laparoscopy.

• The hysteroscope is withdrawn.

• This procedure usually takes 30 minutes to 1 hour, but can take longer if extensive surgery is required.

Risks and Complications

• If gas was used to distend the uterus, you may experience transient pain in the upper abdomen and shoulder and shortness of breath (as gas passes into the abdominal cavity).

• Rare complications include infection, inadvertent perforation of the uterus (which requires surgical repair), and bleeding.

• If general anesthesia is used, the procedure carries the associated risks.

After the Test

• You will remain in the doctor's office or hospital until you recover from the effects of anesthesia (usually for about 1 to 2 hours). During this time, your vital signs will be monitored, and you will be observed for any signs of complications.

• Arrange for someone to drive you home.

• If you experience any pain in the upper abdomen and shoulder and shortness of breath (due to the passage of instilled gas from the uterus to the abdominal cavity), it should subside within 24 to 36 hours.

• You may experience mild abdominal cramping and slight vaginal bleeding for 1 or 2 days. You may be given a pain reliever, if needed.

• Contact your doctor immediately if you develop severe abdominal pain, excessive vaginal bleeding or discharge, or fever.

Estimated Cost: $$

Hysteroscopy continued

Immersion Oil Preparation

Description
• In this test, which is used to diagnose parasitic skin infections such as scabies or lice infestation, a specimen of the suspected parasite is obtained and then viewed under a microscope.

Purpose of the Test
• To determine whether a skin disorder marked by itching is caused by parasites that live on the surface of the skin, such as lice or the mites that cause scabies.

Who Performs It
• A physician.

Special Concerns
• If the test is performed on a lesion that contains no parasites, a false-negative result (see page 35) is possible. In scabies, for example, only a small proportion of sores actually contain mites.

Before the Test
• No special preparation is needed.

What You Experience
• If scabies is suspected, the doctor pours a drop of immersion oil on one of your sores and then uses a scalpel to scrape out the lesion. The immersion oil helps the mite stick to the scalpel blade.
• If a lice infestation is suspected, the doctor locates the lice with a magnifying glass and then picks them up using a forceps. The doctor may also obtain specimens of lice eggs by plucking or cutting the hairs to which they are attached.
• The test takes about 1 to 2 minutes.

Risks and Complications
• You may experience minor discomfort or pain if your skin is scraped.

After the Test
• You may resume your normal activities.

Estimated Cost: $

Results
▼

➡ The specimen is usually examined right at the doctor's office. If microscopic inspection identifies a specific parasite, appropriate medications will be initiated. (For more on microscopic examination, see Chapter 1.)

➡ If no parasite is found but scabies is still suspected, your doctor may prescribe a trial of antiscabies therapy.

Intravenous Pyelography
(IVP, Excretory Urography)

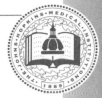

Description
• A contrast dye is injected into a vein in the arm, and a series of x-ray films is taken at timed intervals as the material flows through the kidneys, ureters, and bladder (illustrated on page 26). The dye delineates these structures on the x-ray images and reveals any abnormalities. Intravenous pyelography (IVP) is the most common imaging test for the evaluation of the urinary system. (For more on contrast x-rays, see Chapter 2.)

Purpose of the Test
• To evaluate the size, shape, structure, and function of the kidneys, ureters, and bladder.
• To aid in the diagnosis of urinary tract disorders, such as kidney stones, tumors, recurring infections, cysts, congenital abnormalities, or traumatic injury.
• To evaluate blood flow to the kidney and aid in the diagnosis of renovascular hypertension (increased blood pressure due to narrowing of the artery that leads to the kidney).

Who Performs It
• A physician or a radiology technician.

Special Concerns
• This test may not produce adequate visualization of the urinary tract in people with abnormal kidney function (due to poor uptake of the contrast agent by the kidney).
• IVP may not be safe for people with dehydration, significantly impaired kidney function, diabetes, or multiple myeloma (a type of cancer) because the contrast dye can worsen kidney function and may cause renal failure.
• People who have an allergy to shellfish or iodine may experience an allergic reaction to the contrast dye.
• Pregnant women should not undergo this test because exposure to ionizing radiation may harm the fetus.

• The presence of feces, gas, or residual barium from recent contrast x-rays can interfere with visualization of the urinary tract.

Before the Test
• Inform your doctor if you have an allergy to iodine or shellfish or if you've ever had an adverse reaction to x-ray contrast dyes. You may be given preventive medication to reduce the risk of an allergic reaction.
• Blood tests will be done to evaluate your kidney function (see page 311).
• You will be given an oral laxative on the night before the test, and an enema or laxative suppository on the morning of the test, to clean the intestines and provide a clearer view on the x-rays.
• Avoid solid foods for 8 hours before the test.
• At the testing facility, you will be given adequate fluids either orally or through an intravenous (IV) line to prevent dye-induced kidney damage.
• You will be asked to disrobe, remove any jewelry, and put on a hospital gown.

Results
▼

➡ The doctor will examine the x-ray films for evidence of any abnormalities in the kidneys and urinary tract.

➡ If a definitive diagnosis can be made, your doctor will recommend an appropriate course of medical or surgical treatment.

➡ In many cases, additional diagnostic tests—such as a kidney ultrasound (see page 80), a kidney CT scan (see page 76), cystoscopy (see page 170), or retrograde pyelography (see page 315)—may be needed to further evaluate abnormal results.

Intravenous Pyelography

Intravenous Pyelography continued

• Empty your bladder just before the procedure.
• A lead shield may be placed over the testes in men to block excess radiation. (However, in women it is not possible to shield the ovaries without obscuring the view of the bladder.)

What You Experience
• You will lie on your back on an x-ray table.
• A preliminary x-ray film is taken to ensure that there are no major abnormalities of the kidneys or urinary tract, and that no residual stool obscures visualization of these structures.
• Contrast dye is injected into a vein in your arm. You may feel a brief burning sensation and metallic taste in your mouth after the dye is injected. Report any other symptoms, such as flushing, nausea, or difficulty breathing, to your doctor.
• X-ray films are taken at regular intervals (usually at 1, 5, 10, 15, 20, and 30 minutes after dye injection) to follow the course of the dye as it is filtered from the bloodstream by the kidneys, and then passes through the ureters into the bladder. You may be instructed to change positions to promote the flow of the dye. Remain still as each x-ray is taken to avoid blurring the pictures.
• In some cases, a sequence of x-ray films (a technique called tomography) is used to produce cross-sectional images, or "slices," through the kidney.
• For several minutes, an inflatable belt may be wrapped around your abdomen and tightened to compress your ureters and keep the dye in your kidneys. This makes it easier to view the collecting systems within the kidney, and causes no discomfort.
• Finally, you will be taken to a bathroom and asked to urinate. A final x-ray film is then taken immediately to visualize the empty bladder and urethra.
• The entire procedure takes about 1 hour to complete.

Risks and Complications
• X-ray exams involve minimal exposure to radiation.
• Some people may experience an allergic reaction to the iodine-based contrast dye, which can cause symptoms such as nausea, sneezing, vomiting, hives, and occasionally a life-threatening response called anaphylactic shock. Emergency medications and equipment are kept readily available.
• Patients who are dehydrated or those with impaired kidney function may experience acute renal failure from infusion of the contrast dye. Adequate hydration before the test can reduce this risk.

After the Test
• You are encouraged to drink clear fluids to avoid dehydration and help flush the contrast dye out of your system. You may also receive IV fluids for several hours.
• Elderly or debilitated individuals may experience weakness as a result of fasting and the use of laxatives during test preparation, and may need to be assisted when first walking after the test.
• If there are no complications, you are free to leave the testing facility and resume your normal diet and activities.
• Delayed allergic reactions to the contrast dye, such as hives, rash, or itching, may appear 2 to 6 hours after the procedure. If this occurs, your doctor will prescribe antihistamines or steroids to ease your discomfort.
• Blood may collect and clot under the skin (hematoma) at the injection site; this is harmless and will resolve on its own. For a large hematoma that causes swelling and discomfort, apply ice initially; after 24 hours, use warm, moist compresses to help dissolve the clotted blood.

Estimated Cost: $$

Iron Tests

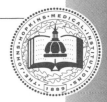

Description

Iron is an essential trace element—primarily derived from dietary sources—that is necessary for the formation of red blood cells. Iron deficiency will lead to anemia (low levels of red blood cells), while persistently high levels can be toxic to the body's organs. The following blood tests are used to measure iron levels in the blood, the amount of iron stored in the body, and the body's capacity to absorb iron.

• **Ferritin**—the major iron-storage protein—is measured to determine the amount of iron stored in the body.

• **Iron level** is determined by measuring the quantity of iron bound to the protein transferrin. Transferrin, which is formed in the liver, is the major carrier of iron in the bloodstream.

• **Total iron-binding capacity (TIBC)** measures all of the proteins available for transporting iron; since transferrin is the primary carrier, this test indirectly measures transferrin levels.

• **Transferrin saturation**—which is determined by dividing TIBC into the blood iron level—is the percentage of transferrin that is saturated with iron. If less than 20% of transferrin is iron-saturated, delivery of iron to developing red cells is impaired; if greater than 60% is saturated, iron may be deposited in organs other than the bone marrow, causing organ damage.

Purpose of the Test

• To detect or evaluate abnormalities of iron metabolism.

• To determine the cause of anemia and to monitor patients with chronic anemia.

• To detect or evaluate iron overload (hemochromatosis is the most common iron overload disease), and to monitor iron removal in people with hemochromatosis.

Who Performs It

• A nurse or a technician will draw the blood sample.

Special Concerns

• Taking iron supplements can affect the results of these tests.

• A nuclear medicine scan (see page 46) performed within the last 4 days may affect the results, because blood samples may be analyzed with a laboratory technique that also utilizes a radioactive isotope (radioimmunoassay).

• Blood samples should be taken early in the morning for the iron level test, since iron levels vary throughout the day.

• While no fasting is required before a ferritin test, recent ingestion of a meal containing a high iron content (from red meat, for example) can cause elevated levels.

Before the Test

• Tell your doctor if you have had any recent procedures, such as a nuclear scan, that intro-

Results

▼

➡ Your blood sample is sent to a laboratory for analysis. A doctor will review the results for evidence of iron deficiency, iron overload, or another problem. (For more on laboratory testing, see Chapter 1.) Abnormal results on iron tests can be caused by many conditions (including bleeding, malnutrition, malabsorption, excessive iron absorption, different types of anemia, liver disease, cancer, infection, and inflammation), as well as by blood transfusions.

➡ If an abnormality is found and the doctor can make a definitive diagnosis, appropriate treatment will begin.

➡ In many cases, abnormal results on one or more iron tests will necessitate additional tests to pinpoint the cause of the problem.

Iron Tests

duce radioactive material into your bloodstream, or if you have had a recent blood transfusion.

• Inform your doctor of any medications, herbs, or supplements that you regularly take.

• Do not eat or drink anything for 12 hours before a blood test for iron level, TIBC, or transferrin. No fasting is necessary before a test for ferritin levels.

What You Experience

• A sample of your blood is drawn from a vein in your arm and sent to a laboratory for analysis. (For more on venipuncture, see page 32.)

Risks and Complications

• None.

After the Test

• Immediately after blood is drawn, pressure is applied (with cotton or gauze) to the puncture site.

• You may return home and resume your normal activities.

• Blood may collect and clot under the skin (hematoma) at the puncture site; this is harmless and will resolve on its own. For a large hematoma that causes swelling and discomfort, apply ice initially; after 24 hours, use warm, moist compresses to help dissolve the clotted blood.

Estimated Cost: $

Joint Biopsy
(Synovial Membrane Biopsy)

Description
• A tissue sample from the synovial membrane—a thin layer of tissue that lines most of the body's joints—is extracted with a needle from a diseased joint and sent to a laboratory for microscopic examination. The procedure can be performed on any major joint, such as the knee, shoulder, elbow, hip, ankle, or wrist. It is typically done only when the results of less invasive tests, such as arthrocentesis (see page 97), are abnormal or inconclusive.

Purpose of the Test
• To aid in the diagnosis of disorders that damage the joints, such as joint infection, osteoarthritis, rheumatoid arthritis, systemic lupus erythematosus, and gout.
• To monitor the progression of certain joint disorders.

Who Performs It
• A physician.

Special Concerns
• This procedure must be performed with caution in people with a bleeding disorder.

Before the Test
• Tell your doctor if you regularly take anticoagulants or nonsteroidal anti-inflammatory drugs (such as aspirin, ibuprofen, or naproxen). You will be instructed to discontinue them for some time before the test.
• A blood sample will be obtained and coagulation studies (see page 157) will be performed to ensure you are a proper candidate for this test.
• Before the procedure begins, your doctor may administer a sedative injection.

What You Experience
• You are asked to remove any clothing covering the joint to be biopsied.

• The skin at the biopsy site is shaved and cleansed with an antiseptic, and a local anesthetic is injected to numb the area (you may still feel a brief pain as the biopsy needle is inserted).
• A trocar (sharp, tubelike instrument) is inserted into the joint space, and the biopsy needle is inserted through the trocar and into the joint.
• The needle is twisted to cut off a small piece of the synovial membrane. Several samples may be taken.
• The needle and trocar are withdrawn. Pressure is placed on the injection site until bleeding has stopped, and a small bandage is applied.
• The procedure usually takes 30 minutes.

Risks and Complications
• The most common aftereffects are swelling and tenderness at the needle insertion site. Serious complications, such as bleeding into the joint or infection, are rare.

After the Test
• You may be given pain-relieving medication.
• Rest the joint for at least 1 day before resuming normal activities.
• Call your doctor if you develop severe swelling or tenderness.

Estimated Cost: $$$

Results
▼

➡ Tissue samples are sent to a pathology laboratory and examined under a microscope for abnormal cells. (For more on microscopic examination, see Chapter 1.)
➡ A definitive diagnosis can usually be made. Appropriate treatment will be initiated, depending on the problem.

Joint Biopsy

Kidney, Ureter, Bladder X-ray
(KUB Radiography)

Description
• X-ray beams are passed through the abdomen, producing images of the kidneys, ureters, and bladder (illustrated on page 26) on a special type of film. This basic imaging test is often used as a first step in diagnosing problems of the urinary system, and is usually done in conjunction with intravenous pyelography, which is described on page 225. (For more on how x-rays work, see Chapter 2.)

Purpose of the Test
• To determine the size, shape, and position of the kidneys and bladder.
• To detect obvious abnormalities of the urinary system, such as kidney stones.
• To help differentiate between urologic and gastrointestinal diseases, which both produce abdominal pain.

Who Performs It
• A radiologist or a qualified technician.

Special Concerns
• Pregnant women should not undergo this test because exposure to ionizing radiation may harm the fetus.
• The presence of severe obesity, gas or feces in the intestine, or residual barium in the abdomen from a recent contrast x-ray study may interfere with clear visualization of the urinary system.

Before the Test
• You will be asked to disrobe, remove any jewelry or metal objects, and put on an x-ray gown.
• In men, the testes may be covered with a lead apron to prevent irradiation.

What You Experience
• You will be positioned on your back or stomach on a table, with your arms overhead, under an x-ray machine.

• You will be asked to take a deep breath and hold it while the x-ray is being taken, in order to provide a clear view of the abdomen. It is important to remain still throughout the procedure because any motion can distort the image.
• The procedure takes several minutes.

Risks and Complications
• X-ray exams involve minimal exposure to radiation.

After the Test
• You may return home and resume your usual activities.

Estimated Cost: $$

Results
▼
➥ X-ray films are usually ready shortly after the test is completed. A radiologist will examine the images for abnormalities.
➥ A definitive diagnosis can rarely be made based on a KUB study alone. In most cases, additional tests—such as ultrasound (see page 80) or intravenous pyelography—are required in order to establish a diagnosis and determine the extent of the problem.

KOH Preparation

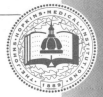

Description
• This test is used to identify fungal organisms in the skin, hair, or nails. The doctor obtains a tissue sample using a scalpel or another instrument. Heat and potassium hydroxide (KOH) are then applied to the sample to dissolve keratin—a fibrous protein that is a major component of skin, hair, and nails—as well as the skin cells that make keratin. Once these substances have been removed, fungal elements can be detected under a microscope.

Purpose of the Test
• To determine whether itchy, red, or scaly conditions of the skin, hair, and nails are caused by a fungal infection.

Who Performs It
• A physician.

Special Concerns
• If the sample is too small or is taken from an area in which there is no fungus, false-negative results (see page 35) may be obtained.
• Previous use of antifungal drugs may also lead to false-negative results.

Before the Test
• No special preparation is required.

What You Experience
• If your skin is the site of the suspected infection, the doctor scrapes the outer layer of abnormal skin with a scalpel.
• When the scalp is affected, the doctor gently removes diseased hairs with a forceps and also scrapes the scalp with a scalpel.
• For nail infections, the examiner scrapes the inner surface of the nail below the tip or clips off the portion of the nail that appears abnormal.
• You may experience some minor discomfort while the sample is being collected.

• Sample collection takes about 1 minute, and the results are usually available within 10 minutes.

Risks and Complications
• There are no risks or complications associated with this test.

After the Test
• You may resume your normal activities after the test.

Estimated Cost: $

Results
▼

➡ If fungal organisms are detected under a microscope, your doctor will prescribe appropriate antifungal medication. In some cases, a fungal culture (see page 166) may be performed to confirm the results or identify the specific type of fungus. (For more on laboratory testing, see Chapter 1.)

➡ If results are negative, your doctor may take a second sample or order a fungal culture to be done.

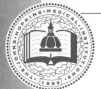

Lactose Tolerance Tests

Lactose Tolerance Tests

Description

• This test measures blood glucose levels after ingestion of a dose of lactose, a sugar typically found in dairy products. Normally, lactose is broken down by the intestinal enzyme lactase into the sugars glucose and galactose for absorption by the intestines. This test is used to identify people who are unable to digest lactose because of deficient levels of lactase, a condition known as lactose intolerance.

• In addition to or instead of the blood test, hydrogen levels in the breath may be measured after ingesting a dose of lactose. The concentration of hydrogen in exhaled air is directly proportional to the amount of lactose that remains undigested.

Purpose of the Test

• To detect lactose intolerance in people with typical symptoms of the condition, such as abdominal cramping and bloating, flatulence, and diarrhea.

Who Performs It

• A physician, a nurse, or a technician will conduct the test.

Special Concerns

• A false-positive result may be caused by engaging in strenuous exercise prior to the test or the presence of an intestinal malabsorption disease other than lactose malabsorption.

• People with diabetes mellitus may experience a rise in blood glucose levels despite lactose intolerance, yielding a false-negative result. (For more on false-positives and false-negatives, see page 35.)

Before the Test

• Do not eat or drink anything and avoid strenuous exercise for 8 hours before the test.

• Inform your doctor if you regularly take any medications, herbs, or supplements. Some of these agents may affect blood glucose levels and must be briefly discontinued before the test.

• Do not smoke before the test.

What You Experience

• An initial blood sample is drawn from a vein, usually one in your arm. (For more on this procedure, called venipuncture, see page 32.)

• The examiner then instructs you to drink a solution containing a specified dose of lactose dissolved in water.

• Three additional blood samples will be taken after 30, 60, and 120 minutes.

Results
▼

➡ Your blood glucose levels are analyzed. If lactase is deficient, lactose will not be broken down and the glucose levels will not rise as expected.

➡ The presence of accompanying symptoms such as cramping and diarrhea further suggest, but do not confirm, a diagnosis of lactose intolerance.

➡ In order to confirm that the presence of lower-than-expected blood glucose levels is due to lactose intolerance, you may need to undergo an oral glucose tolerance test (see page 210).

➡ If the test results indicate the presence of a severe lactase deficiency, there may be a variety of culprits, including inflammatory bowel disease and malabsorption syndromes. Additional testing will usually be done to identify the precise cause.

• If the hydrogen breath test is being conducted, you will also be asked to exhale into a special device at these times.

• The procedure takes about 2 hours.

Risks and Complications

• None.

After the Test

• Immediately after blood is drawn, pressure is applied (with cotton or gauze) to the puncture site.

• You may leave the testing facility promptly after the test is completed.

• If you are lactose intolerant, you may experience symptoms such as flatulence, bloating, diarrhea, or gas pains.

• You may resume your normal diet and any medications withheld before the test.

• Blood may collect and clot under the skin (hematoma) at the puncture site; this is harmless and will resolve on its own. For a large hematoma that causes swelling and discomfort, apply ice initially; after 24 hours, use warm, moist compresses to help dissolve the clotted blood.

Estimated Cost: $$

Lactose Tolerance Tests continued

Laparoscopy
(Pelvic Endoscopy, Peritoneoscopy)

Description
• In this surgical procedure, a rigid viewing tube (called a laparoscope) is inserted through a small incision in the abdomen, just below the navel. Fiberoptic cables permit a doctor to visually inspect the abdominal and pelvic organs for abnormalities. In addition, various instruments may be passed through the scope or inserted through other incisions to obtain fluid or tissue samples for laboratory examination or to perform therapeutic procedures.

Purpose of the Test
• To determine the cause of acute or chronic abdominal or pelvic pain or fluid accumulation in the abdomen.
• To detect and evaluate abnormalities affecting the female reproductive organs in the pelvis (see page 28); these include endometriosis (invasion of endometrial tissue, which lines the uterus, outside of the uterine cavity), ectopic pregnancy, pelvic inflammatory disease, and abnormal growths (tumors, cysts, adhesions, or fibroids).
• To detect and evaluate problems affecting the abdominal organs, such as tumors and cysts.
• To detect pelvic abnormalities that prevent pregnancy and test for patency of the fallopian tubes as part of an infertility evaluation.
• To obtain a tissue biopsy in order to confirm suspected cancer of an abdominal or pelvic organ, or to assess the severity of diagnosed cancer.
• Used therapeutically to perform procedures including appendectomy (removal of the appendix), tubal ligation (cutting and tying off of fallopian tubes), removal of the gallbladder, and hernia repair.

Who Performs It
• Depending on the purpose of the procedure, laparoscopy may be performed by a gynecologist, a gastroenterological surgeon, or a general surgeon.

Special Concerns
• The procedure may not be possible in people who have had multiple abdominal surgeries. Scar tissue may have formed, making it difficult to perform the procedure safely.
• Suspected internal bleeding (hemorrhage) may be a reason to postpone laparoscopy. Blood can obscure the view through the scope.
• Certain laparoscopic procedures can be performed with local anesthesia, but most require the use of general anesthesia (especially if extensive surgery is anticipated).

Before the Test
• Other tests, such as an electrocardiogram (see page 174) and a chest x-ray (see page 156), may be ordered to ensure that general anesthesia is safe for you.

Results

▼

➡ During the visual inspection of your abdominal cavity and pelvic region, the doctor will note any abnormalities. Any photographs taken during the procedure will later be reviewed.

➡ If tissue or fluid samples were taken, specimen containers may be sent to several different laboratories for examination. For example, biopsied tissue may be inspected under a microscope for the presence of unusual cells, or may be cultured (see page 166) for infectious organisms. (For more on laboratory testing, see Chapter 1.)

➡ This test usually results in a definitive diagnosis. Your doctor will recommend appropriate medical or surgical treatment, depending on the specific problem.

• Tell your doctor if you regularly take anticoagulants or nonsteroidal anti-inflammatory drugs (such as aspirin, ibuprofen, or naproxen). You may be instructed to discontinue them for 1 to 2 weeks before the procedure.

• Do not eat or drink anything after midnight on the day before the procedure.

• You will be asked to disrobe and put on a hospital gown.

• Empty your bladder just before the test.

• If local anesthesia is being used, you may be given a sedative before the test to relax you.

• If general anesthesia is required, the medication is administered through an intravenous (IV) needle or catheter inserted into a vein in your arm.

What You Experience

• You will lie on your back on an operating table.

• The hair surrounding your navel is shaved (if necessary) and the area is cleansed with an antiseptic. (If applicable, a local anesthetic is injected.)

• A small incision is made below the navel and a hollow, blunt-tipped needle is inserted through the incision into the abdominal cavity. Gas (carbon dioxide or nitrous oxide) is pumped through the needle to distend the abdominal walls so that the organs within are easier to see. The needle is withdrawn.

• The laparoscope is inserted through the incision. Magnifying devices permit the doctor to directly inspect the abdominal cavity and pelvic area, and images of the area may also be transmitted onto a TV screen. Photographs may be taken for later examination, and the scope may be moved to different locations as needed. (If you are conscious, you may be asked to perform certain simple maneuvers to improve the view of certain structures.)

• Following this visual inspection, the doctor may insert surgical instruments through the scope or through other small incisions to remove tissue or fluid samples for laboratory analysis or to perform therapeutic measures.

• The laparoscope is withdrawn, the insufflated gas is allowed to escape, and the incision is closed with stitches or staples.

• Depending on the extent of the procedure, laparoscopy may take from 30 minutes to several hours.

Risks and Complications

• Most patients experience temporary pain or cramping in the abdomen and referred pain in the shoulder (as a result of the instilled gas) for 24 to 36 hours.

• Rare complications include infection, inadvertent perforation of the bowel (which requires surgical repair), and bleeding. Call your doctor if you have severe pain, bleeding from the incision, or fever.

• If general anesthesia is necessary, the procedure carries the associated risks.

After the Test

• You will remain in the hospital until you recover from the effects of anesthesia. (Usually an overnight stay is not required, but overnight admission may be considered if extensive surgery was performed.) During this time, your vital signs will be monitored and you will be observed for any signs of complications.

• You may be given a pain reliever, if needed, to relieve any postoperative pain in the abdomen or shoulder.

• You may return home. After general anesthesia, you should arrange for someone else to drive you.

• You may resume your regular diet. However, your doctor may recommend that you avoid carbonated beverages for a few days, since they may adversely interact with the gases that were pumped into the abdominal cavity during the procedure.

• Your doctor may instruct you to restrict your activity for 2 to 7 days.

Estimated Cost: $$$

Laparoscopy continued

Laryngoscopy
(Direct or Fiberoptic Laryngoscopy)

Description

• In flexible laryngoscopy, a thin, flexible viewing tube (called a laryngoscope) is passed through the nose and guided to the vocal cords, or larynx (illustrated on page 22). Fiberoptic cables permit a physician to directly inspect the nose, throat, and larynx for abnormalities. This test is typically performed in a doctor's office using local anesthesia.

• Alternatively, a rigid viewing tube may be passed through the mouth for a more thorough inspection, a procedure called rigid laryngoscopy. Instruments may be passed through the scope to obtain tissue samples for microscopic examination, or to perform therapeutic procedures. Rigid laryngoscopy is done in an operating room under general anesthesia.

Purpose of the Test

• To detect laryngeal abnormalities, such as inflammation, lesions, or narrowed passages (strictures).

• To obtain a tissue biopsy in order to confirm suspected cancer of the larynx, or to assess the severity of diagnosed cancer.

• Used therapeutically to remove foreign objects or benign lesions such as polyps from the larynx.

Who Performs It

• A physician, usually an ear, nose, and throat specialist (otolaryngologist) or a surgeon.

Special Concerns

• This procedure may be combined with bronchoscopy (see page 134) and esophagogastroduodenoscopy (see page 194) to fully evaluate some people with known head-and-neck cancer; this variation is known as panendoscopy.

Before the Test

• Tell your doctor if you regularly take anticoagulants or nonsteroidal anti-inflammatory drugs (such as aspirin, ibuprofen, or naproxen). You may be instructed to discontinue these agents before the test.

• Do not eat or drink anything for 12 hours before the test if you are undergoing general anesthesia, or 8 hours if you are receiving local anesthesia.

• You will be instructed to remove contact lenses, dentures, and jewelry and to empty your bladder before the test begins.

• Before you receive general anesthesia, an intravenous (IV) needle or catheter is inserted into a vein in your arm.

• If local anesthesia is to be used, you may be given a sedative medication before the test, but you will remain conscious throughout the procedure. You may also be given a drug called atropine to help dry up your saliva. These drugs may be given orally or through an IV line.

Results
▼

➥ During the visual inspection of your mouth, throat, and larynx, the doctor will note any abnormalities. In some cases, this examination is sufficient to provide a diagnosis.

➥ If tissue or fluid samples were taken, specimen containers may be sent to several different laboratories for examination. For example, biopsied tissue may be inspected under a microscope for the presence of unusual cells, or may be cultured (see page 166) for infectious organisms. (For more on laboratory testing, see Chapter 1.)

➥ This test usually results in a definitive diagnosis. Your doctor will recommend appropriate medical or surgical treatment, depending on the specific problem.

What You Experience

Flexible laryngoscopy:

• You will sit upright in an exam chair in your doctor's office.

• Relax and breathe through your nose. A local anesthetic is sprayed into the back of your nose and throat to numb these areas and suppress the gag reflex (however, you may still gag and feel some discomfort when the laryngoscope is first inserted).

• The doctor inserts the scope through one nostril and closely inspects your nose, throat, and larynx.

• Photographs may be taken with a tiny camera attached to the scope.

• This procedure usually takes 5 to 10 minutes, though the anesthetic may last up to an hour.

Rigid laryngoscopy:

• You will lie on your back on an operating room table, and general anesthesia is administered.

• A rigid laryngoscope is inserted into your mouth and the doctor inspects your throat and larynx. Instruments may be passed through the scope to remove tissue samples for laboratory analysis. (In some cases, a special blue dye may be applied to suspicious areas in order to stain abnormal cells and identify areas for biopsy.)

• Photographs may be taken of the larynx with a tiny camera attached to the scope.

• If necessary, therapeutic procedures, such as removal of polyps, may also be done with a rigid scope and specialized instruments.

• This procedure usually takes 30 minutes to 1 hour.

Risks and Complications

• Most patients experience temporary hoarseness and a sore throat. Rare complications include inadvertent injury of the mouth or throat, bleeding, and infection.

• If the procedure was performed under general anesthesia, it will carry all the associated risks.

After the Test

• You will lie down in a recovery room to recuperate from the effects of anesthesia or sedation. (If you received general anesthesia, you will be placed with your head slightly elevated to prevent aspiration of foreign contents into your lungs.) During this time, your vital signs will be monitored, and you will be observed for any signs of complications.

• At first, you will be given a basin and asked to spit out your saliva rather than swallow it. If you had a biopsy, you will also be advised to avoid coughing, clearing your throat, and smoking until it is clear there are no complications.

• You may be given an ice collar to minimize any throat swelling.

• You may be given pain-relieving medication, if needed.

• If you received local anesthesia, you will not be allowed to eat or drink until your gag reflex returns, usually in a few hours. (Touching the back of the throat with a tongue depressor tests for this reflex.)

• You will likely be able to return home in 4 hours if local anesthesia was used; general anesthesia may necessitate an overnight hospital stay. You may then resume your usual activities and (according to your doctor's instructions) any medications withheld before the test.

• You may feel hoarse or have a sore throat for several days. Lozenges or a warm saline gargle may provide some relief. You may also cough up small amounts of blood for several days.

• Contact your doctor immediately if you develop excessive bleeding or a high fever after the test.

Estimated Cost: $$ to $$$$

Laryngoscopy continued

Lipid Profile
(Cholesterol Test)

Lipid Profile

Description

• Measuring levels of various blood fats, or lipids, in a blood sample can provide important information about the condition of arteries in the body (as well as the presence of liver disease and other conditions). The underlying cause of coronary artery disease (CAD) and most other cardiovascular diseases is atherosclerosis—the narrowing of large arteries by plaques made up of lipids such as cholesterol, as well as smooth muscle cells, collagen and other proteins, and calcium deposits. A lipid profile may contain the following components.

• **Total cholesterol.** The accumulation of the lipid cholesterol on artery walls plays a primary role in the development of atherosclerosis. Cholesterol is carried through the bloodstream on proteins, called lipoproteins, that are named according to their density properties. Total cholesterol levels include both LDL and HDL cholesterol.

• **LDL cholesterol.** Most cholesterol is transported on low-density lipoprotein, and is thus termed LDL cholesterol. Because LDL cholesterol is the major contributor to atherosclerosis and the most important risk factor for CAD, it is sometimes known as "bad" cholesterol.

• **HDL cholesterol.** Transported on high-density lipoprotein, HDL cholesterol helps to protect against atherosclerosis by removing cholesterol from artery walls and returning it to the liver for disposal. Thus, HDL cholesterol is commonly known as "good" cholesterol; high HDL levels may help to offset the negative impact of high total and LDL cholesterol levels.

• **Triglycerides.** Another major blood lipid that is primarily carried through the bloodstream on very-low density lipoprotein (VLDL), triglycerides serve as a storage source for energy. High levels also contribute to atherosclerosis, and are almost always accompanied by low HDL cholesterol levels.

Purpose of the Test

• To evaluate the risk of cardiovascular disease (particularly CAD).

Results

➡ Chemical tests are performed to measure lipids levels in your blood sample. (For more on laboratory testing, see Chapter 1.)

➡ The National Cholesterol Education Program (NCEP) recommends that total cholesterol levels be kept below 200 milligrams per deciliter (mg/dL).

➡ LDL cholesterol should ideally be kept below 100 mg/dL; between 100 and 129 mg/dL is classified as near or above optimal; between 130 and 159 mg/dL is borderline high; and 160 mg/dL and over is considered high.

➡ HDL cholesterol levels of less than 40 mg/dL are considered a risk factor for CAD. On the other hand, levels of 60 mg/dL or higher are considered protective against CAD.

➡ A normal triglyceride level is defined as less than 150 mg/dL; between 150 and 199 mg/dL is considered borderline high; between 200 and 499 mg/dL is classified as high; and 500 mg/dL or above is labeled very high.

➡ If this test was performed to assess CAD risk and your lipid levels are high, your doctor will set target levels and prescribe lifestyle measures (such as diet and exercise) and/or lipid-lowering medications to achieve them.

➡ If this test was done for another reason, your doctor will consider your lipid levels along with your history, your symptoms, and the results of other tests in order to make a diagnosis.

• To monitor lipid levels in people with known cardiovascular disease.

• To confirm a diagnosis of nephrotic syndrome (a kidney disorder), inflammation of the pancreas (pancreatitis), liver disease, and overactive or underactive thyroid gland (hyper- or hypothyroidism); all of these conditions can affect fat metabolism and are characterized by elevated blood lipid levels.

Who Performs It

• A nurse or a technician.

Special Concerns

• The results of this test may be affected by pregnancy, menopause, a wide variety of medications, smoking, current illness, recent surgery, alcohol, and failure to follow pre-test dietary restrictions.

• HDL levels vary according to age and gender.

Before the Test

• Report to your doctor any medications, herbs, or supplements you are taking. You may be advised to discontinue certain of these agents before the test.

• Since dietary intake affects cholesterol levels, be sure to follow your typical diet for at least a week before the test to maximize the accuracy of results.

• Do not consume alcohol for 24 hours before the test.

• Your doctor will instruct you to avoid eating or drinking anything for 12 to 14 hours before the test (water is permitted). For cholesterol testing, the last meal before the fast should be a low-fat one.

• If HDL cholesterol is being measured, you should also avoid exercise for 12 to 14 hours.

What You Experience

• A sample of your blood is drawn from a vein, usually in your arm, and sent to a laboratory for analysis. (For more on this procedure, called venipuncture, see page 32.)

Risks and Complications

• None.

After the Test

• Immediately after blood is drawn, pressure is applied (with cotton or gauze) to the puncture site.

• You may resume your normal diet and any medications withheld before the test.

• Blood may collect and clot under the skin (hematoma) at the puncture site; this is harmless and will resolve on its own. For a large hematoma that causes swelling and discomfort, apply ice initially; after 24 hours, use warm, moist compresses to help dissolve the clotted blood.

Estimated Cost: $

Lipid Profile continued

Liver Biopsy
(Needle Biopsy of the Liver)

Description

• A thin needle is used to extract a tissue sample from the liver, and this specimen is sent to a laboratory for analysis. A liver biopsy may be performed to obtain a specimen from a particular area of the liver that appears altered due to disease (focal defect), or to obtain a representative sample of tissue in order to diagnose disease that is present throughout the liver.

Purpose of the Test

• To diagnose or confirm the presence of liver disease, such as hepatitis, damage to the liver due to drugs, or cirrhosis.
• To distinguish between benign or malignant (cancerous) tumors that were detected on an imaging test, such as a CT scan.
• To determine the cause of unexplained liver enlargement, jaundice (yellowing of the skin), or persistently elevated liver enzyme levels (see page 111) when less invasive tests have proven inconclusive.

Who Performs It

• A gastroenterologist or a radiologist.

Special Concerns

• This procedure is not appropriate for people with infections near the biopsy site (such as in the lung), jaundice caused by a bile duct obstruction, or ascites (excess fluid in the abdomen); those who have difficulty remaining still and holding their breath; some people with anemia; and some patients with bleeding disorders.
• Blood coagulation studies (see page 157) are needed before the biopsy is done to ensure it can be performed safely.
• Obtaining the tissue sample may be difficult in obese patients.
• Rarely, a liver biopsy may be performed via laparoscopy (see page 234) rather than needle biopsy.

Before the Test

• Tell your doctor if you regularly take anticoagulants or nonsteroidal anti-inflammatory drugs (such as aspirin, ibuprofen, or naproxen). You will be instructed to discontinue them for some time before the test. Also mention any herbs or supplements that you take.
• Do not eat or drink anything after midnight on the day before the test.
• If needed, your doctor may give you a sedative injection to reduce anxiety.
• Empty your bladder before the test.
• You will be asked to disrobe above the waist and put on a hospital gown.

What You Experience

• You will lie down on your back with your right hand behind your head.
• The skin above the liver is cleansed with antiseptic, and a local anesthetic is injected to numb the area. (You may still experience some discomfort when the biopsy is taken.)
• The doctor will ask you to exhale completely and hold your breath. (You may practice this several times.)
• While you are holding your breath, the doctor quickly inserts the biopsy needle through the chest wall into the liver and withdraws a thin core of tissue; this takes about 1 second.

Results

▼

➡ The tissue sample is sent to a pathology laboratory and examined under a microscope for abnormalities such as scarring (cirrhosis), inflammation (hepatitis), or tumors. (For more on microscopic examination, see Chapter 1.)
➡ This test usually results in a definitive diagnosis. Treatment will be initiated, depending on the specific problem.

• In many cases, ultrasound imaging, CT scanning, or MRI (see Chapter 2) is used to guide placement of the needle in order to precisely target a specific lesion.

• Pressure is placed on the biopsy site until bleeding has stopped, and a small bandage is applied.

• The procedure usually takes about 10 to 15 minutes.

Risks and Complications

• Possible serious complications include bleeding, infection (peritonitis) caused by inadvertent puncture of a bile duct and subsequent bile leakage, and pneumothorax (leakage of air outside the lungs and into the pleural cavity, resulting in a collapsed lung) due to improper needle placement in the chest cavity.

After the Test

• You will lie on your right side in a recovery area for 1 to 2 hours after the procedure. (This compresses the liver against the chest wall, reducing the risk of bleeding or bile leakage.) You may be instructed to place a small pillow under your side during this period to provide additional pressure. During this time, your vital signs will be monitored and you will be observed for signs of complications.

• Drink only clear fluids (such as water or apple juice) for the first several hours. After this period, you may resume your regular diet.

• You may be given pain-relieving medication to allay any discomfort around the biopsy site.

• You should rest in bed for up to 24 hours.

Estimated Cost: $$

Liver Biopsy continued

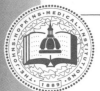

Lower Lip Biopsy
(Labial Salivary Gland Biopsy)

Lower Lip Biopsy

Description
• In this test, several tiny salivary glands from the lower lip are removed and sent to a laboratory for microscopic examination. This procedure is typically performed when the results of other tests, such as antibody testing (see page 89), suggest a diagnosis of Sjögren's syndrome (an autoimmune disorder marked by dryness of the eyes and mouth) or are inconclusive.

Purpose of the Test
• To confirm or rule out a diagnosis of Sjögren's syndrome.

Who Performs It
• A surgeon.

Special Concerns
• Lower lip biopsy should be performed with caution in people with blood clotting disorders. Blood tests to evaluate clotting function, or coagulation studies (see page 157), may be needed to ensure the biopsy can be done safely.
• The procedure may be performed in a hospital or an outpatient setting.
• The presence of mouth sores or infection may lead to false-positive results (see page 35).

Before the Test
• Tell your doctor if you regularly take anticoagulants or nonsteroidal anti-inflammatory drugs (such as aspirin, ibuprofen, or naproxen). You will be instructed to discontinue these agents for some time before the test. Also mention any other medications, herbs, or supplements that you take.

What You Experience
• You will sit in a dental chair.
• A local anesthetic (such as lidocaine) will be injected into your lower lip.

• When the anesthetic has taken effect, the doctor makes a small horizontal incision in the inner portion of the lip and removes at least 5 salivary glands. (Because they are so small, evidence of Sjögren's syndrome may not be present in all glands.)
• The incision is sutured closed.
• The procedure usually takes about 1 hour.

Risks and Complications
• Extremely rare complications include excessive bleeding or lip numbness at the biopsy site.

After the Test
• You may leave the testing facility and return to your normal activities.
• It may be difficult to eat solid foods for several hours after the procedure.
• You may be given pain-relieving medication to allay any discomfort around the biopsy site.
• Resume taking any medications that were discontinued before the test, according to your doctor's instructions.
• A follow-up examination may be scheduled to check the healing of the incision site.

Estimated Cost: $$$

Results
▼
➡ The tissue samples are sent to a pathology laboratory for microscopic examination. The presence of large clumps of inflammatory cells indicates Sjögren's syndrome. (For more on laboratory testing, see Chapter 1.)
➡ If a diagnosis of Sjögren's syndrome is confirmed, treatment for the condition will be initiated.

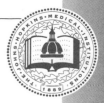

Lumbar Puncture
(Spinal Tap, Cerebrospinal Fluid Analysis)

Description
• In this test, a thin needle is inserted through the lower (lumbar) region of the back and into the spinal canal to measure the pressure and obtain a sample of the cerebrospinal fluid (CSF). CSF is a clear fluid that cushions the brain and spinal cord, transports many vital nutrients through the central nervous system, and carries out waste products. The fluid sample is then sent to a laboratory for analysis.

Purpose of the Test
• To measure the pressure of the CSF and help to detect obstruction of CSF circulation.
• To aid in the diagnosis of disorders affecting the brain or spinal cord, including infections such as meningitis or encephalitis, inflammation, tumors, bleeding, neurosyphilis, and multiple sclerosis.
• Used therapeutically to administer drugs into the spinal canal or to lower the pressure of the CSF.

Who Performs It
• A doctor, sometimes with the assistance of a nurse or a technician.

Special Concerns
• In some cases—for example, in people who cannot assume the curled position required for lumbar puncture or those with an infection near the standard puncture site—an alternative procedure may be performed, in which CSF is drawn from the upper spinal canal via a needle in the back of the neck (cisternal puncture).
• Lumbar puncture is not appropriate for individuals with increased pressure within the skull (intracranial pressure) or severe arthritis in the lumbar spine.

Before the Test
• Prior to lumbar puncture, you must undergo a CT scan (see page 121) to detect increased

pressure within the skull, which may make the procedure too dangerous to perform. You will also be given a basic neurologic assessment to evaluate your strength, sensation, and movement (especially in your legs).
• You will be advised to empty your bladder and bowels before the test.
• You will be asked to disrobe and put on a hospital gown.

What You Experience
• You will either lie on your side on a bed or table, with your knees drawn to your abdomen and your chin on your chest (someone may

---

Results
▼

➡ In some cases, your doctor will be able to immediately identify abnormalities in your CSF based on its appearance. For example, bloody fluid may indicate bleeding in the brain or spinal cord, while cloudiness may be a sign of an infection such as meningitis. High CSF pressure may suggest swelling, bleeding, or a tumor, while low pressure may indicate a blockage in the spinal canal above the puncture site.

➡ At the laboratory, your CSF sample will be analyzed for any abnormality, such as blood, bacteria, antibodies, cancer cells, or excessive protein or white blood cells. (For more on laboratory testing, see Chapter 1.)

➡ If a definitive diagnosis can be made, appropriate treatment will be initiated.

➡ In some cases, further imaging studies, such as skeletal CT scan or MRI (see pages 325 and 327), may be needed to clarify abnormal results.

Lumbar Puncture continued

help you maintain this position), or the procedure is done while you are seated and leaning forward at the waist.

• The skin at the puncture site is cleansed and draped, and the area is numbed with a local anesthetic. You may feel a brief stinging as it is injected.

• It is important to lie very still during the procedure. You should relax and take deep, slow breaths through your mouth.

• The doctor inserts a long, thin needle through your lower back and into the subarachnoid space, which is located between membranes that surround the spinal cord. You may feel some brief discomfort as the needle is inserted and repositioned. If you do, tell your doctor. He or she may be able to move the needle so you are more comfortable.

• Once the needle is properly positioned, a device called a manometer may be attached to it in order to read the pressure of the CSF. You may be asked to straighten your legs before the pressure is read.

• A sample of CSF is collected (which takes about 5 minutes). After measuring the CSF pressure again, the doctor withdraws the needle. Pressure is placed on the site and a small adhesive bandage is applied.

• Lumbar puncture takes 20 to 30 minutes.

Risks and Complications

• Lumbar puncture is generally safe. The most common side effect is a headache, which typically subsides with bed rest. In rare cases (less than 1%), a severe headache develops and you must stay at the testing facility until the pain subsides. In addition, transient back pain or tingling in the legs may occur.

• Rare but serious complications include persistent CSF leak, inadvertent introduction of bacteria into the CSF leading to meningitis, herniation (rupture) of the brain due to decreased CSF pressure, and accidental puncture of the spinal cord or a major blood vessel.

After the Test

• You may leave the testing facility. Avoid strenuous exercise or activity for 24 hours after the test.

• Drink plenty of fluids during the 24 hours after the test to replace the CSF lost by your body.

• If a headache develops, it is usually relieved by bed rest.

• Call your doctor immediately if you develop a fever, stiff neck, persistent headache, numbness, or weakness—which may indicate infection or another serious reaction.

Estimated Cost: $$

Lung Biopsy
(Needle or Open Lung Biopsy)

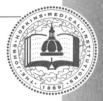

Description

• A tissue sample is extracted from the lung for laboratory analysis; the specimen is taken from an area that appears altered due to disease (lesion). Several techniques may be used, including **needle biopsy,** in which a long needle is passed through the chest wall and into the lung, and **open biopsy,** which accesses the lung surgically through a small incision. Tissue specimens may also be obtained by passing a tube-like viewing instrument called an endoscope through the airways (bronchoscopy; see page 134) or chest wall (thoracoscopy; see page 352).

Purpose of the Test

• To confirm a diagnosis of lung disease, such as inflammatory conditions, infection, or cancer—especially after a chest x-ray (see page 156), CT scan (see page 152), and bronchoscopy have failed to provide a conclusive diagnosis.

Who Performs It

• Needle biopsy is conducted by a physician assisted by a radiology technician.
• Open biopsy is performed by a chest surgeon and surgical team.

Special Concerns

• This procedure is not appropriate for some patients with pulmonary hypertension or serious bleeding disorders, as well as those with lung cysts or blisters, lung blood vessel abnormalities, respiratory insufficiency (as may occur with emphysema), and some types of heart disease.
• Chest x-rays, a CT scan, and certain blood tests, such as coagulation studies (see page 157), may be needed before the biopsy is done.
• Open biopsy, which requires general anesthesia, is performed less frequently than needle biopsy. It is generally done in cases where less invasive tests have been inconclusive, a large piece of tissue is needed to confirm a

diagnosis, or the lesion is well-defined and may require complete removal.

Before the Test

• Tell your doctor if you regularly take anticoagulants or nonsteroidal anti-inflammatory drugs (such as aspirin, ibuprofen, or naproxen). You will be instructed to discontinue them for some time before the test. Also mention any herbs or supplements that you take.
• Do not eat or drink anything for 12 hours before the procedure. (Sometimes clear fluids are allowed the morning of the test.)
• At the testing facility, you will be asked to disrobe and put on a hospital gown.
• Before undergoing a needle biopsy, the doctor may give you a sedative, if necessary.
• Immediately before open biopsy, an intravenous (IV) needle or catheter is inserted into a vein in your arm, and you are placed under general anesthesia. A thin tube attached to a breathing machine is inserted through your windpipe to ensure you breathe properly during the procedure.

Results
▼

➥ With an open lung biopsy, the doctor may be able to make a diagnosis by examining the structures in the chest.

➥ Tissue samples are sent to a pathology laboratory and examined under a microscope for unusual cells. They may also be sent to a microbiology lab and cultured (see page 166) for infectious organisms. (For more on laboratory testing, see Chapter 1.)

➥ This test usually results in a definitive diagnosis. Treatment will be initiated, depending on the specific problem.

Lung Biopsy

What You Experience

Needle biopsy:

• You are asked to either sit with your arms supported on a table or lie down on your stomach or back. The doctor will advise you to remain still and avoid coughing during the procedure to reduce the risk of needle damage to the lung.

• A local anesthetic is injected to numb the area where the biopsy needle will be inserted. (You may still experience a pinching pain when the biopsy is taken.)

• The doctor inserts a thin biopsy needle through the chest wall into the lung (sometimes through a small incision made with a scalpel). Fluoroscopic imaging or CT scanning (see Chapter 2) is used to guide the placement of the needle.

• You may be asked to hold your breath during needle insertion. A tissue specimen is obtained and the needle is withdrawn.

• Pressure is placed on the incision site until bleeding has stopped, and a small bandage is applied.

• The procedure takes 30 to 60 minutes.

Open biopsy:

• You are positioned on your back or side, and an incision is made in your chest.

• A portion of lung tissue is removed with surgical instruments, and the lung is sutured closed.

• A chest tube is left in place for about 24 hours, in order to drain fluid and air from the chest.

• An open lung biopsy can take 2 to 4 hours.

Risks and Complications

• Possible serious complications include bleeding in the lungs, infection, inadvertent needle-induced damage to the lung, or pneumothorax. (Pneumothorax, the collection of air in the pleural cavity that surrounds the lungs, always occurs after open biopsy. It is relieved by the chest tube left in place after surgery.)

• Open biopsy carries all the risks associated with general anesthesia.

After the Test

• You will remain in a recovery room for up to 3 hours after a needle biopsy; you may be hospitalized for 3 to 7 days after an open biopsy. During this time, your vital signs will be monitored and you will be observed for any signs of complications.

• You may be given pain-relieving medication to allay any discomfort around the biopsy site.

• You may cough up small amounts of blood temporarily. If it persists for more than 72 hours, notify your doctor.

• A chest x-ray is done after a needle biopsy to ensure that a pneumothorax has not developed.

• Arrange for someone to drive you home after you have recovered.

• Upon returning home after a needle biopsy, avoid strenuous activity for at least 24 hours.

• Go to the nearest emergency room if you experience chest pain or difficulty breathing.

Estimated Cost: $$$

Lung Nuclear Scan
(Ventilation/Perfusion Scan, Pulmonary Scintigraphy)

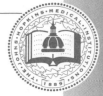

Description

• Nuclear scanning of the lungs includes two imaging procedures—ventilation scans and perfusion scans—that may be performed either separately or together. For the ventilation scan, you must inhale a radioactive gas; the perfusion scan is done by injecting a radioactive tracer into your bloodstream. A special camera then records the movement and uptake of the radioactive material in your breathing passages, air sacs, and pulmonary blood vessels (see the illustration on page 23). The resulting images indicate which portions of your lungs are receiving air and blood. (For more on nuclear imaging, see Chapter 2).

Purpose of the Test

• To help diagnose pulmonary embolism, a blood clot in an artery in the lung.
• To identify areas of the lung that are capable of ventilation (taking in air).
• To evaluate the function of different parts of the lung prior to lung surgery.
• To assess growths in the lungs before and after therapy.

Who Performs It

• A physician or a technician who specializes in nuclear medicine.

Special Concerns

• If you have had other recent nuclear imaging tests, such as a thyroid or bone scan, the results of this test may not be accurate.
• This test should not be performed in pregnant women because of possible risks to the fetus.
• The presence of conditions such as pneumonia, emphysema, pleural effusion (excess fluid in the space that surrounds the lungs), or tumors may interfere with interpretation of the results.

Before the Test

• A chest x-ray may be performed within 12 hours prior to this test or immediately afterward to detect any abnormalities that might affect the results of the scan.
• Immediately before the test, you will be asked to disrobe above the waist. (Women may wear a loose-fitting hospital gown that opens in the front.)

What You Experience
Ventilation scan:

• You are seated and the examiner places a breathing mask over your nose and mouth.
• The examiner asks you to follow specific instructions about inhaling and exhaling as you breathe in a mixture of air and radioactive gas.
• A large scanning camera takes pictures of your chest, recording the gamma rays emitted by the radiotracer.

Perfusion scan:

• The examiner injects a small amount of radioactive material into a vein in your hand

Results
▼

➡ A physician analyzes the results of the ventilation and perfusion scans for evidence of a specific disorder, such as pulmonary embolism or pneumonia.

➡ If a definitive diagnosis can be made, appropriate therapy will be started, depending on the specific problem.

➡ In some cases, additional diagnostic tests, such as pulmonary angiography or arteriography (see page 302), may be needed to clarify the results.

Lung Nuclear Scan

or arm. Other than this injection, the procedure is painless.

• A large scanning camera takes pictures of your chest from various angles as you are sitting or lying down and breathing freely.

• The combined ventilation/perfusion scan takes approximately 30 to 60 minutes.

Risks and Complications

• The trace amount of radioactive material used in this test is not associated with significant risks or complications.

• In extremely rare cases, patients may be hypersensitive to the radiotracer and may experience an adverse reaction.

After the Test

• Drink extra fluids to aid in the excretion of the radioactive material.

• You may leave the testing facility and resume your normal activities.

• After a perfusion scan, blood may collect and clot under the skin (hematoma) at the injection site; this is harmless and will resolve on its own. For a large hematoma that causes swelling and discomfort, apply ice initially; after 24 hours, use warm, moist compresses to help dissolve the clotted blood.

Estimated Cost: $$

Lymph Node Biopsy

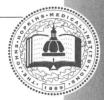

Description
• In this test, samples of lymph node tissue are taken from one or more locations; the specimens are sent to a laboratory for microscopic examination. (The lymphatic system is illustrated on page 19.) The following techniques may be used:
• **Fine needle biopsy,** which is done with local anesthesia, uses a long, thin needle to withdraw (aspirate) a specimen.
• **Excisional biopsy** is a surgical procedure performed to completely excise one or a group of lymph nodes through a small incision. This is the method of choice when lymphatic cancer (lymphoma) is suspected. It is usually done with local anesthesia, but may require general anesthesia and hospitalization (for example, to obtain deeper nodes).
• **Sentinel lymph node (SLN) biopsy** is a new technique that is increasingly used in cancer patients. Cancer cells can use the lymphatic system to spread (metastasize) throughout the body. Until this test, it was common to remove all lymph nodes nearest to a malignant tumor along with the tumor itself. But the so-called sentinel lymph node is the first one to receive lymphatic fluid draining from a cancer site; examining this node alone therefore indicates whether cancer has spread. Thus, surgeons can predict whether cancer is likely to be found in the rest of the lymphatic system without removing all of the nearby nodes. If the sentinel node contains no cancer cells, the other lymph nodes are likely to be clear, and a complete lymph node dissection may be unnecessary. If the sentinel node tests positive for cancer, however, all nearby nodes must be removed.

Purpose of the Test
• To distinguish between benign or malignant (cancerous) lymph node tumors, and to help diagnose lymphatic cancers such as Hodgkin's disease and non-Hodgkin's lymphomas.
• To determine whether cancer cells have metastasized to the lymph nodes from a nearby tumor.
• To identify the cause of lymph node enlargement due to nonmalignant conditions, such as infection or rheumatoid arthritis.

Who Performs It
• A physician.

Special Concerns
• This procedure may not be safe in people with bleeding disorders.
• Because SLN biopsy may use a radioactive

Results
▼

➡ Tissue specimens are sent to a pathology laboratory and inspected under a microscope for unusual cells. (For more on microscopic examination, see Chapter 1.)

➡ If the biopsy reveals cancerous cells, your doctor will recommend appropriate medical or surgical treatment based on the findings. For example, after a positive SLN biopsy, surgery will be performed to completely excise the nodal cluster. More tests, such as a chest CT scan (see page 152) and a bone scan (see page 329), may also be performed to determine if the cancer has spread. Hodgkin's and non-Hodgkin's lymphomas are typically treated with radiation therapy or chemotherapy.

➡ If findings are unclear, additional tests, such as a biopsy of deeper lymph nodes taken during mediastinoscopy (see page 357), may be required.

➡ If no cancer is present, periodic testing may be recommended.

tracer, this procedure should not be done in women who are pregnant or breastfeeding.

Before the Test
• If general anesthesia is being used, do not eat anything after midnight on the day before the test. You may drink only clear liquids.
• Depending on the biopsy site, you may be asked to disrobe and put on a hospital gown.

What You Experience
Fine needle biopsy:
• The skin over the biopsy site is cleansed with an antiseptic solution, and a local anesthetic is injected to numb the area (this injection may cause brief discomfort).
• You will be positioned differently according to the selected biopsy site.
• A thin biopsy needle is inserted into the lymph node, and a specimen is obtained. The tissue is sent to a laboratory for analysis.
• The needle is withdrawn. Pressure is placed on the biopsy site until bleeding has stopped, and a small bandage is applied.
• The procedure takes less than 15 minutes.

Excisional biopsy:
• The skin over the biopsy site is cleansed with an antiseptic solution, and a local anesthetic is injected to numb the area.
• You will be positioned differently according to the selected biopsy site.
• Once the local anesthetic has taken effect, the doctor or surgeon will make a small incision in the skin over the node.
• The selected node or cluster of nodes is removed and sent to a laboratory for analysis.
• The incision is sutured closed, and a sterile dressing is applied.
• Alternatively, this procedure is done while you are in an operating room under general anesthesia.
• The procedure takes 15 to 30 minutes.

SLN biopsy:
• The skin over the site of your primary tumor is cleansed with an antiseptic solution, and a

local anesthetic is injected to numb the area (this injection may cause brief discomfort).
• To determine which node is the sentinel, a radioactive tracer, a blue dye, or a combination of the two is injected into the tumor.
• When the tracer or dye enters the lymph duct system, it flows from the tumor and drains into the nearest, or sentinel, node.
• Once it is located, the surgeon will make a small incision and remove the entire sentinel node. The tissue is sent to a laboratory for analysis.
• The incision is sutured closed and a bandage is applied.
• The procedure takes 60 to 90 minutes.

Risks and Complications
Fine needle biopsy:
• Rarely, bleeding or infection may occur.

Excisional biopsy:
• A possible complication is lymphedema, a buildup of lymph fluid that causes uncomfortable, chronic swelling and stiffness around the biopsy site.
• Rarely, bleeding or infection may occur.
• If general anesthesia is used, the procedure carries the associated risks.

SLN biopsy:
• This procedure is less invasive and initially produces less pain and discomfort than excisional biopsy. However, lymphedema, bleeding, and infection may still occur.

After the Test
• If you received general anesthesia, you must remain in the hospital until you recover from its effects. Otherwise, you may return home and resume your normal activities.
• The biopsy site may remain sore for about 2 to 3 days. You may be given pain-relieving medication to allay any discomfort.
• If you experience bleeding, tenderness, or redness around the biopsy site, call your doctor.

Estimated Cost: $$

Lymphangiography
(Lymphography)

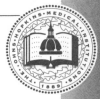

Description
• In this test, a contrast dye is injected into lymph vessels in your feet or hands (see the illustration on page 19). Filled with dye, these vessels can be visualized on x-ray film. Continuous x-ray imaging, or fluoroscopy (see page 205), is used to track the flow of dye through the lymphatic circulation; plain x-ray films are also obtained to record any abnormalities. Lymphangiography is especially useful for evaluating patients with suspected cancers of the lymphatic system, such as Hodgkin's disease and non-Hodgkin's lymphomas. (For more on contrast x-rays, see Chapter 2.)

Purpose of the Test
• To diagnose and determine the stage of lymphomas, and to identify metastatic cancer (spread from other areas of the body) involving the lymph nodes.
• To evaluate the effectiveness of chemotherapy or radiation therapy for lymphomas.
• To evaluate suspected cases of lymphedema— an accumulation of lymph fluids resulting in swelling of the arms and legs, which may be primary (caused by a lymph vessel defect of unknown origin) or secondary (caused by tumors, inflammation, infection, or removal of the lymph nodes).

Who Performs It
• A radiologist.

Special Concerns
• Pregnant women should not undergo this test because exposure to ionizing radiation may harm the fetus.
• People with allergies to iodine or shellfish may experience an allergic reaction to iodine-based contrast dyes.
• This test is not appropriate for people with severe chronic lung, heart, kidney, or liver disease because the lipid-containing contrast dye

may further damage these organs.
• Because the dye remains in the lymph nodes for up to 2 years, subsequent x-rays can be used to assess the progress of any lymphatic disease and the effectiveness of treatment.

Before the Test
• Inform your doctor if you have an allergy to iodine or shellfish. You may be given a combined antihistamine-steroid preparation to reduce the risk of an allergic reaction.
• You may be given a sedative before the test.
• Empty your bladder just before the test.

What You Experience
• You will lie on your back on an examination table.
• The skin on your feet is cleansed with an antiseptic, and a blue contrast dye is injected into the web of skin between several of the toes on both feet. (Less often, this is done between fingers in both hands instead.) These injections will cause a brief sting.
• After about 15 to 30 minutes, the lymphatic vessels will appear as small blue lines on the upper surface of the instep of each foot.
• A local anesthetic is then injected into both

Results
▼

➡ A doctor will examine the x-ray films for evidence of any abnormality.

➡ If a definitive diagnosis can be made, appropriate treatment will be initiated, depending on the specific problem.

➡ In some cases, additional tests, such as a lymph node biopsy (see page 249), may be needed to establish a diagnosis and determine the extent of the problem.

Lymphangiography

feet (this injection may cause brief discomfort). Once the area is numb, a thin needle is inserted through a small incision into a lymphatic vessel in each foot; the needle is attached to a tube (cannula). Contrast dye is infused into the vessels at a slow rate; it usually takes 60 to 90 minutes for the infusion to be completed. Remain as still as possible during this time to avoid dislodging the needles.

• As the dye is being infused, its progress may be followed with fluoroscopy, which projects real-time x-ray images onto a viewing screen. The infusion is stopped when the dye reaches about waist level.

• The needles are removed, the incisions sutured closed, and sterile dressings are applied.

• Next, x-ray films are taken of your chest, abdomen, pelvis, and legs to demonstrate filling of the lymph nodes.

• The entire procedure usually takes about 3 hours.

• You must return in 24 hours so that additional x-ray films can be taken.

Risks and Complications

• Although radiation exposure is minimal, you receive a higher dose than during standard x-ray procedures.

• Possible complications include infection and lipoid (or lipid) pneumonia, which can occur if the contrast dye penetrates the thoracic duct and causes tiny pulmonary blood clots (emboli); these clots typically disappear after several weeks or months.

• Some people may experience an allergic reaction to the iodine-based contrast dye, which can cause symptoms such as nausea, sneezing, vomiting, hives, and occasionally a life-threatening response called anaphylactic shock. Emergency medications and equipment are kept readily available.

After the Test

• You must rest in a hospital bed for 24 hours, with your feet elevated to help reduce swelling. Your vital signs will be monitored periodically and you will be observed for signs of complications.

• Ice packs can be applied to the incision sites to help reduce swelling, and you may be given a pain reliever.

• The blue dye may cause a bluish tinge to your skin and vision and may also discolor your urine and stool for 48 hours.

• Call your doctor if you notice redness, pain, and swelling at the infusion sites.

• Do not immerse your feet in water until the sutures have been removed—about 7 to 10 days after the procedure.

Estimated Cost: $$

Magnetic Resonance Angiography
(MRA)

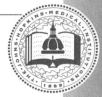

Description

• MRA—a type of magnetic resonance imaging (MRI) study that is obtained with the same scanning machine—uses a strong magnetic field combined with radiofrequency waves to create highly detailed images of blood vessels in the body. (The test is most often used to examine vessels in the brain, neck, kidneys, and legs.) The resulting scans, which provide information about blood flow and the condition of blood vessel walls, may then be saved on a computer or on film and examined for abnormalities. To provide better definition of blood vessels on the images, a weakly magnetic contrast dye, such as gadolinium, is sometimes injected into a vein in the arm. (For more on how MRA and MRI work, see Chapter 2.)

Purpose of the Test

• To evaluate people with symptoms of a stroke.
• To diagnose lesions that significantly disrupt blood flow in the carotid and vertebral arteries leading to the brain, such as blockages or dissection (leakage of blood between layers of the blood vessel wall).
• To detect and evaluate blood vessel abnormalities within the brain, including aneurysm (abnormal outpouching that is prone to rupture), dilation, inflammation, and arteriovenous malformation (a congenital blood vessel defect).
• To detect and evaluate blood vessel abnormalities in the legs, kidneys, and other parts of the body.
• To define the blood supply to malignant (cancerous) vascular tumors in the brain.

Who Performs It

• A radiologist or a qualified technician.

Special Concerns

• MRA is expensive and is often unavailable outside of large cities and major medical centers.
• People who experience claustrophobia may find it difficult to undergo this test, which takes place in a narrow, tunnel-like structure.
• This test may not be possible for severely overweight individuals (over 300 lbs).
• Because the MRI generates a strong magnetic field, it cannot be performed on people who have certain internally placed metallic devices, including pacemakers, inner ear implants, or intracranial aneurysm clips.
• The test should not be done in pregnant women because the long-term effects of MRI on the fetus are unknown.

Before the Test

• Tell your doctor if you suffer from claustrophobia. He or she may administer a sedative to help you tolerate the procedure.
• Empty your bladder before the test.
• Remove any metallic objects, including watches, hair clips, belts, credit cards, and jewelry. You may be asked to disrobe and put on a hospital gown.

What You Experience

• You will lie down on a narrow padded bed that slides into a large, enclosed cylinder con-

---

Results
▼

➥ A radiologist will examine the MRA images for evidence of any abnormality.

➥ If a definitive diagnosis can be made, appropriate treatment will be initiated, depending on the specific problem.

➥ In some cases, additional tests, such as a CT scan (see page 121) or a PET scan (see page 298) of the brain, may be needed to establish a diagnosis and determine the extent of the problem.

taining the MRI magnets. You must remain still throughout the procedure because any motion can distort the scan.

• If a contrast dye is to be used, it is injected intravenously, and imaging begins shortly after the injection.

• There is a microphone inside the imaging machine, and you may talk to the technician performing the scan at any time during the test.

• You will hear loud thumping sounds as the scanning is performed. To block out the noise, you can request earplugs or listen to music on earphones.

• The entire procedure takes 10 to 20 minutes, or twice that long if contrast dye is used.

Risks and Complications

• MRA does not involve exposure to ionizing radiation and is not associated with any risks or complications.

After the Test

• Sedated patients may be monitored for a short period until the effects of the sedative have worn off.

• You may leave the testing facility and resume your normal activities.

• Blood may collect and clot under the skin (hematoma) at the injection site; this is harmless and will resolve on its own. For a large hematoma that causes swelling and discomfort, apply ice initially; after 24 hours, use warm, moist compresses to help dissolve the clotted blood.

Estimated Cost: $$$$

Mammography
(Mammogram)

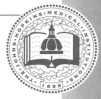

Description
• In this test, x-ray beams are passed through the breasts, producing images of the internal tissue on a special type of film. Periodic mammography is used as a screening tool to detect breast cancer earlier than is possible with physical examination of the breasts. It is considered to be the best, most cost-effective method of finding abnormal growths within the breast. (For more on how x-rays work, see Chapter 2.)

Purpose of the Test
• To screen for tumors (benign or malignant) and cysts before they can be detected with a physical examination.
• To evaluate any abnormalities detected in a physician or self-administered breast exam.
• To monitor women with breast cancer who have been treated with surgery and radiation.

Who Performs It
• A radiologist or a qualified technician.

Special Concerns
• There is considerable debate regarding when women should begin to have screening mammograms. Most experts agree that periodic mammograms are beneficial in women age 50 and older; the value of regular mammography in women age 40 to 50 is more controversial. (See Chapter 3 for more discussion on the use of mammography as a screening tool.)
• Mammography is of limited usefulness in younger women, since their breasts contain more dense, glandular tissue. Since glandular tissue and tumors both appear white on x-ray film, it can be difficult to distinguish between them, increasing the possibility of a false-positive result (see page 35) that could lead to unnecessary biopsies. (Older women have less glandular and more fatty tissue,

which appears gray on an x-ray, so potential tumors are more readily detectable.) Thus, ultrasound (see page 130) is preferred for examining breast tissue in younger women.
• Pregnant women should not undergo this test because exposure to ionizing radiation may harm the fetus.

Before the Test
• You will be asked to disrobe from the waist up, remove any jewelry or metal objects, and put on an x-ray gown.
• Do not put talcum powder, lotion, or perfume on your breasts or use deodorant on the day of the test.
• Tell your doctor if you have breast implants or have previously undergone breast surgery. These factors may obscure the x-ray images.

Results
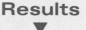

➡ A radiologist who specializes in mammography will examine the x-ray images for the presence of any unusual or suspicious shadows, masses, distortions, and differences between the two breasts. Mammography can detect lesions as small as one-quarter inch—too small to be felt during a physician breast exam.

➡ If abnormalities are detected, additional tests will be required, such as another mammogram, breast ultrasound, or a breast biopsy (see page 125), in order to reach a definitive diagnosis and determine the extent of the problem.

➡ If the films are normal, your physician will advise you on when to return for another mammogram, usually in 1 to 2 years.

What You Experience

• You will stand in front of the mammography unit.

• A technician will position the breast being examined between two compression plates.

• In order to obtain as clear an image as possible, the breast is compressed and flattened between the plates. This pressure will be slightly uncomfortable, but lasts only for a brief time.

• Two x-ray photographs are taken, one from above and one from the side.

• The same procedure is then repeated with the other breast.

• Mammography takes only about 10 to 15 minutes to perform.

Risks and Complications

• This procedure involves minimal exposure to radiation.

After the Test

• You may be asked to wait while the films are developed to ensure they are readable. After that, you may return home and resume your usual activities.

Estimated Cost: $$

Mediastinoscopy

Description
• In this surgical procedure, a flexible or rigid viewing tube (mediastinoscope) is inserted through a small incision in the chest. Fiberoptic cables permit direct visualization of the lymph nodes located in the area between the lungs (mediastinum). A biopsy forceps may be passed through the scope to obtain lymph node tissue samples for laboratory examination. This analysis can help to detect lung diseases (since the lymph nodes receive drainage from the lungs) and diseases of the mediastinum.

Purpose of the Test
• To help diagnose lung infections, sarcoidosis (a systemic disease that causes inflammation of the lungs), lymphatic or lung cancers, and some other uncommon diseases.
• To determine the stage of cancer (the extent to which it has spread) in people with known lung cancer, and to assess the appropriateness of surgical treatment.

Who Performs It
• A chest surgeon and a surgical team.

Special Concerns
• A prior mediastinoscopy may be a contraindication for a second one.

Before the Test
• Tell your doctor if you regularly take anticoagulant drugs. You will be instructed to discontinue them for some time before the test.
• Do not eat or drink anything for 12 hours before the test.
• Immediately before the procedure begins, an intravenous (IV) line is inserted into a vein in your arm, and you are placed under general anesthesia.
• A thin tube that is attached to a breathing machine may be passed into your windpipe to ensure that you breathe properly during the procedure.

What You Experience
• You will be lying down on a table in an operating room.
• A small incision is made between your collarbones, and the doctor inserts the scope into the mediastinum.
• After a close visual inspection of the lymph nodes, the doctor may pass a biopsy forceps through the scope to obtain tissue specimens

Results
▼
➡ During the visual inspection of the mediastinum, the doctor will note any abnormalities.
➡ Tissue samples are inspected under a microscope for the presence of unusual cells, or may be cultured (see page 166) for infectious organisms. (For more on laboratory testing, see Chapter 1.)
➡ In some cases, biopsied tissue is examined immediately via frozen section (see page 39). If this inspection reveals lung cancer that has not spread to the lymph nodes, surgery may be performed immediately to remove all or part of the affected lung. If lung cancer or any other malignancy is detected in the lymph nodes, surgery is usually contraindicated; nonsurgical treatments (such as radiation) may be begun.
➡ If a definitive diagnosis can be made, appropriate treatment will be initiated.
➡ If the doctor cannot make a diagnosis, additional tests, such as open lung biopsy (see page 245), may be needed.

Mediastinoscopy

from any suspicious areas.

• The scope is withdrawn, and the incision closed with sutures.

• The procedure takes about 1 hour.

Risks and Complications

• You may experience temporary chest pain, tenderness at the incision site, or a sore throat (due to the breathing tube).

• Rare complications include infection; bleeding; unintentional puncture of the esophagus, trachea, or great blood vessels; pneumothorax (leakage of air outside the lungs and into the pleural cavity, resulting in a collapsed lung); and damage to the laryngeal nerve of the vocal cords.

• Mediastinoscopy requires general anesthesia, and thus carries the associated risks.

After the Test

• You will remain in the hospital for 1 or 2 days until you recover from the effects of anesthesia. During this time, your vital signs will be monitored, and you will be observed for any signs of complications.

• You may be given a pain reliever, if needed.

• You may return home and resume your regular activities.

• If you develop a cough or shortness of breath, inform the doctor immediately.

Estimated Cost: $$

Modified Barium Swallow

Description

• In this test, you ingest foods and liquids containing barium sulfate, a contrast dye that sharply outlines your mouth, throat, and esophagus (illustrated on page 24) on x-ray film. Using real-time x-rays, or fluoroscopy (see page 205), a physician and a speech pathologist observe the movement of the barium through these structures on a television monitor. This test is specifically aimed at evaluating the swallowing process in individuals who have difficulty speaking or swallowing food without inhaling, or aspirating, it into the windpipe. Spot x-ray films may be taken of specific abnormalities, and the entire test may be recorded on videotape for later viewing. (For more on how contrast x-rays and fluoroscopy work, see Chapter 2.)

Purpose of the Test

• To identify the cause of difficult or impaired swallowing (dysphagia).
• To help determine the most appropriate treatment or management techniques for swallowing problems.

Who Performs It

• An ear, nose, and throat specialist (otolaryngologist), a radiologist, and a speech pathologist may all be present.

Special Concerns

• People who aspirate saliva are not suitable candidates for this test.
• Pregnant women should not undergo this test because exposure to ionizing radiation may harm the fetus.
• Failure to remain still while the procedure is being performed may interfere with the accuracy of the results.

Before the Test

• You may be instructed to refrain from eating

or drinking anything for several hours before the procedure.
• At the testing facility, you will be asked to remove your clothes and eyeglasses and to put on a hospital gown.

What You Experience

• You will either be strapped to an x-ray table that tilts vertically, or you will be seated in a chair.
• You will consume a barium-containing meal. The consistency of the items in the meal varies, ranging from thin liquid to semisolid foods (for example, applesauce) or solid foods (such as a cookie).
• As you swallow different amounts of the meal

Results

➡ The doctor will try to identify the nature and origin of your swallowing problem on the viewing monitor during the test. Swallowing difficulties may be caused by a wide variety of conditions, including structural abnormalities, such as tumors or inflammation, or neurologic (nerve) disorders, such as Parkinson's disease or post-stroke syndrome.

➡ If possible, the speech pathologist will recommend specific corrective actions to help you resolve the swallowing problem during the test, and no further testing or treatment is needed.

➡ If the test findings are still not definitive after the recorded x-rays and video have been reviewed, or if the test reveals abnormalities that require further evaluation, additional tests such as esophagogastroduodenoscopy (see page 194) may be ordered.

Modified Barium Swallow

items, the examiners use fluoroscopic imaging to observe the swallowing process on a television screen in order to determine which foods are difficult for you to swallow and which structures are responsible for the problem. The swallowing process may be observed at normal speed or in slow motion.

• Other than chewing and swallowing, you must remain still during the procedure.

• A speech pathologist is also normally present during the test to evaluate your swallowing ability and, if possible, to suggest some possible corrective actions.

• The test usually takes from 30 minutes to 1 hour depending on the findings.

Risks and Complications

• Although radiation exposure during this test is minimal, you will receive a higher dose than during standard x-ray procedures.

After the Test

• You may leave the testing facility immediately and resume your normal diet and activities.

• Drink plenty of fluids to help eliminate the barium from your system.

• Your stool will be chalky and light-colored initially, but it should return to normal color after 1 to 3 days.

Estimated Cost: $$

Muscle Biopsy

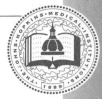

Description

• In this test, a tissue sample is extracted from a muscle and sent to a laboratory for microscopic examination. Several techniques may be used, including **needle biopsy,** which uses a long, thin needle to withdraw a specimen, and, less often, **open biopsy,** which accesses the muscle surgically through a small incision.

Purpose of the Test

• To diagnose some muscle diseases, including muscular dystrophy (progressive atrophy of muscles) and myositis (inflammation of the muscles).

• To help distinguish between nerve and muscle disorders.

• To diagnose certain diseases of the blood vessels and connective tissues, such as generalized vasculitis (inflammation of blood vessels).

• To diagnose infections that affect the muscles, such as trichinosis or toxoplasmosis.

Who Performs It

• A physician.

Special Concerns

• Preliminary tests, including laboratory studies and electromyography (EMG; see page 177), should be done first to determine if a muscle biopsy is necessary and to identify an appropriate biopsy site. The biopsy is usually performed only to confirm a suspected diagnosis.

• Open biopsy is typically done only in cases where a larger piece of tissue is needed to confirm a diagnosis, or when the condition is believed to be localized or found in patches.

• Muscle biopsy should not be performed on sites that have recently undergone EMG or areas affected by preexisting conditions such as nerve compression.

Before the Test

• You may be asked to wear loose clothes or to remove your clothes and put on a hospital gown, depending on the biopsy site.

What You Experience

Needle biopsy:

• You will be positioned differently according to the selected procedure site.

• The skin at the biopsy site is cleansed with an antiseptic solution, and a local anesthetic is injected to numb the area. You may feel a brief stinging sensation for a few seconds after the anesthetic is injected, and you may still feel pressure or a pulling sensation when the biopsy is taken.

• The doctor inserts a thin needle through the skin into the muscle, and withdraws a small plug of tissue. Sometimes several samples are taken.

• Pressure is placed on the needle insertion site until bleeding has stopped, and a small

Results

▼

➡ A pathologist examines the muscle specimens under a microscope for the presence of muscle fiber abnormalities or unusual cells. In some cases, chemical analysis may also be done, for example, to examine the activity of various enzymes responsible for producing energy in the muscle. (For more on laboratory tests, see Chapter 1.)

➡ In many cases, a definitive diagnosis can be made and treatment will be initiated.

➡ A negative biopsy does not exclude the presence of a suspected disease—for example, if the biopsy site was not selected properly. In such cases, the procedure may need to be repeated.

Muscle Biopsy

bandage is applied.
• The procedure usually takes about 1 hour.

Open biopsy:
• You will be positioned differently according to the selected procedure site.
• The skin at the biopsy site is shaved and cleansed with an antiseptic, and a local anesthetic is injected to numb the area (you may still experience brief discomfort when the biopsy is taken). You may feel a brief stinging sensation for a few seconds after the anesthetic is injected.
• A small incision is made with a scalpel, the skin is pulled back, and surgical scissors are used to extract several small pieces of muscle tissue.
• The incision is stitched closed and covered with a sterile dressing.
• An open muscle biopsy takes about 1 hour to perform.

Risks and Complications
• The most common aftereffect is soreness. In addition, after a needle biopsy, swelling or discoloration may develop due to collection of blood under the skin (hematoma) at the needle insertion site; this is harmless, but may cause some discomfort. Serious complications are rare.

After the Test
• The biopsy site may remain sore for about 1 week. You may be given pain-relieving medication to allay any discomfort.
• For a large hematoma that causes swelling and discomfort, apply ice initially; after 24 hours, use warm, moist compresses to help dissolve the clotted blood.
• Resume your normal activities when it is comfortable to do so.

Estimated Cost: $$

Myelography
(Myelogram)

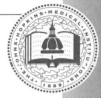

Description
• Myelography is the x-ray examination of the spinal canal after administration of a contrast dye to provide definition on the images. To perform this test, the contrast dye is injected into the subarachnoid space—the compartment surrounding the spinal cord and brain that contains the cerebrospinal fluid (CSF). Because the contrast agent is heavier than CSF, it flows through the spinal canal to selected areas as an examining table is tilted up or down. Continuous x-ray imaging, or fluoroscopy (see page 205), is used to track the movement of the dye and visualize the contents of the spinal canal. Any abnormalities, such as narrowed areas, may then be recorded on x-ray film or by a CT scanning machine. (For more on contrast x-rays and CT scanning, see Chapter 2.)

Purpose of the Test
• To diagnose abnormalities affecting the spinal cord—such as tumors, herniated disks, arthritic bone spurs, or an abscess—in people with severe back pain or neurologic symptoms that suggest problems in the spinal canal.
• To assess abnormalities in the spinal cord prior to surgery.
• To identify injuries to the nerve roots that branch off from the spinal cord.
• To detect tumors in the lower part of the brain.

Who Performs It
• A radiologist.

Special Concerns
• Pregnant women should not undergo this test because exposure to ionizing radiation may harm the fetus.
• Myelography is not appropriate for individuals who have increased intracranial pressure, infection at the site of the needle insertion, or multiple sclerosis.
• Different types of contrast dyes—either oil-based or water-soluble—may be used for this procedure. Oil-based dyes must be withdrawn after myelography before the needle is removed; this is not necessary with water-soluble dyes, which are absorbed by the body and excreted through the kidneys.
• People with allergies to iodine or shellfish may experience an allergic reaction to iodinated, oil-based contrast dyes.
• Certain drugs can increase the risk for seizures in patients receiving a water-soluble contrast agent, such as metrizamide.
• People who experience claustrophobia may find it difficult to undergo a CT scan, which takes place in a narrow, tunnel-like struc-

Results
▼

➡ The doctor will examine the x-ray or CT images and other test data for evidence of abnormalities, such as blocked or narrowed areas, affecting the spinal canal or the base of the brain.

➡ If a sample of CSF is taken, it will be sent to a laboratory for analysis to provide further diagnostic information. (For more on laboratory tests, see Chapter 1.)

➡ If a definitive diagnosis can be made, your doctor will recommend an appropriate course of medical or surgical treatment, depending on the specific problem.

➡ In some situations, additional diagnostic tests, such as a skeletal MRI (see page 327), may be needed to further evaluate abnormal results.

Myelography

Myelography continued

ture. In addition, the CT scan may not be possible for severely overweight individuals (over 300 lbs).

Before the Test

• If iodinated dye is to be used, inform your doctor if you have an allergy to iodine or shellfish. You may be given a combined antihistamine-steroid preparation to reduce the risk of an allergic reaction.

• Tell your doctor if you are taking any medications, herbs, or supplements. You may be advised to discontinue certain of these agents before the test.

• Do not eat or drink anything for 8 hours before the test.

• You will be advised to empty your bladder and bowels before the test.

• You may be given an anticholinergic drug, such as atropine, in addition to a sedative to reduce swallowing during the procedure.

• You will be asked to remove your clothes and any metal objects (including watches, hair clips, and jewelry) and put on a hospital gown.

What You Experience

• You will lie on your side on a table or bed, with your knees drawn up toward your chest and your forehead bent toward your knees. (Less often, the procedure is done while you are sitting.)

• The needle insertion site on your lower back is cleansed with an antiseptic solution, and a local anesthetic is injected to numb the area. You may feel a brief stinging during this injection.

• Next, a long needle is carefully inserted into the spinal canal. Fluoroscopic imaging is used to guide it into the subarachnoid space, which is located between membranes that surround the spinal cord. You may feel some pressure as the needle is inserted.

• Once the needle is in place, a small amount of CSF may be removed for laboratory analysis (a procedure called lumbar puncture that is described on page 243).

• A contrast dye is then injected through the needle into the spinal canal. You may feel a transient flushing sensation, warmth, a headache, a salty taste, or nausea after the material is injected.

• With the needle in place, you will be positioned on your stomach and strapped in place with a foot support and shoulder brace or harness. Your chin will be hyperextended outward with a towel or sponge placed underneath for comfort.

• The flow of the contrast agent is followed using fluoroscopy, and representative x-ray films are obtained of any abnormalities. (Alternatively, you will be advanced into a CT scanning machine.)

• To move the dye to selected areas, the table may be adjusted so that your head is tilted down during parts of the test, which may be uncomfortable.

• Once the procedure has been completed, the needle is removed. (If an oil-based contrast dye was used for the test, as much dye as possible must be aspirated through the needle before it is withdrawn. This may cause some discomfort.)

• The puncture site is cleansed with an antiseptic solution and a dressing is applied.

• The procedure usually takes about 1 hour.

Risks and Complications

• Radiation exposure is minimal, but if the test includes a CT scan, you will receive a higher dose of radiation than during standard x-ray procedures.

• Headache or soreness in the back may occur for a short time after the procedure. Rarely, serious complications such as meningitis or (when water-based dye is used) seizures may develop.

• Some people may experience an allergic reaction to the iodine-based contrast dye, which can cause symptoms such as nausea, sneezing, vomiting, hives, and occasionally a life-threatening response called anaphylactic shock. Emergency medications and equipment are kept readily available.

• If a lumbar puncture is performed, it carries the associated risks.

After the Test

• If an oil-based contrast agent was used, you must lie flat in bed for up to 12 hours after the procedure. If a water-based dye was used, you must rest with your head elevated for about 6 to 8 hours.

• Your blood pressure and other vital signs will be checked periodically and you will be monitored for signs of complications.

• You may return home. If there are no complications or adverse reactions, you may resume your normal diet and activities the day after the test.

• You are encouraged to drink clear fluids to avoid dehydration and to help flush the contrast dye out of your system. (If a lumbar puncture was done, extra fluids also help to speed the replacement of CSF.)

• Delayed allergic reactions to the contrast dye, such as hives, rash, or itching, may appear 2 to 6 hours after the procedure. If this occurs, your doctor will prescribe antihistamines or steroids to ease your discomfort.

Estimated Cost: $$

Myelography continued

Nasal or Sinus Endoscopy
(Rhinoscopy)

Nasal or Sinus Endoscopy

Description
• A thin, flexible or rigid viewing tube (endoscope) is passed through the nasal passages. Fiberoptic cables permit direct visualization of the nasal passages, sinuses, and throat. In addition, various instruments may be passed through the scope to obtain fluid or tissue samples for laboratory examination, and to perform therapeutic procedures.

Purpose of the Test
• To visually inspect the nasal passages, sinuses, septum (the wall of tissue dividing the nasal cavity), vocal cords (larynx), and nearby structures for abnormalities, such as structural defects, nasal polyps, a blockage, or a laryngeal injury.
• To diagnose recurrent or resistant sinus infections (sinusitis).
• To drain the sinuses, dispense antibiotics, or remove polyps from the nose and throat.

Who Performs It
• An allergist or an ear, nose, and throat specialist (otolaryngologist).

Special Concerns
• People who experience frequent nosebleeds or those with a severe bleeding disorder may not be suitable candidates for this procedure.

Before the Test
• No special preparation is necessary.

What You Experience
• You will sit in a chair with a headrest.
• A local anesthetic is sprayed into your nose, and may also be applied to the back of your throat to suppress the gag reflex.
• The doctor inserts the scope into a nostril and then closely inspects your nasal passages, sinuses, larynx, and nearby structures, looking for any abnormalities.

• If appropriate, a suction device may be used to remove fluid, or instruments may be passed through the scope to obtain tissue samples.
• If an infection is suspected or there is a buildup of mucus, the doctor may administer antibiotics or suction the mucus away.
• This procedure generally takes only 10 to 15 minutes.

Risks and Complications
• This is a safe procedure. You may experience a nosebleed, nasal discomfort, and coughing.

After the Test
• You will be given a gauze pad to absorb any blood or fluid that may drain from your nose.
• Do not eat or drink until your gag reflex returns, usually in a few hours.
• You may resume your usual activities.

Estimated Cost: $$

Results
▼

➡ During the visual inspection, the doctor will note any abnormalities such as inflammation, blood, secretions, or growths. This examination may be sufficient to provide a definitive diagnosis.

➡ If tissue or fluid samples were taken, specimen containers may be sent to several different laboratories for examination. (For more on laboratory tests, see Chapter 1.)

➡ If a definitive diagnosis can be made, appropriate treatment will be initiated.

➡ If further evaluation is necessary, a CT scan (see page 212) or an MRI (see page 214) of the head may be recommended.

Octreotide Scan

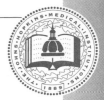

Description

• This nuclear imaging test is used to visualize hormone-producing tumors of the nervous and endocrine systems, or neuroendocrine tumors (see pages 16 and 18 of the body atlas). Most tumors of this nature contain cells with a receptor for the hormone somatostatin. In this test, octreotide, an analogue of somatostatin, is labeled with a radioactive tracer and injected intravenously; the radioactive octreotide attaches to somatostatin receptors on the tumor cells and can then be observed with a special scanning camera. A variation of nuclear scanning, called single-photon emission computed tomography, or SPECT, enhances the sensitivity of the test. (For more on nuclear imaging and SPECT, see Chapter 2.)

Purpose of the Test

• To identify and pinpoint the location of benign or malignant (cancerous) neuroendocrine tumors prior to their surgical removal; this test can identify both primary cancer and cancer that has metastasized (spread) from other locations.
• To monitor the effectiveness of therapy for neuroendocrine tumors and to detect recurrences or progression of disease.

Who Performs It

• A technician trained in nuclear medicine.

Special Concerns

• This test should not be performed in women who are pregnant or breastfeeding because of possible risks to the fetus or infant.
• Patients with an allergy to shellfish or iodine could experience a severe allergic reaction to radioactive iodine; another type of radiotracer should be used.
• The presence of residual barium due to recent contrast x-rays of the gastrointestinal tract can cause defects in the scan that may

be misinterpreted as growths. In addition, various abnormalities other than neuroendocrine tumors can also pick up octreotide, including certain infections, rheumatoid arthritis, and nonhormonal cancers. These factors may lead to false-positive results (see page 35).

Before the Test

• Inform your doctor if you have an allergy to shellfish or iodine so that a noniodinated radiotracer can be used.
• If an iodinated dye is being used, you will receive iodine for 3 days prior to the test to preclude uptake of the radiotracer by the thyroid gland.
• If you have been receiving octreotide as a form of anticancer therapy, the agent will be discontinued for 2 weeks prior to the scan.

What You Experience

• The examiner injects radioactive octreotide into a vein in your arm or hand. Other than this injection, the procedure is painless.
• One hour after the injection, you will lie on a table under a large camera that records the gamma rays emitted by the radioactive material. You may be asked to assume various positions—on your back, side, and stomach—as the camera scans the length of your body.
• A computer translates signals from the scan-

Results

▼

➡ A physician trained in nuclear medicine interprets the results of the scans.
➡ If no abnormality is found, no further testing may be necessary.
➡ If surgery is to be performed to remove neuroendocrine tumors, the scans will be used to help plan the procedure.

Octreotide Scan

ner into images that are recorded on film. (More detailed images may also be obtained using SPECT.)

• About 2 hours after the octreotide injection, you will usually be given a fatty meal to help clear the radioactive material from your gallbladder.

• After 4 hours, you will be given a strong laxative to clear the octreotide from your bowel.

• Nuclear scanning is repeated at periodic intervals—for example, 2, 4, 24, and 48 hours after the octreotide is administered.

• You are free to go home in between scanning sessions.

Risks and Complications

• The trace amount of radioactive material used in this test is not associated with any significant risks or complications.

After the Test

• Drink plenty of fluids to help your kidneys excrete the radioactive octreotide.

• You may leave the testing facility and resume your normal activities.

• Blood may collect and clot under the skin (hematoma) at the injection site; this is harmless and will resolve on its own. For a large hematoma that causes swelling and discomfort, apply ice initially; after 24 hours, use warm, moist compresses to help dissolve the clotted blood.

Estimated Cost: $$$

Ocular and Orbit Ultrasound
(Ocular and Orbit Ultrasonography)

Description

• In this procedure, a device called a transducer directs high-frequency sound waves (ultrasound) through the eye and the orbit (the bony cavity that contains the eye). The sound waves are reflected back to the transducer and electronically converted into graphic representations of internal structures that are displayed on a viewing monitor. (For more on how ultrasound imaging works, see Chapter 2.)

• Two techniques are used for this test, often together: An **A-scan** converts the ultrasound echoes into waveforms that correspond to the positions of different structures, while a **B-scan** converts the echoes into two-dimensional images of ocular structures. These images can then be saved on film or video and reviewed for abnormalities.

Purpose of the Test

• To detect abnormalities of the eye and orbit, such as vitreous hemorrhage (leakage of blood in the eye resulting from a ruptured blood vessel); detachment of the retina; ocular tumors or cysts; the presence of foreign bodies; or alterations in corneal or ocular shape due to disease, surgical procedures, or trauma.

• To evaluate the internal structures of the eye prior to planned surgical procedures, such as cataract removal with intraocular lens implantation.

• To examine the eye when previous surgery, scarring, a cataract, or other factors preclude visual examination with an ophthalmoscope.

Who Performs It

• An ophthalmologist or a technician trained in ultrasound.

Special Concerns

• None.

Before the Test

• If you wear contact lenses, remove them before the test.

• The examiner will administer topical anesthetic eye drops 5 to 10 minutes prior to the procedure.

What You Experience
A scan:

• You will lie down on an examination table.

• A clear plastic eye cup is placed directly on your eyeball.

• A water-soluble gel is applied to the eye cup to enhance sound wave transmission.

• The transducer is placed on the eye cup and moved over its surface.

• The echoed sound waves are converted into waveforms on a viewing monitor and recorded for later analysis.

• The test takes about 5 minutes.

B scan:

• You will lie down on an examination table.

• You are asked to close your eyes.

• A water-soluble gel is applied to your eyelid to enhance sound wave transmission.

Results
▼

➡ A physician reviews the recorded ultrasound images for evidence of any abnormality in the eye or orbit.

➡ If a definitive diagnosis can be made based on these findings, your doctor will recommend appropriate treatment.

➡ In some cases, additional tests, such as a CT scan (see page 212) or an MRI (see page 214), may be necessary to further evaluate any abnormal results.

• The examiner moves a transducer back and forth over the surface of your eyelid to obtain various views of the targeted structures on a video monitor. You may be instructed to move your eye or change your gaze to provide different views.

• Once clear images are obtained, they are recorded on film or video for later analysis.

• The test takes about 5 minutes.

Risks and Complications

• Ultrasound is painless, noninvasive, and involves no exposure to radiation. There are no associated risks.

After the Test

• Immediately after the test, the examiner removes the eye cups and/or the conductive gel from your eyelids.

• You are free to leave the testing facility and resume your normal activities.

• If anesthetic eye drops were administered, do not rub your eyes for at least 30 minutes to avoid injuring the cornea.

• Do not reinsert your contact lenses for at least 2 hours after the test.

Estimated Cost: $$

Oculoplethysmography
(OPG)

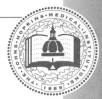

Description
• Oculoplethysmography (OPG) is a procedure that gives an estimation of blood pressure in the ophthalmic arteries of the eye. This information is used as an indirect means to assess blood flow in the carotid arteries in the neck, which supply the eyes and brain (see the illustration on page 20 of the body atlas). The detection of impaired blood flow in the ophthalmic arteries indicates carotid artery narrowing, which is a major risk factor for stroke.

Purpose of the Test
• To aid in the evaluation of patients with suspected carotid artery narrowing or blockage due to the buildup of plaques (atherosclerosis).
• To monitor the effectiveness of carotid endarterectomy, a surgical procedure to remove plaques from carotid artery walls.

Who Performs It
• A doctor, a nurse, or a trained technician.

Special Concerns
• OPG is not appropriate for people who recently had eye surgery or artificial lens implantation; those who have experienced retinal detachment; or individuals who take anticoagulant medications such as warfarin (Coumadin, Panwarfin).

Before the Test
• If you wear contact lenses, remove them before the test.
• If you have glaucoma, continue to take your usual eye drops or oral medications before the test.
• The doctor will administer topical anesthetic eye drops to the eyes 5 to 10 minutes prior to the procedure. Your eyes may burn slightly after the drops are instilled.

What You Experience
• You will lie on your back on a bed or table.
• The examiner will take your blood pressure in both arms.
• ECG leads (see page 174) may be applied to your arms or legs to detect any abnormal heart rhythms.
• Eye cups resembling contact lenses are placed directly on the surface of each eye. These sensors detect and record pulsatile changes in the pressures of the eyes. (This information is translated into a graphic recording for later review.)
• Next, vacuum suction is applied to the eye cups, and gradually increased until the pressure in the eye (intraocular pressure) is higher than the arterial pressure, causing pulsation to stop in the arteries. (This may cause a pulling sensation and brief loss of vision.)
• The suction is then released, and the time needed for the arterial pulsation to reappear is recorded.

Results
➡ The OPG test data are reviewed by a physician. If the arterial pulse pressures in the eye are reduced or there is a delay in pulsation, a carotid artery may be blocked or narrowed.
➡ If a carotid blockage is suspected based on the results of OPG, additional tests—such as carotid Doppler ultrasound (see page 149) or arteriography (see page 95)—will be necessary to establish the location and degree of any plaques.
➡ If no carotid blockage is indicated, no further testing is needed.

Oculoplethysmography

• The procedure generally takes about 20 to 30 minutes.

Risks and Complications
• Possible rare complications of this test include bleeding from the conjunctiva (the mucous membrane that lines the eye surface), corneal abrasion, and temporary sensitivity to light.

After the Test
• You may experience temporary blurred vision or mild burning in the eyes as the anesthetic drops wear off, and your eyes may be bloodshot for several hours. Artificial tears may be instilled to soothe any irritation.
• You are free to leave the testing facility. Arrange for someone to drive you.
• Do not rub your eyes for at least 2 hours after the test.
• If you use contact lenses, do not reinsert them for at least 2 hours after the test.
• If your eyes feel sensitive to light, wear sunglasses.
• Report any severe burning, pain, or prolonged sensitivity to light to your doctor.

Estimated Cost: $$

Oncoscint Scan

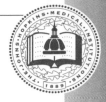

Description

• The Oncoscint scan is a nuclear imaging test that is used to detect recurrences of ovarian or colorectal cancer. For this test, you receive an intravenous injection of a radioactive tracer bound to a specific protein (monoclonal antibody) that is attracted to the cell surface of colorectal and ovarian cancer cells. A special scanning camera records the movement and distribution of this radioactive material throughout your body; areas of increased uptake may represent ovarian or colorectal cancer cells. The camera data are then translated by computer into two-dimensional images that are recorded on film. (For more on nuclear imaging, see Chapter 2.)

Purpose of the Test

• To identify and locate recurrent ovarian or colorectal cancer in people with elevated blood levels of certain tumor markers (see page 370).

Who Performs It

• A physician or a technician who specializes in nuclear medicine.

Special Concerns

• This test should not be performed in pregnant or breastfeeding women because of possible risks to the fetus or infant.
• Because the radiotracer may concentrate in areas of degenerative joint disease, abdominal aortic aneurysms, abdominal inflammatory processes, or inflammatory bowel disease, false-positive results may occur if these disorders are not identified before the test.
• This scan may also give false-negative results up to 30% of the time. (For more on false-positives and false-negatives, see page 35.)
• Because the monoclonal antibody used for this test is derived from a mouse, up to 40% of people who undergo this scan develop human antimurine antibodies (HAMA). These antibodies may cause falsely elevated levels of certain tumor markers (CEA and CA 125) on later blood tests.

Before the Test

• An abdominal CT scan (see page 76) is usually performed before the test to identify other conditions that could produce increased uptake of the radioactive material and distort the test results.

What You Experience

• A physician injects the radiotracer-antibody combination into a vein in your hand or arm.
• You may go home after the injection. You will be asked to return 48 to 72 hours later for the scanning procedure.
• You will lie on a padded table. A large scanning camera, which records the gamma rays being emitted by the radioactive material, is passed over the front and back sides of your chest, abdomen, and pelvis.
• Additional scans may be performed 24 and 48 hours later.
• If a significant amount of radioactive material is observed in your bowel on the scans, you may be given a laxative or enema to provide a

Results

▼

➡ A physician analyzes the recorded images for evidence of recurrent colorectal or ovarian cancer.

➡ If no abnormality is found, your doctor will recommend careful monitoring of your condition.

➡ If cancer recurrence is detected, appropriate therapy will be started.

Oncoscint Scan

better view of the rest of the abdomen and aid in the interpretation of the images.

• The scanning procedure takes about 1 hour each time, for 1 to 4 days.

Risks and Complications

• The trace amount of radioactive material used in this test is not associated with significant risks or complications.

• Fewer than 4% of patients react to the monoclonal antibody used in this test by developing a slight fever, a rash, low blood pressure, or a headache. Rarely, chest or joint pain may occur.

After the Test

• You may leave the testing facility and resume your normal activities.

• Drink extra fluids to help your body eliminate the radioactive material.

• Blood may collect and clot under the skin (hematoma) at the injection site; this is harmless and will resolve on its own. For a large hematoma that causes swelling and discomfort, apply ice initially; after 24 hours, use warm, moist compresses to help dissolve the clotted blood.

Estimated Cost: $$$$

Ophthalmodynamometry
(ODM)

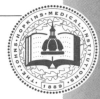

Description

• Ophthalmodynamometry (ODM) gives an approximate measurement of blood pressures in the central retinal arteries of the eye. As pressure is applied to the surface of the eye with a plunger-like device, an ophthalmologist uses a hand-held magnifying instrument (ophthalmoscope) to observe blood flow through the retinal arteries. This test is used as an indirect means to assess blood pressure in the carotid arteries in the neck, which supply the eyes and the brain. Reduced retinal artery pressure indicates carotid artery narrowing (a risk factor for stroke).

Purpose of the Test

• To aid in the evaluation of patients with suspected carotid artery narrowing or blockage due to the buildup of plaques (atherosclerosis).

Who Performs It

• An ophthalmologist.

Special Concerns

• This test is not appropriate for people who have recently had eye surgery.

Before the Test

• If you wear contact lenses, remove them before the test.
• The doctor will administer topical anesthetic eye drops 5 to 10 minutes prior to the procedure. Your eyes may burn slightly after the drops are instilled.

What You Experience

• A plunger-like device is used to apply gradual pressure to the surface of one eye, while the doctor observes pulsations in the central retinal artery through an ophthalmoscope.
• The retinal artery pressures are recorded.
• This procedure is repeated in the other eye.
• The test takes 5 to 15 seconds for each eye.

Risks and Complications

• This test may result in corneal discomfort or abrasion and slight bleeding under the conjunctiva (the mucous membrane lining the front of the eye and eyelid).

After the Test

• Do not rub your eyes for at least 30 minutes (until the anesthesia wears off) to avoid injuring the cornea.
• If you wear contact lenses, do not reinsert them for at least 2 hours after the test.

Estimated Cost: $

Results

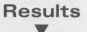

➥ An ophthalmologist reviews the test data. Retinal artery pressures are compared to systemic blood pressure, and pressures are also compared between eyes. A difference of more than 20% in retinal artery pressures between the two eyes indicates impaired blood flow in the carotid artery on the side with the lower reading.

➥ If no carotid blockage is indicated, no further testing is needed.

➥ If a carotid blockage is suspected, additional tests, such as carotid Doppler ultrasound (see page 149) or arteriography (see page 95), will be needed to establish the location and extent of any plaques.

Ophthalmodynamometry

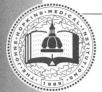

Oral Food or Drug Allergy Test
(Oral Challenge Test, Oral Provocation Test)

Oral Food or Drug Allergy Test

Description
• For this test, you ingest a food or drug in a capsule or in its natural form, and a physician observes you for the development of typical allergic symptoms. Food allergies can usually be detected using various dietary methods, in which the suspected food is excluded from the diet for a certain period of time and then reintroduced to see if symptoms appear. This test is typically ordered only if the results from such dietary techniques—as well as from blood and skin allergy tests (see pages 110 and 335)—are inconclusive or negative, but an allergy or intolerance is still suspected.

Purpose of the Test
• To confirm a suspected allergy or intolerance to a particular food or food additive.
• To confirm a suspected allergy or intolerance to certain medications, such as nonsteroidal anti-inflammatory drugs.

Who Performs It
• A physician.

Special Concerns
• If you are currently experiencing a severe cold, diarrhea, or other digestive problems, the test should be postponed until your condition improves.
• This test should not be performed if you have previously experienced a severe, life-threatening allergic reaction to the food or drug in question.
• Risky challenge tests are often done in special research units or hospitals.

Before the Test
• Avoid all of the foods or drugs that are suspected of causing an allergic reaction for 1 to 2 weeks prior to testing, according to your doctor's instructions.
• Stop taking antihistamines or other drugs that might suppress your allergic response prior to the test, according to your doctor's instructions.

What You Experience
• You will be asked to swallow liquid or solid foods or test capsules containing the suspected food or drug at specific time intervals.
• You will then be observed for any evidence of an allergic reaction to the test substance. Possible responses include hives; itching; wheezing; swelling of the eyes, lips, face, or tongue; nasal irritation; or gastrointestinal symptoms such as nausea, diarrhea, and abdominal pain.
• To ensure objective results, the test may be performed twice. One of these times, you will ingest a placebo capsule containing a harmless substance, usually sugar. (A third party labels the capsules so that neither you nor your physician knows which of the test capsules is the placebo.)
• Depending on the nature and the severity of the expected allergic reaction, you may be

Results
▼

➥ The doctor will assess your response to the various test substances. This test is considered positive if you develop typical allergic symptoms after ingesting the potential allergen, but not after taking the placebo capsule.

➥ If a specific allergy is diagnosed, your doctor will advise you to avoid the food or drug that is causing your symptoms.

➥ A negative result with this test is usually considered conclusive, and no further tests are needed.

observed for a period ranging from few minutes to several hours.

Risks and Complications

• There are several serious risks associated with this test, including a life-threatening response called anaphylactic shock (characterized by symptoms such as respiratory distress, decreased blood pressure, and shock); acute asthma; urticaria (hives or wheals); and angioedema (a sudden swelling involving the lips and skin, mucous membranes, and sometimes the abdominal organs).

• In the event that complications arise, emergency medications and equipment are kept readily available.

After the Test

• You will be asked to remain at the testing facility until the risk of an acute allergic reaction has passed.

• If this test does result in allergic symptoms, they may persist for several hours or even days.

• Inform your doctor immediately if you develop any symptoms after leaving the testing area.

Estimated Cost: $$$

Oral Food or Drug Allergy Test continued

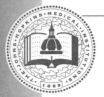

Oximetry

Description

• A sensor, attached to a device called a pulse oximeter, is clipped to your finger or ear, and then directs a beam of light through the tissue. The device is able to monitor oxygen saturation in the blood by measuring the amount of light absorbed by oxygenated hemoglobin (the oxygen-carrying pigment in red blood cells).

Purpose of the Test

• To monitor oxygen levels in patients at risk for decreased oxygen saturation in the blood (hypoxemia), including those who are undergoing surgery, cardiac stress testing (see page 147), or pulmonary function tests (see page 306); people who are heavily sedated, severely injured, or using a mechanical ventilation machine; and individuals undergoing studies in a sleep laboratory (see page 337).

Who Performs It

• A doctor, a nurse, or a technician.

Special Concerns

• A variety of factors may interfere with the results, including extreme changes in temperature, movement of the fingers, severe anemia, and fingernail polish.

Before the Test

• If you wear nail polish, remove it from at least one fingernail.

What You Experience

• The person performing the test will rub your fingertip or ear to increase blood circulation, and attach the monitoring sensor.
• The procedure is painless and noninvasive, and takes a few minutes.

Risks and Complications

• None.

After the Test

• No special aftercare is needed.

Estimated Cost: $

Results
▼

➡ If your oxygen levels are insufficient, you may be given supplemental oxygen through a face mask or small prongs that fit in the nose. Additional tests, such as arterial blood gases (see page 93), may be needed to determine the cause.

➡ If you are recovering from surgery with general anesthesia, the results of oximetry will help determine when you are ready for discharge.

➡ Decreased oxygen levels during sleep studies may indicate sleep apnea.

Pap Smear
(Pap Test, Papanicolaou Test)

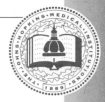

Description

• In this test, a sample of loose cells is gently scraped from the cervix (the lower part of the uterus that opens into the vagina), spread on a glass slide, and sent to a laboratory for microscopic examination. A Pap smear is often done as part of a routine gynecologic examination in women, and is able to detect precancerous and cancerous conditions in their early and most treatable stages. (The female reproductive system is illustrated on page 28.)

• Alternatively, a new technique known as a liquid-based smear involves placing the scraped specimen into a vial of liquid. This liquid-based material is then studied under a microscope.

Purpose of the Test

• Performed regularly in women after age 18 to 21 (or in younger women who are sexually active) to screen for cancer of the vagina, cervix, and uterus. (For more on screening tests, see Chapter 3.)

• To detect benign cervical abnormalities, such as inflammation of the cervix.

Who Performs It

• A gynecologist or a nurse practitioner.

Special Concerns

• The test should not be performed during your menstrual period, since the presence of blood may interfere with the results.

• The best time to schedule a Pap smear is two weeks after the start of your last menstrual period.

• The presence of vaginal or cervical infection or inflammation may result in an abnormal Pap smear in the absence of any malignant or precancerous condition; this is known as a false-positive result (see page 35) and may lead to unnecessary follow-up tests.

Before the Test

• Be sure to inform your doctor of any medications that you regularly take, including oral contraceptives.

• You will be asked to disrobe from the waist down and to put on a drape or hospital gown.

• You will be instructed to empty your bladder before the test.

What You Experience

• You will lie on your back on an examination table, with your knees bent and your feet raised and resting in stirrups.

Results
▼

➡ A pathologist will examine the Pap smear under a microscope for the presence of unusual cells. In addition, several computer programs are currently available to help recognize and classify any abnormal cells. (For more on microscopic examination, see Chapter 1.)

➡ In many cases, you will not be notified of your Pap smear results unless further evaluation is needed.

➡ If your Pap smear is normal, the test will typically be repeated annually, depending on your age, your risk factors, and any abnormalities found on the previous Pap smear.

➡ If abnormal cells are detected, you may need to undergo further testing—such as colposcopy with a cervical punch biopsy (see page 162), or pelvic or transvaginal ultrasound (see page 285)—to establish a diagnosis and determine the extent of the problem.

Pap Smear

Pap Smear continued

• A small metal or plastic instrument, called a speculum, is inserted into your vagina. (Insertion may cause slight discomfort, but is not painful.) The speculum holds the walls of the vagina open so that the examiner can view the upper vagina and cervix. Relax and breathe through your mouth to ease the insertion.

• The examiner then wipes a cotton swab, tiny brush, or thin wooden spatula over the cervix to collect cells.

• You may feel some mild discomfort as the sample is obtained.

• The cells are spread on a glass slide and sent to a laboratory for microscopic analysis.

• The speculum is withdrawn.

• The test usually takes about 2 to 3 minutes to perform.

Risks and Complications

• There are no risks or complications associated with this test.

After the Test

• You may dress and leave the doctor's office promptly after the test is completed.

Estimated Cost: $

Paracentesis
(Peritoneal Fluid Analysis)

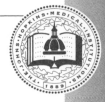

Description
• In this test, a needle is used to withdraw (aspirate) fluid from the peritoneal cavity, which surrounds the organs of the abdomen. The fluid sample is sent to a laboratory for analysis to identify the cause of ascites (excess fluid in the abdomen). This procedure may also be performed as a therapeutic measure to remove this excess peritoneal fluid.

Purpose of the Test
• To determine the cause of ascites and help select an appropriate treatment.
• To relieve excessive pressure on the organs in the abdomen, which causes discomfort and interferes with the ability to eat and digest properly.

Who Performs It
• A physician.

Special Concerns
• Paracentesis should not be performed in people with untreated bleeding disorders or in those who have had prior extensive abdominal surgery.

Before the Test
• Tell your doctor if you are taking any antimicrobial drugs, such as antibiotics.
• Your weight and abdominal girth may be measured.
• You will be instructed to empty your bladder before the procedure begins.

What You Experience
• You are asked to remove your shirt and lie down on a table or bed, or to sit in a chair with your feet placed flat on the floor or supported by a stool. You must remain still during the procedure.
• The skin at the site of injection (usually about 1 to 2 inches below the navel) is shaved and cleansed with an antiseptic solution. A local anesthetic is injected to numb the area.
• If a small amount of fluid is being withdrawn, an aspiration needle is inserted through the abdominal wall and into the peritoneal cavity. If larger amounts must be drained, a small incision is made and a larger needle and thin tube (cannula) are used instead.
• CT scanning or ultrasound imaging (see Chapter 2) may be used to guide the placement of the needle.
• You will feel pressure and slight pain as the needle is inserted and will hear an audible sound as it penetrates the tough membrane that lines the abdominal cavity (peritoneum).
• Fluid is withdrawn through the needle and placed into multiple specimen containers.
• The procedure takes 5 to 20 minutes.

Results
▼

➤ The specimen containers may be sent to several different laboratories for examination. The fluid may be analyzed for the presence of white blood cells, bacteria, protein, amylase (a type of enzyme secreted by the pancreas), and other components. (For more on laboratory testing, see Chapter 1.)

➤ Your doctor will diagnose the cause of the peritoneal effusion based on results from these laboratory tests. Possible causes include congestive heart failure, tuberculosis, cancer, cirrhosis and other liver diseases, pancreatitis (inflammation of the pancreas), infection, and various fungal or parasitic diseases.

➤ Appropriate treatment will be initiated, depending on the specific problem.

Paracentesis continued

Risks and Complications
• Potentially dangerous complications of this procedure include unintentional injury of internal organs or blood vessels with the needle, bleeding, edema (swelling), infection, and hypotension (low blood pressure). Emergency equipment is readily available if such complications arise.
• The risk of complications is reduced if CT scanning or ultrasound is used to guide needle insertion.

After the Test
• The needle is withdrawn and pressure is placed on the puncture site with sterile gauze pads for 3 to 5 minutes. A bandage is then applied.
• Your blood pressure and vital signs will be monitored periodically, and the puncture site will be observed for signs of bleeding or inflammation, usually for a few hours.
• Your weight and abdominal girth may be measured again and compared to your pretest values.
• If no complications develop and you have no health problems that require hospitalization, you are free to leave the testing facility.

Estimated Cost: $$

Patch Test

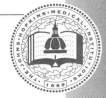

Description

• In this test, common allergens—substances known to produce an allergic reaction in susceptible individuals—are applied to skin on the back, in order pinpoint the cause of recurrent skin irritation (dermatitis). Since some allergens only cause a reaction in combination with ultraviolet (UV) light, application of the potential allergens is sometimes followed by exposure to UV light; this variation is called a photopatch test.

Purpose of the Test

• To determine whether dermatitis—characterized by itching, redness, and other skin irritation—is caused or aggravated by a contact allergy, and to identify the substance responsible for the problem. Common culprits include perfume, cosmetics, nickel in jewelry, and latex.

Who Performs It

• A doctor or a nurse.

Special Concerns

• A variety of conditions may make it difficult to interpret the results. These include using very high or low concentrations of allergen extracts, impurities in the extracts, examining the test sites too early or too late, and placing patches on already inflamed skin.

• Use of high-dose oral steroids or topical steroid cream or ointment, or recent intense sun or suntan parlor exposure of the test sites, may produce false-negative results.

• Even in the absence of interfering factors, the accuracy of testing may vary. You may react to an allergen during testing but not during normal exposure; conversely, you may have a negative test result and still be allergic to a substance.

Before the Test

• On your initial visit to the doctor before the test, bring any items you suspect might be causing the allergic reaction, such as jewelry, perfume, cosmetics, or items of clothing.

• Do not tan outdoors or go to a tanning parlor before the test.

• Do not apply steroid cream or ointment to the skin that will be used for the test.

What You Experience

• Small amounts of the selected allergens are first applied to small disks and then taped to the skin on your back. (Usually 20 to 60 separate allergens are used.) This process takes less than 30 minutes.

• The patches should remain in place undisturbed for the next 48 hours. Because the patch sites must be kept dry, you cannot bathe or shower during this time, and you should also avoid strenuous exercise in order to prevent heavy sweating.

Results

▼

➡ For a routine patch test, a finding of redness, bumps, blisters, or other skin abnormalities at a specific patch site suggests that you are allergic to the tested substance. Your doctor will recommend that you avoid that allergen.

➡ In the photopatch test, the presence of a reaction at the site that was exposed to UV light—but not at the corresponding protected site—indicates that you have a photoallergic reaction to that particular substance. Your doctor will recommend that you avoid that allergen.

➡ If the initial test is negative, your doctor may order additional tests in an effort to identify the cause of your dermatitis.

Patch Test

• If you experience severe itching or pain at any of the sites, remove the patch by cutting it out and inform your doctor immediately.

• The patches are removed in the doctor's office, and the test sites are examined at this time and again in another 1 to 5 days.

• For a photopatch test, duplicate patches are applied to your back for each allergen and taped in place with opaque material. After 24 to 48 hours, one allergen site from each pair is uncovered and exposed to UV light, while the other site remains covered.

Risks and Complications

• Mild skin irritation may occur at the test sites.

• Infrequently, the dermatitis that prompted the test may flare up, or several or many sites may turn red ("angry back"). If this occurs, the test will be discontinued.

After the Test

• If some of the test sites itch, the doctor may prescribe a steroid ointment or cream for relief.

• Skin on some of the test sites may remain slightly dark for several weeks, but the discoloration will fade eventually.

Estimated Cost: $$ to $$$

Pelvic or Transvaginal Ultrasound

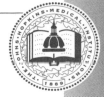

Description

• In these procedures, a device called a transducer is used to direct high-frequency sound waves (ultrasound) at the organs and structures within the pelvic region—typically the uterus and ovaries in women. The transducer may either be passed over the surface of the abdomen (pelvic ultrasound) or inserted into the vagina (transvaginal ultrasound). The sound waves are reflected back to the transducer and electronically converted into images displayed on a viewing monitor. These images can be saved on film or video and then reviewed for abnormalities. (For more on how ultrasound works, see Chapter 2.)

Purpose of the Test

• To determine the size, shape, and position of organs in the pelvic region.

• To evaluate pain, abnormal bleeding, or other menstrual problems in women.

• To detect abnormalities affecting the ovaries and uterus, such as tumors, abscesses, cysts, fibroids, and inflammation.

• To evaluate infertility problems.

• To monitor follicle development in the ovaries of an infertility patient receiving ovulation-inducing drugs (fertility drugs) or undergoing in vitro fertilization.

• To monitor the health and development of the fetus and placenta in pregnant women, and to detect problems such as ectopic (tubal) pregnancy. (Transvaginal ultrasound is more often used early in pregnancy, and pelvic ultrasound later in pregnancy.)

Who Performs It

• A doctor or a radiology technician.

Special Concerns

• Because transvaginal ultrasound places the transducer closer to the internal pelvic structures, it can produce more detailed images than external pelvic ultrasound. It may also be more comfortable because it doesn't require a full bladder. However, an external exam is better for viewing structures in the upper pelvis (especially in pregnant women); giving an overall picture of pelvic organs in relation to one another; and examining obese patients, since fat may interfere with transmission of sound waves.

• Because residual barium and gas in the colon can distort sound waves and affect the test results, this exam should be done before any barium contrast x-rays are performed.

Before the Test

• External pelvic ultrasound requires a full bladder to displace the bowel from the pelvic cavity and push the uterus and ovaries outward, making them easier to see on the scan. Your doctor will instruct you to drink 3 to 4 glasses of water or other liquid about 1 hour before the test; do not urinate until the procedure is complete. (This step is not necessary, however, late in pregnancy.)

• Empty your bladder before a transvaginal ultrasound exam.

• Your clothes will be arranged so as to expose

Results

▼

➡ A radiologist reviews the recorded images and video for evidence of any abnormality.

➡ If a definitive diagnosis can be made, appropriate treatment will be initiated.

➡ If ultrasound fails to yield a definitive diagnosis, other diagnostic tests, such as a sonohysterogram (see page 342), may be needed to provide more specific information or to further evaluate abnormal findings.

your lower abdomen before a pelvic ultrasound exam. You must disrobe from the waist down and put on a drape before transvaginal ultrasound.

What You Experience

Pelvic ultrasound:

• You will lie on your back on an examination table.

• A water-soluble gel is applied to the skin on your lower abdomen to enhance sound wave transmission.

• The examiner then moves the transducer back and forth over the surface of your pelvic region to obtain different views of the targeted organs on a viewing monitor.

• Once clear images are obtained, they are recorded on film or video for later analysis.

• The test takes about 20 minutes.

Transvaginal ultrasound:

• You will assume a position similar to the one used for a pelvic exam—lying on your back with your knees bent and feet placed in stirrups.

• A sterile latex condom is placed over a special oblong transducer (which is slightly smaller than a tampon), and a small amount of water-soluble gel is applied to the device.

• The transducer is gently inserted (either by the examiner or yourself) into the vagina and rested against the cervix.

• The examiner rotates the transducer to one side, then the other, to obtain different views of the targeted organs on a viewing monitor.

• Once clear images are obtained, they are recorded on film or video for later analysis.

• The transducer is gently withdrawn.

• The test takes less than 10 minutes.

Risks and Complications

• Ultrasound is painless, noninvasive, and involves no exposure to radiation. There are no associated risks.

After the Test

• After pelvic ultrasound, the examiner removes the conductive gel from your skin.

• You may urinate and resume your normal diet and activities.

Estimated Cost: $

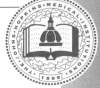

Percutaneous Transhepatic Cholangiography (PTHC)

Description

• In this test, a contrast dye is injected directly into a bile duct in the liver, and a series of x-ray films is taken as the material flows through the biliary system. The dye delineates the biliary tract on the x-ray images and reveals any significant abnormalities. This test is usually ordered after less invasive tests, such as CT scanning or ultrasound, fail to provide a definitive diagnosis. (For more on contrast x-rays, see Chapter 2.)

Purpose of the Test

• To evaluate the cause of jaundice (yellowing of the skin); in particular, to determine whether impaired bile flow is caused by a bile duct obstruction or nonobstructive liver disease.
• To identify the location and extent of any mechanical obstruction in a bile duct.
• To determine the cause of upper abdominal pain that persists after the gallbladder has been removed.

Who Performs It

• A radiologist.

Special Concerns

• Endoscopic retrograde cholangiopancreatography (see page 187) is used more frequently than PTHC to visualize the biliary system because it is associated with fewer complications. However, PTHC is the only method that can be used to examine the bile ducts after most gastric surgeries.
• People with allergies to iodine or shellfish may experience an allergic reaction to the iodine-based contrast dye.
• Pregnant women should not undergo this test because exposure to ionizing radiation may harm the fetus.
• This test is not suitable for patients with infection of the bile ducts (cholangitis), a large amount of ascites (excess fluid in the abdomen), or certain bleeding disorders. Blood coagulation studies (see page 157) may be necessary to ensure you are a proper candidate for the test.
• Severe obesity or the presence of residual barium in the abdomen from recent contrast x-rays of the digestive tract may interfere with visualization of the bile ducts.

Before the Test

• Inform your doctor if you have an allergy to iodine or shellfish. You may be given a combined antihistamine-steroid preparation to reduce the risk of an allergic reaction, or an alternative noniodinated contrast agent may be used.
• Do not eat or drink after midnight on the day before the test.
• You may be asked to take a laxative on the night before the test, and you may receive a cleansing enema on the morning of the test.
• If necessary, you may receive intravenous

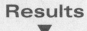

Results

➡ The doctor will examine the x-ray films to determine whether the bile ducts are dilated (indicating an obstruction) or normal size (indicating nonobstructive jaundice caused by liver disease). Obstruction can be caused by gallstones, tumors, cysts, inflammation, or stricture (narrowing).

➡ If a bile duct obstruction is present, your doctor may recommend treatment, such as insertion of a temporary catheter or stent, to drain the biliary tract.

➡ If liver disease is suspected, another test, such as a liver biopsy (see page 240), may be needed to identify the cause.

antibiotic injections on the day before the test to prevent infection.

• The doctor may give you a sedative before the procedure.

What You Experience

• You will lie on your back on an x-ray table. The skin on your right upper abdomen is cleansed with an antiseptic solution, and a local anesthetic is injected to numb the area overlying the liver and the liver itself. You may feel brief discomfort when the needle penetrates the liver.

• Under the guidance of fluoroscopy (see page 205), which transmits continuous, moving x-ray images to a viewing screen, the doctor advances a thin, flexible needle through your skin and into the liver. You are instructed to exhale completely and hold your breath as the needle is inserted.

• When the needle is positioned in a bile duct, contrast dye is injected. You may feel a sensation of abdominal pressure and fullness, as well as transient pain in your upper back on the right side.

• A series of x-ray films is obtained. At various points, the table may be rotated, and you may be asked to assume several different positions. You must remain perfectly still as the films are taken.

• After the x-rays are completed, the needle is withdrawn slowly.

• The procedure takes about 45 to 60 minutes.

Risks and Complications

• Some people may experience an allergic reaction to the iodine-based contrast dye, which can cause symptoms such as nausea, sneezing, vomiting, hives, and occasionally a life-threatening response called anaphylactic shock. Emergency medications and equipment are kept readily available.

• Serious risks include peritonitis (infection or inflammation of the membrane lining the abdominal cavity) caused by passage of bile outside of the liver; bleeding caused by unintentional puncture of a large blood vessel in the liver; inflammation of the bile ducts (cholangitis); and blood poisoning (septicemia) or infection (bacteremia).

After the Test

• You must remain in bed for at least 6 hours after the test, preferably lying on your right side, to help prevent bleeding (hemorrhage). Pain medication is provided if needed. A sandbag may be placed over the injection site to help control any bleeding.

• While you recover, your vital signs are monitored periodically, and you will be checked for any signs of complications, such as bleeding or swelling at the injection site, chills, fever, and abdominal pain, tenderness, or distention.

• You may resume your normal diet and gradually return to your normal activities.

Estimated Cost: $$$

Pericardiocentesis
(Pericardial Fluid Analysis)

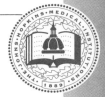

Description

• A needle is used to aspirate fluid from the pericardial sac, which surrounds the heart. The fluid sample is sent for laboratory analysis to identify the cause of pericardial effusion (excess fluid around the heart). This procedure may also be performed as an emergency therapeutic measure to relieve increased pressure on the heart.

Purpose of the Test

• To determine the cause of pericardial effusion and help select an appropriate treatment.
• Used as a treatment to relieve excessive pressure on the heart, known as cardiac tamponade, which can interfere with the contractions of the heart.

Who Performs It

• A physician.

Special Concerns

• Tell your doctor if you have a bleeding disorder; if so, pericardiocentesis should not be done.
• This procedure must be performed in a cardiac catheterization laboratory, an operating room, or an emergency room.

Before the Test

• If this is an elective procedure, restrict your fluid and food intake for 6 hours before the test.
• Your doctor may ask if you are taking any antimicrobial drugs, such as antibiotics.

What You Experience

• After removing your shirt, you will lie down on a table. You must remain still during the procedure.
• An intravenous (IV) line will be inserted into a vein in your arm to administer fluid, medications, or a sedative, if necessary.

• ECG leads (see page 174) may be used to monitor your heart rate and rhythm during the procedure.
• The skin at the site of needle insertion (just below and to the left of the sternum) is swabbed with an antiseptic solution, and then a local anesthetic is administered to numb the area.
• The aspiration needle is inserted through the chest wall into the pericardial sac; you will feel pressure during insertion, but there will be no other discomfort.
• You may be asked to hold your breath briefly to make it easier for the doctor to accurately place the needle.
• Once the needle is inserted, a clamp is attached to hold it in place, and fluid is withdrawn through the needle into multiple specimen containers.
• The procedure takes 10 to 20 minutes.

Results
▼

➡ The specimen containers may be sent to several different laboratories for examination. The fluid will be analyzed for the presence of blood, bacteria, malignant cells, and other components. (For more on laboratory testing, see Chapter 1.)

➡ Your doctor will diagnose the cause of the pericardial effusion based on results from these laboratory tests. Possible causes include acute heart attack, pericarditis, tuberculosis, cancer, rheumatoid disease, systemic lupus erythematosus, hypothyroidism, and infection.

➡ Appropriate treatment will be initiated, depending on the problem.

Pericardiocentesis

Pericardiocentesis continued

• A pericardial catheter may be left in place to drain continuously for 1 to 3 days.

Risks and Complications
• Potentially dangerous complications of this procedure include unintentional laceration of a coronary artery or the heart muscle; a life-threatening arrhythmia called ventricular fibrillation; cardiac arrest; pleural (lung) infection; and accidental puncture of the lung, liver, or stomach. Emergency equipment is available if such complications arise.
• The risk of complications is reduced if echocardiography (see page 365) or fluoroscopy (see page 205) is used to visualize the heart and guide needle insertion.

After the Test
• When the test is completed, the needle is withdrawn.
• Pressure is applied to the needle insertion site with sterile gauze pads for 3 to 5 minutes. A bandage is then applied.
• Your blood pressure and vital signs will be monitored periodically for a few hours after the procedure.

Estimated Cost: $$

Phototesting

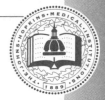

Description
• These tests are used to evaluate skin abnormalities—such as rash, itching, blisters, and hives—that are either caused or exacerbated by exposure to sunlight. In standard phototests, small areas of skin are irradiated with different doses of long- and short-wave ultraviolet (UVA and UVB) and visible light, and then observed for a reaction.
• The photopatch test (described on page 283) is used when light-induced skin reactions are believed to be linked to a particular contact allergy (such as a fragrance or cosmetic).

Purpose of the Test
• To confirm a diagnosis of photosensitivity (sensitivity to light) and to assess its severity.
• To determine the particular wavelengths of light that elicit a skin reaction.
• To evaluate the effectiveness of treatment.
• To follow the development of a light-induced skin disorder over time.

Who Performs It
• A technician or a nurse at a dermatologist's office.

Special Concerns
• Some photosensitivity reactions occur only after ingestion of certain drugs or after the skin is exposed to a particular substance. If these agents are not present, a false-negative result may occur (see page 35).
• Blood tests are necessary to confirm a diagnosis in some light-induced skin disorders.

Before the Test
• No special preparation is needed before this procedure.

What You Experience
• The examiner shines UVA, UVB, and visible light on different small areas of skin, such as on the back or forearms. The portion of the body that is exposed to light, the type of light, and the dose and duration of exposure—ranging from a few minutes to less than one hour—vary depending on the suspected diagnosis.
• The examiner assesses the skin reaction immediately after exposure, 24 hours later, and then periodically thereafter for up to three weeks.
• The minimal erythema dose (MED) at 24 hours is noted; this is the lowest dose of UVA or UVB radiation that produces a clearly identifiable pink mark on the skin.

Results
▼

➡ If you have a positive skin reaction, your doctor will try to diagnose the cause of your disorder based on your symptoms, history, and the results of other tests.

➡ A variety of conditions may be responsible for skin photosensitivity, including a common condition of unknown origins called polymorphous light eruption (PLE); a rare disorder called solar urticaria; and the generalized autoimmune disease systemic lupus erythematosus (SLE).

➡ Sensitivity to sunlight may also be a side effect of certain medications (drug-induced photosensitivity).

➡ If the doctor can make a definitive diagnosis, appropriate medications or ointments will be prescribed.

➡ If the test results are negative, the doctor may order additional tests in an effort to determine the cause of the problem.

Phototesting

• When drug-induced photosensitivity is the suspected diagnosis, the testing procedure is done two times—once while you are taking the medication and again after you have discontinued it and the drug has been cleared from your system—to confirm the disappearance of photosensitivity.

Risks and Complications
• A positive reaction to phototesting may cause pain, itching, blisters, or redness at the tested sites. Fever and malaise may also occur.

After the Test
• You will be instructed to avoid exposing the irradiated skin areas to sunlight until the testing process is completed (that is, after the final examination is performed).
• If any lesions or irritation develops on the exposed areas of skin, the doctor may prescribe a steroid cream or lotion to help control the reaction.
• If you develop a skin reaction at a test site after testing has been completed, let your doctor know immediately; this information is crucial for the correct diagnosis of your skin disorder.

Estimated Cost: $

Pituitary Hormone Tests

Description

• The pituitary—a small, oval gland located at the base of the brain—is sometimes called the master gland because it regulates and controls the secretions of other endocrine glands and various body processes by producing a variety of hormones. (The endocrine system is illustrated on page 18.) Measuring blood levels of the following pituitary hormones can provide valuable information about the function of the pituitary and the other glands controlled by these hormones.

• **Growth hormone (GH),** as its name implies, plays a central role in regulating the body's growth. If a blood test indicates an elevated level of GH, a **GH suppression test,** which measures GH levels in response to glucose (a sugar that normally suppresses GH secretion) is done to confirm the finding. If the blood level of GH is low, a **GH stimulation test** is performed to measure GH levels in response to substances that normally stimulate GH secretion (such as the hormone insulin, the amino acid arginine, or growth hormone-releasing hormone, or GHRH).

• **Insulin-like growth factor-1 (IGF-1)** is not a hormone but a substance secreted by the liver that is often measured to assess GH secretion by the pituitary. GH accomplishes its effects on many tissues through somatomedins, a group of proteins that include IGF-1. Because GH is produced in several bursts during the day and may be affected by a variety of factors such as food intake and exercise, measuring IGF-1 may in fact be a more accurate reflection of average GH levels than a direct blood test.

• **Prolactin** is a pituitary hormone that helps to prepare the mammary glands for lactation during pregnancy and stimulates milk production after a woman gives birth. Prolactin levels are measured in people suspected of having pituitary tumors, which are known to secrete excessive amounts of this hormone.

• **ACTH,** or corticotropin, is a pituitary hormone that stimulates the adrenal gland to release cortisol and other hormones (see page 83). Measuring ACTH levels in the blood can aid in the diagnosis of adrenal gland abnormalities, such as Cushing's syndrome (overproduction of cortisol) and Addison's disease (a form of adrenal insufficiency marked by underproduction of cortisol). To help diagnose Cushing's syndrome, the **dexamethasone suppression test** may be performed to measure the effect that dexamethasone, a drug similar to cortisol, has on cortisol levels. Alternatively, to evaluate adrenal insufficiency the **ACTH stimulation test** is used to measure the adrenal response to ACTH administration.

• **Luteinizing hormone (LH),** produced by the pituitary, acts on the ovary in women and the testis in men. In women, a surge in LH secretion at mid-menstrual cycle causes ovulation and helps to maintain the specialized portion of the ovary that produces the female sex hormone progesterone. In men, LH secretion stimulates specialized cells in the testis to

Results

▼

➥ Your blood samples are sent to a laboratory for analysis. A physician will review the results for evidence of any pituitary hormone disorder or other problem. (For more on laboratory testing, see Chapter 1.)

➥ If an abnormality is found and the doctor can make a definitive diagnosis, appropriate treatment will be initiated.

➥ In many cases, abnormal results on one or more of the pituitary hormone tests will necessitate additional tests to establish a definitive diagnosis.

Pituitary Hormone Tests

release the male sex hormone testosterone. LH levels are measured in the evaluation of infertility in both women and men.

• **Follicle-stimulating hormone (FSH)** is a pituitary hormone that also helps to control the activity of the ovary and testis. In women, FSH stimulates the development of the ovarian follicles for ovulation. In men, FSH stimulates and helps to maintain sperm production. FSH measurements can aid in the evaluation of infertility and disorders of menstruation.

Purpose of the Test
Growth hormone and IGF-1 tests:
• To aid in the diagnosis of acromegaly (a disease marked by enlargement of the bones of the extremities, face, and jaw).
• To help identify tumors affecting the pituitary or the hypothalamus in the brain.
• To aid in the monitoring of human growth hormone therapy.

Prolactin test:
• To diagnose and monitor pituitary tumors.
• To evaluate patients with amenorrhea (absence of menstruation) or galactorrhea (abnormal secretion of milk).

ACTH tests:
• To aid in the diagnosis and evaluation of adrenal abnormalities, such as Addison's disease and Cushing's syndrome.

LH and FSH tests:
• To aid in the diagnosis of infertility in both men and women.
• To help evaluate disorders of menstruation, including amenorrhea.
• To determine the onset of menopause.
• To monitor infertility treatments designed to induce ovulation.

Who Performs It
• A doctor, a nurse, or a technician.

Special Concerns
• A wide range of factors—including medica-

tions and nutritional supplements, exercise, sleep, stress, nutrition, and the menstrual cycle—may alter the results of the various tests. In particular, these variables cause a significant overlap between normal and abnormal results when GH is measured directly.
• A nuclear scan performed within the previous week may affect the results of these tests, because pituitary hormones are often measured with a laboratory technique that utilizes a radioactive isotope (radioimmunoassay).
• Certain individuals, including those with epilepsy, cerebrovascular disease, or a recent heart attack, should not undergo the GH stimulation test because it produces low blood sugar and may cause serious complications.
• Blood levels of ACTH vary during the day, peaking in the early morning (from 6 to 8 AM) and declining in the evening (from 6 to 11 PM). This pattern differs in people who work nights and sleep during the day; this fact must be taken into account when interpreting the test results.

Before the Test
• You may be asked to fast, limit your physical activity, and reduce stress levels for variable periods before these tests.
• Report to your doctor any medications, herbs, or supplements you are taking. You may be advised to discontinue certain of these agents before the test.
• Tell your doctor if you've had any recent procedures, such as a nuclear scan, that introduce radioactive material into your bloodstream.

What You Experience
Direct blood test for pituitary hormones:
• A sample of your blood is drawn from a vein, usually in your arm, and sent to a laboratory for analysis. (For more on this procedure, called venipuncture, see page 32.)
• The blood sample may need to be taken at a specific time during the day.

GH stimulation test:
• A special type of intravenous (IV) catheter is inserted into a vein in your arm. It allows both

administration of medications and withdrawal of blood samples.

• A blood sample is taken so that pre-test blood levels of GH, glucose, and cortisol can be measured.

• Arginine, insulin, or GHRH is then infused through the IV line, and blood samples are obtained at several intervals over the next 2 hours.

• When insulin is used, you will be monitored continuously for signs of hypoglycemia (weakness, restlessness, hunger, sweating, nervousness) and low blood pressure.

• You may be given ice chips to chew to alleviate thirst.

GH suppression test:
• Blood samples are drawn between 6 AM and 8 AM using venipuncture (see page 32) to record pre-test GH levels.

• You are asked to drink a glucose solution. It will taste very sweet. Drink it slowly to avoid nausea.

• Additional blood samples are drawn at several intervals over the next 2 hours so that they can be analyzed for GH levels in response to the glucose.

ACTH stimulation test:
• Blood samples are drawn using venipuncture (see page 32) to record pre-test cortisol levels.

• Less than 30 minutes later, an ACTH analogue (cosyntropin) is injected into a vein, usually in the arm, over a 2-minute period.

• Blood samples are taken 30 and 60 minutes after the injection so they can be analyzed for cortisol levels in response to cosyntropin.

Dexamethasone suppression test:
• At 11 PM, you are given 1 mg of dexamethasone by mouth, together with milk or an antacid to prevent gastric irritation.

• At 8 AM the next morning, blood samples are taken by venipuncture (see page 32) to measure your cortisol level before you arise.

• If no cortisol suppression is observed, you will be given a higher dose of dexamethasone (8 mg) to suppress ACTH production.

Risks and Complications
• Severe hypoglycemia may develop during the GH stimulation test, but this complication is unlikely to occur under close observation.

• The other tests entail no significant risks.

After the Test
• Resume your normal diet and any medications that were withheld before the test, according to your doctor's instructions.

• After the GH stimulation test, you will be given cookies and punch or an IV glucose infusion to restore your normal blood sugar levels.

• After the ACTH suppression test, you will be evaluated for signs of gastric irritation as well as steroid-induced side effects by monitoring your weight, glucose level, and potassium level.

• Blood may collect and clot under the skin (hematoma) at the site of needle puncture or IV insertion; this is harmless and will resolve on its own. For a large hematoma that causes swelling and discomfort, apply ice initially; after 24 hours, use warm, moist compresses to help dissolve the clotted blood.

Estimated Cost: $ to $$

Pituitary Hormone Tests continued

Plethysmography

Plethysmography

Description

• This noninvasive technique uses blood pressure cuffs or other sensors attached to an instrument called a plethysmograph (or pulse volume recorder) to measure changes in the volume of a limb (or extremity). Because these volume changes are directly related to the amount of blood flowing through the limb, this test helps to identify problems affecting blood circulation.

• **Arterial plethysmography** may be used to rule out blockage of an artery in the leg or to identify problems in the smaller arteries in the hands, fingers, feet, and toes (such as Raynaud's disease, a condition marked by abnormal constriction of blood vessels in the extremities upon exposure to cold or emotional distress).

• **Venous plethysmography** helps to identify problems in blood flow through the veins in a limb or limbs. This test is most often performed to help identify or rule out a blood clot in a calf vein (deep vein thrombosis or DVT). It may also be used to detect dysfunction of important valves in the venous system causing blood to run backwards rather than forwards with exercise.

Purpose of the Test

• To detect or rule out blockages (occlusion) and other circulatory problems in the extremities.

Who Performs It

• A technician trained in vascular studies.

Special Concerns

• Venous plethysmography complements venous duplex scanning (see page 385) for identifying DVT in a calf vein.

• Venous plethysmography is less accurate than venography (see page 382) for detecting DVT in general, but it is often done as an initial test to rule out DVT because it is noninvasive and easy to perform.

• Arterial plethysmography is not as accurate as arteriography (see page 95) for detecting arterial blockages, but has the advantage of being noninvasive and easy to perform.

Before the Test

• Do not smoke cigarettes for at least 30 minutes before the test begins, since nicotine constricts the peripheral blood vessels and can interfere with the accuracy of the results.

• You will be instructed to remove all clothing from the limb or limbs being examined.

What You Experience
Arterial plethysmography:

• You will be placed in a reclining position. You must remain still during the procedure.

• Blood pressure cuffs or other sensors are placed at different locations on the arms, legs, fingers, and/or toes. (If cuffs are used, they are partially inflated to make them more sensitive to small changes in the circumference of the limbs corresponding to blood flow.)

• The sensors record the pulse waves that occur with each heart beat. (This data is translated into a graphic recording for later review.)

• In some cases, the test also records changes in pulsation under various conditions, such as exposure to cold or temporary stoppage of blood flow to the limb (which is done by inflat-

Results

▼

➡ A physician will review the test data for evidence of abnormal blood circulation in the extremities.

➡ If an abnormality is found, your doctor may recommend more invasive tests, such as arteriography or venography, to provide more information and establish a diagnosis.

ing a blood pressure cuff in the upper region of the limb until the blood vessels collapse).

• The test usually takes about 30 minutes.

Venous plethysmography:

• You will lie down on a bed or table. You must remain still during the procedure.

• Blood pressure cuffs or other sensors are placed at different locations on one or both legs or arms. (If cuffs are used, they are partially inflated to make them more sensitive to small changes in the circumference of the limbs corresponding to blood flow.)

• The sensors measure the volume of the limb before, during, and after blood flow is halted temporarily by inflating the uppermost cuff in the limb until the blood vessels collapse. (This data is translated into a graphic recording for later review.)

• You may be asked to stand and perform certain stepping procedures as further recordings are taken.

• The test usually takes about 30 minutes.

Risks and Complications

• This test is noninvasive and is not associated with any risks or complications.

After the Test

• You may resume your normal activities.

Estimated Cost: $$

Positron Emission Tomography
(PET Scan)

Description

• Positron emission tomography (PET) combines the techniques of nuclear scanning and biochemical analysis to assess body processes like blood flow and metabolism in certain organs. In this test, a radioactive tracer is tagged to a biologically active molecule—such as glucose, oxygen, carbon monoxide, hormones, or neurotransmitters—and introduced into the body, usually by injection. After you enter a special scanning machine, radiation detectors record the emissions of the radioactive material. This information is relayed to a computer, which constructs color-coded, cross-sectional images depicting which areas of the organ are active. PET scanning can provide valuable information not only about the structure of particular organs, but also about how they work. (For more on PET scanning, see Chapter 2.)

Purpose of the Test

• To assess various body processes—particularly brain activity, but also activity in the heart, lungs, and other tissues and organs.
• To evaluate neurologic illnesses, including epilepsy, Alzheimer's disease, and other types of dementia.
• To help determine heart muscle function in patients with heart disease and distinguish between viable and dead cardiac tissue during the early stages of a heart attack.
• To detect cancerous tumors, determine the stage of cancer, and evaluate the effectiveness of cancer therapy.

Who Performs It

• A specially trained radiologist or technician.

Special Concerns

• PET scanning is very costly (because the positron-emitting radiotracers used for this test must first be generated by a particle accelerator, or cyclotron), and is not routinely performed outside of major medical institutions.
• This test should not be performed in pregnant or breastfeeding women because of possible risks to the fetus or infant.
• Extreme obesity may limit the accuracy of PET scans of the heart or lung.
• Drugs such as tranquilizers and sedatives as well as recent use of caffeine, alcohol, or tobacco may alter the test results.
• When radiolabeled glucose is used, the presence of diabetes may affect the results. Blood sugar levels must be monitored during testing in most patients.

Before the Test

• Do not ingest alcohol, caffeine, tobacco, sedatives, or tranquilizers for 24 hours before the procedure.
• If you have diabetes, you will be asked to take your pretest dose of insulin at a meal 3 to 4 hours before the test.
• Two intravenous (IV) lines may be placed in veins in your arms, one for infusing the radioactive tracer and the other for taking a series of blood samples.
• Empty your bladder before the test.

What You Experience

• You will lie down on a table.

Results

▼

➡ A radiologist reviews the PET scan data for evidence of abnormalities.
➡ If a definitive diagnosis can be made, appropriate therapy will be initiated.
➡ In some cases, additional tests, such as magnetic resonance angiography (see page 253), may be needed to establish a diagnosis and determine the extent of the problem.

Positron Emission Tomography

• The radioactive tracer is either injected through one of the IV lines or inhaled in the form of a radioactive gas.

• You enter into the PET scanning machine, and the gamma rays emitted by the radiotracer are recorded by a circular array of detectors. The resulting images are displayed on a computer.

• You must lie very still during the procedure.

• If you are undergoing a PET scan of the brain, special cushions may be placed against your head to hold it in place. You may be asked to perform various cognitive activities, such as doing a mathematical calculation or remembering a sequence of words. To minimize external stimuli, you may be asked to wear a blindfold and earplugs.

• The procedure can take from 1 to 2 hours.

Risks and Complications

• The radioactive tracers used in PET scans are short-lived and rapidly cleared from the body. They are not associated with any significant risks or complications.

After the Test

• You may be advised to stand up slowly after the procedure to avoid feeling faint or dizzy.

• You are free to leave the testing facility and resume your normal activities.

• Drink plenty of fluids to help flush the radioactive material from your body.

• Blood may collect and clot under the skin (hematoma) at the IV needle insertion site(s); this is harmless and will resolve on its own. For a large hematoma that causes swelling and discomfort, apply ice initially; after 24 hours, use warm, moist compresses to help dissolve the clotted blood.

Estimated Cost: $$$

Positron Emission Tomography continued

Prostate Biopsy

Description

• In this test, a thin needle is used to extract tissue samples from the prostate gland (illustrated on page 28); the specimens are sent to a laboratory for microscopic examination. Two techniques may be employed. In the majority of cases, an ultrasound probe is used to guide a needle through the rectum and into the prostate (transrectal approach). Rarely, a thin needle may be inserted through the perineum, the patch of skin located between the anus and scrotum, into the prostate (perineal approach). A biopsy is considered the only definitive way to confirm prostate cancer in men who have high PSA levels (see page 55) or a lump detected by a urologist during a digital rectal exam (DRE).

Purpose of the Test

• To establish a diagnosis of prostate cancer.

Who Performs It

• A urologist or a specially trained radiologist.

Special Concerns

• The perineal approach is considered less accurate, and is usually done only in cases where a prostate has a specific nodule or obvious diffuse abnormality.
• In some cases, prostate cancer may be diagnosed incidentally after a transurethral resection of the prostate (TURP), a surgical procedure to remove excess prostate tissue in men with benign prostate enlargement (known as benign prostatic hyperplasia, or BPH). In this procedure, the prostate is accessed with a thin viewing tube (resectoscope) that is passed through the urethra; a wire is passed through the instrument to remove excess prostate tissue, and samples are routinely sent to a laboratory for microscopic examination.
• In some cases, a biopsy may fail to detect cancer cells, resulting in a false-negative result (see page 35). The more tissue specimens that are taken, the smaller the risk of missing cancer.

Before the Test

• Before a transrectal biopsy, antibiotics will be prescribed to prevent infection.
• You may receive a cleansing enema before a transrectal biopsy to clear your intestine and provide better visibility during the test.
• You will be asked to disrobe and put on a hospital gown.
• Just before the biopsy, you may be given a mild sedative to relax you.

What You Experience

Transrectal approach:
• You are asked to lie on your side on a table.

Results

▼

➡ A pathologist inspects the tissue samples under a microscope for the presence of unusual cells. In most cases, a definitive diagnosis can be made and appropriate treatment will be initiated. (For more on laboratory testing, see Chapter 1.)

➡ If cancer is present, treatment decisions are based on the extent and aggressiveness of the cancer—as determined by your biopsy results, DRE, and PSA levels, and sometimes by additional tests such as a bone scan (see page 329).

➡ If the biopsy is negative, a repeat biopsy may be necessary—especially when PSA levels are very high, have risen rapidly, the DRE is very suspicious for cancer, or the initial biopsy shows cells suspicious for cancer or a precancerous condition.

While you may feel some discomfort during the biopsy, anesthesia is not commonly used.

• A thin, cylindrical ultrasound probe (see page 45) may be gently inserted into your rectum. This device transmits an image of your prostate to a video screen, so the doctor can precisely guide needle insertion into the gland.

• To obtain the prostate specimens, the doctor may use a spring-loaded biopsy device to push a tiny needle through the wall of the rectum and into the prostate, and remove a small core of tissue. Alternatively, a thin biopsy guide is inserted into your rectum, and a long, thin needle is inserted through the guide and rotated to withdraw tissue (this method may cause pain as the specimens are obtained).

• The doctor typically extracts 6 to 12 specimens from various areas in the prostate for microscopic examination.

• The procedure takes about 20 minutes.

Perineal approach:

• You will be positioned on an examining table—either on your side; on your knees and chest with your arms outstretched before you; or on your back with your feet raised and resting in stirrups.

• The skin over the perineum is cleansed with an antiseptic, and a local anesthetic is injected to numb the area.

• The doctor gently inserts a finger into the rectum to immobilize the prostate.

• A thin needle is inserted through the perineum into the prostate, rotated to secure a sample, and withdrawn. Several more samples may be obtained by reinserting the needle at other angles.

• Pressure is placed on the puncture site until bleeding has stopped, and a small bandage is applied.

• The procedure usually takes less than 30 minutes.

Risks and Complications

• The most common aftereffects are soreness, temporary blood in the urine (hematuria), minor rectal bleeding, and blood in the semen. These effects are temporary and typically harmless.

• Rare but serious complications include excessive bleeding and infection.

After the Test

• The biopsy site may remain sore for about 2 to 3 days. You may be given pain-relieving medication to allay any discomfort.

• You may be prescribed antibiotics after a transrectal biopsy to further reduce the risk of infection.

• Resume your normal activities when it is comfortable to do so.

• You should expect to see blood in your urine and stool for 2 to 3 days and in your semen for 2 to 4 weeks. This is harmless.

• Notify your doctor immediately if you develop a fever, persistent bleeding, or severe redness or swelling at the biopsy site.

Estimated Cost: $$$

Prostate Biopsy continued

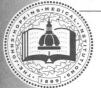
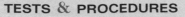
Pulmonary Angiography
(Pulmonary Arteriography)

Pulmonary Angiography

Description
• A doctor inserts a catheter into a vein in your groin or arm, and carefully threads it into the heart's right upper chamber (atrium), through the right lower chamber (ventricle), and into the main pulmonary artery, which brings blood from the heart to the lungs (see the illustration on page 21). The catheter records blood pressures in these areas. A contrast dye is then injected through the catheter to help delineate your pulmonary blood vessels on x-ray images. (For more on angiography, see Chapter 2.)

Purpose of the Test
• To detect a pulmonary embolism (a blood clot in an artery in the lung)—especially after a lung nuclear scan (see page 247) has proven inconclusive.
• To evaluate pulmonary blood circulation abnormalities.
• To evaluate pulmonary circulation prior to surgery in those with congenital heart disease.
• To determine the location of a large pulmonary embolism prior to its surgical removal.

Who Performs It
• A cardiologist or a radiologist.

Special Concerns
• Pulmonary angiography is typically performed in a hospital catheterization laboratory. In critically ill patients, the procedure may be done in the intensive care unit.
• People who have a serious bleeding disorder or who are extremely agitated cannot undergo this procedure.
• People who have an allergy to shellfish or iodine may experience an allergic reaction to the contrast dye. Preventive medication may be administered, or a special form of the dye may be used.
• Pregnant women should not undergo this test because exposure to ionizing radiation may harm the fetus.

Before the Test
• Tell your doctor if you regularly take anticoagulant drugs. You must discontinue them for some time before the test.
• Inform your doctor if you regularly take nonsteroidal anti-inflammatory drugs (such as aspirin, ibuprofen, or naproxen), herbs, or nutritional supplements; these agents may need to be discontinued before the test.
• Be sure to tell your doctor if you have a known shellfish or iodine allergy or have ever had an adverse reaction to x-ray contrast dyes.
• Do not eat or drink anything for 12 hours before the test.
• Immediately before the test, an intravenous (IV) line is inserted into a vein in your arm. You may be given a mild sedative, but you will remain conscious throughout the procedure.

What You Experience
• You lie on your back on a padded table, and ECG leads (see page 174) are applied to monitor your heart rate and rhythm during the procedure.
• The area of catheter insertion (your groin or arm) is cleansed with an antiseptic to help prevent infection and numbed with a local anesthetic. The doctor then makes a small

---

Results
▼
➥ The doctor will review the test data for evidence of any pulmonary or circulatory abnormalities.
➥ This test is usually definitive. Based on the findings, your doctor will then decide on a course of medical or surgical treatment.

incision and inserts a catheter into the vein; you will feel pressure during insertion, but no other discomfort.

• The doctor threads the catheter through your heart and into your main pulmonary artery, using fluoroscopy (see page 205) to watch its progress on a viewing monitor.

• A contrast dye is administered through the catheter. The dye will circulate through the pulmonary artery and blood vessels in the lung and delineate them on x-rays. You may feel a hot, flushing sensation briefly after injection; some people experience nausea and possibly vomiting.

• The doctor takes several moving and still x-ray pictures (angiograms) of your pulmonary blood vessels for later analysis.

• The procedure takes from 30 minutes to 90 minutes.

Risks and Complications

• Possible complications include abnormal heart rhythms (arrhythmias), blood clot formation, bleeding, blood vessel damage, or infection at the site of catheter insertion.

• Some people may experience an allergic reaction to the iodine-based contrast dye, which can cause symptoms such as nausea, sneezing, vomiting, hives, and occasionally a life-threatening response called anaphylactic shock. Emergency medications and equipment are kept readily available.

After the Test

• Immediately after the test, you will rest in a recovery room. Your vital signs will be monitored, and you will be observed for signs of complications such as delayed reaction to the contrast dye.

• You are encouraged to drink clear fluids to avoid dehydration and help flush the contrast dye out of your system.

• Most people are able to return home after about 6 to 8 hours, though some may require overnight hospitalization. You will need bed rest for about 12 to 24 hours.

• If you develop swelling or discomfort at the catheter insertion site, apply cold compresses.

• You may experience the urge to cough after this procedure.

• Avoid heavy lifting and do only light activities for a few days after the test.

Estimated Cost: $$$

Pulmonary Angiography continued

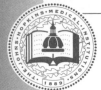

Pulmonary Artery Catheterization
(Right-Heart or Swan-Ganz Catheterization)

Description
• A doctor inserts a catheter into a vein in the arm, neck, or groin, and carefully threads it into the heart's right atrium, through the tricuspid valve, into the right ventricle, and into the main pulmonary artery, which brings blood to the lungs (see the illustration on page 21). The catheter records blood circulation and fluid pressures in these areas. Pulmonary artery pressures can be used to indirectly assess function of the left ventricle—the heart's main pumping chamber—and to measure cardiac output (the amount of blood pumped from the heart).

Purpose of the Test
• To monitor patients for complications after a heart attack, such as cardiogenic shock or fluid in the lungs (pulmonary edema).
• To monitor blood volume and heart valve function in people who are in shock or who have another serious medical condition, such as burns, kidney disease, or pulmonary edema.
• To evaluate the effects of certain cardiovascular medications, such as nitroprusside and dobutamine.
• To monitor patients undergoing open heart surgery, particularly coronary artery bypass procedures.
• To determine the cause of low blood pressure.

Who Performs It
• A cardiologist.

Special Concerns
• If the procedure is elective, it is performed in a hospital catheterization laboratory. In critically ill patients, it may be done in the intensive care unit.
• People who have a serious bleeding disorder or who are extremely agitated cannot undergo this procedure.
• The test cannot be performed in people with an abnormal heart rhythm (arrhythmia) called left bundle branch block because placement of the right-heart catheter may lead to complete heart block.

Before the Test
• Do not eat or drink fluids for 6 to 8 hours before the test.

What You Experience
• Immediately before the test, an intravenous (IV) line is inserted into a vein in your arm. You may be given a mild sedative, but you will remain conscious throughout the procedure.
• You lie on your back on a padded table, and ECG leads (see page 174) are applied to monitor your heart rate and rhythm during the procedure.
• The area of catheter insertion (your arm, neck, or groin) is cleansed with an antiseptic to help prevent infection, and a local anesthetic is injected to numb the area.
• The doctor makes a small incision and inserts a catheter into the selected vein; you will feel pressure during insertion, but no other discomfort.
• The doctor then carefully threads the catheter to your heart. In many cases, fluoroscopy (see page 205) is used to watch its progress on a viewing monitor.

Results
▼
➡ The doctor will review the test data for evidence of cardiac or circulatory abnormalities.
➡ If a definitive diagnosis can be made, appropriate therapy will be initiated, depending on the specific problem.
➡ In some cases, additional tests may be needed to further evaluate abnormal results.

• The position of the catheter tip is verified by a chest x-ray and by monitoring devices that record pressures within the heart.

• Catheter insertion takes from 30 minutes to 1 hour. In critically ill patients, the catheter may remain in place for several days to allow continuous monitoring.

Risks and Complications

• Possible complications include arrhythmias; blood clots; pulmonary embolism (blockage of a pulmonary artery); perforation of the pulmonary artery or heart wall; catheter-induced damage to the vein; infection or blood loss at the insertion site; and low blood pressure. Emergency equipment is available at the catheterization lab.

After the Test

• You will remain hospitalized for a few hours after the procedure (or longer if you are already hospitalized for another medical condition).

• Your blood pressure and other vital signs will be checked periodically, and the catheter insertion site will be monitored for any signs of infection, such as redness, swelling, or discharge.

Estimated Cost: $$$

Pulmonary Artery Catheterization continued

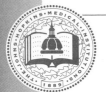

Pulmonary Function Tests

Description
• As you breathe into a mouthpiece that is attached to monitoring equipment, a series of measurements is made to evaluate how well your lungs are functioning and to detect any respiratory abnormalities.

Purpose of the Test
• To determine the cause of breathing difficulties, such as shortness of breath.
• To distinguish between obstructive lung disease (such as asthma or emphysema), which primarily inhibits expiration (breathing out), and restrictive lung disease (such as pulmonary fibrosis, respiratory muscle weakness, or tumors), which primarily inhibits inspiration (breathing in).
• To assess the severity of known lung disease, monitor the course of lung disease, or evaluate the effectiveness of specific treatments (such as bronchodilator medications).
• To evaluate patients before thoracic (chest) or abdominal surgery.

Who Performs It
• A doctor, a respiratory therapist, or a pulmonary lab technician.

Special Concerns
• Pulmonary function testing may not be safe for individuals with unstable asthma or respiratory distress; severe heart disease or a recent heart attack; pneumothorax (leakage of air outside the lungs and into the pleural cavity, resulting in a collapsed lung); or active tuberculosis.
• Pregnancy or a distended stomach may affect test results.
• Accurate results may not be possible in people who cannot follow the examiner's instructions carefully, such as those with chest pain (for example, due to a fractured rib) or mental instability.

Before the Test
• Do not smoke for 4 to 6 hours before the test, and do not eat a heavy meal beforehand.
• Be sure to inform your doctor of all medications you are taking. Certain drugs, including bronchodilators, pain relievers, and sedatives, may affect the results and should be discontinued before the test.
• If you have well-fitted dentures, wear them during the test.
• Wear loose clothing that won't inhibit your breathing.
• Empty your bladder before the test.

What You Experience
• A clip is placed on your nose to prevent air from passing through your nostrils during the procedure.

Results
▼

➡ A physician will assess your lung function by comparing your test values with the average values obtained from healthy individuals of your age, sex, height, and weight. Results are expressed as a percentage; in general, a score lower than 80% is considered abnormal.

➡ Arterial blood gas levels (see page 93), another valuable measure of lung function, are usually also considered when making a diagnosis.

➡ Based on your test results, medical history, and physical exam, your doctor will recommend appropriate treatment, if necessary.

➡ If your results are normal but your symptoms still suggest a diagnosis of asthma, the doctor may recommend a methacholine challenge test (see page 132).

• You are asked to seal your lips tightly around a mouthpiece that is connected by a tube to the monitoring device. At first, you should breathe normally while the examiner makes sure the test equipment is working properly.

• Next, you are instructed to perform a variety of breathing exercises, such as breathing in as deeply as possible, briefly holding your breath, and exhaling as hard as you can. You will repeat these exercises several times. For the most accurate results, follow the examiner's instructions as closely as possible.

• In some cases, you will repeat the tests after inhaling a bronchodilator spray medication, or you may inhale a special mixture of air and carbon monoxide in order to assess how well your lungs deliver oxygen to your blood. Occasionally, breathing tests are performed while you exercise by walking on a treadmill or cycling on a stationary bike.

• If at any point you feel tired or lightheaded, ask for a chance to rest between exercises.

• The total process takes from 20 to 90 minutes, depending on how many tests are done.

Risks and Complications

• Pulmonary function testing is generally safe, though it may temporarily irritate breathing symptoms in those with some types of lung disease.

• Inhalation studies may trigger an asthmatic episode, so bronchodilators are kept available for immediate treatment.

After the Test

• You may leave the testing facility immediately after the test, and resume your normal diet and any medications that were withheld.

• If you feel tired, dizzy, or lightheaded, rest until you are recovered.

Estimated Cost: $

Pulmonary Function Tests continued

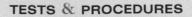

Renal and Mesenteric Doppler Ultrasound

(Renal and Mesenteric Duplex Ultrasound)

Renal and Mesenteric Doppler Ultrasound

Description

• This test uses a technique called Doppler ultrasound to evaluate blood flow through the renal arteries (which supply blood to the kidneys) and/or the mesenteric arteries (which supply the intestine and other abdominal organs). A device called a transducer is passed lightly across different areas of your abdomen or lower back, directing high-frequency sound waves (ultrasound) at the selected arteries. The sound waves are reflected back at frequencies that correspond to the velocity of blood flow, and are converted into audible sounds and graphic recordings.

• **Duplex scanning** combines Doppler ultrasound with real-time ultrasound imaging of the arteries, allowing calculation of the percent of narrowing in the vessels. Images are displayed on a viewing monitor and may also be recorded on film or video. This method is the best initial test to screen for narrowing or blockage of the renal or mesenteric arteries. (For more on Doppler and duplex ultrasound, see Chapter 2.)

Purpose of the Test

• To detect arterial narrowing or blockages that prevent adequate blood flow to the kidneys and abdominal organs.

Who Performs It

• A technician trained in ultrasound.

Special Concerns

• None.

Before the Test

• You will be asked to disrobe and put on a hospital gown.

• Do not eat or drink anything for 8 hours before the test.

What You Experience

• You will either lie on your front or back on a bed or table.

• A small amount of water-soluble gel is applied to the skin of your lower back or abdomen to enhance sound wave transmission.

• The examiner then moves the transducer back and forth over the skin to record blood flow and obtain different views of the blood vessels being studied.

• Once clear images are obtained, they are recorded on film or video for later analysis.

• The test takes about 30 to 45 minutes.

Risks and Complications

• Ultrasound is painless, noninvasive, and involves no exposure to radiation. There are no associated risks.

After the Test

• The examiner removes the conductive gel from your skin.

• You may resume your normal activities.

Estimated Cost: $$

Results

▼

➡ A physician reviews the recorded images and other test data for evidence of any blockages in the renal and/or mesenteric arteries.

➡ In some cases, additional tests, such as arteriography (see page 95), are required to further evaluate abnormal findings and determine the appropriate course of treatment.

➡ If no further tests are warranted, your doctor will recommend an appropriate schedule of follow-up exams and/or treatment.

Renal Biopsy
(Kidney Biopsy)

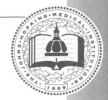

Description

• A doctor inserts a long needle through your skin and into the kidney (see page 27) to obtain a tissue sample for microscopic examination. Fluoroscopy, ultrasonography, or CT scanning may be used to guide placement of the needle. (For more on these imaging techniques, see Chapter 2.) Occasionally, an open renal biopsy—which accesses the kidney surgically through a small incision—is performed instead.

Purpose of the Test

• To diagnose a suspected kidney (renal) disorder (for example, after finding blood or protein in the urine) or unexplained kidney dysfunction.
• To monitor the effectiveness of treatment for renal disease.
• To evaluate a transplanted kidney for signs of organ rejection, as well as to determine the appropriate dose of immunosuppressive drugs.
• To detect a kidney malignancy in patients who are unable to undergo surgery.

Who Performs It

• A nephrologist assisted by a radiologist or a radiology technician.

Special Concerns

• People who have serious bleeding disorders, hydronephrosis (collection of urine in the renal pelvis due to obstructed outflow), urinary tract infections, severe hypertension, or only a single kidney are not candidates for this procedure.
• Individuals with operable kidney tumors should not undergo this procedure, since there is a risk it may disseminate tumor cells.
• Blood coagulation tests (see page 157) are performed to determine whether you have any bleeding abnormalities. If so, the biopsy may be canceled.

Before the Test

• Report to your doctor any medications, herbs, or supplements you are taking. You may be advised to discontinue certain drugs (including nonsteroidal anti-inflammatory drugs, such as aspirin or naproxen) before the test because they can interfere with blood clotting.
• Restrict your intake of food and fluids for 8 hours before the test.
• If you are anxious about undergoing this procedure, your doctor may prescribe a sedative to relax you.
• You will be instructed to empty your bladder just before the test.

What You Experience

• You will lie face down on an examining table with a pillow or sandbag under your abdomen to straighten your spine.
• The skin over your kidney is cleansed with an antiseptic to help prevent infection, and a local anesthetic is injected to numb the area (you may still feel a pinching pain when the biopsy is taken).
• While you hold your breath and remain still to stop kidney motion, the doctor inserts a thin biopsy needle and obtains a specimen, using fluoroscopy, ultrasound, or CT scanning to visualize the kidney. (A small finder needle

Results
▼

➡ A pathologist examines the kidney specimen under a microscope for changes that indicate a specific kidney disorder, malignancy, or transplant rejection. (For more on microscopic examination, see Chapter 1.)
➡ This test usually results in a definitive diagnosis. Appropriate treatment will be initiated, depending on the specific problem.

Renal Biopsy

may be used to correctly locate the kidney prior to using the longer biopsy needle.)

• The doctor may repeat this procedure a few times until an adequate specimen is obtained, and the needle is withdrawn.

• The procedure may take as little as 15 or 20 minutes once the kidney is well visualized.

Risks and Complications

• Many patients experience back pain and some urinary tract bleeding in the first 24 hours after the procedure.

• Possible serious complications include infection, major blood loss and need for transfusion, displacement of the kidney, and, rarely, loss of the kidney or death.

• Rarely, the biopsy needle may inadvertently puncture another organ (such as the liver, lung, or bowel) or a blood vessel (such as the aorta or inferior vena cava).

After the Test

• You are positioned on your back and advised to stay in a hospital bed for 12 to 24 hours. Your vital signs are carefully monitored during this time, and the needle insertion site is checked for signs of bleeding or infection.

• Your urine is examined for blood. Some individuals have visible blood in the urine initially, but this typically subsides after 24 hours.

• You are encouraged to drink plenty of fluids after the procedure to prevent blood clot formation and urine retention. You may resume your normal diet.

• Your doctor may prescribe a pain reliever for any back pain.

• Upon returning home, you should avoid strenuous activities and exercise for at least 2 weeks to prevent possible bleeding.

• Call your doctor if you experience symptoms of kidney hemorrhage (such as worsening back, flank, or shoulder pain or lightheadedness) or urinary tract infection (a fever or burning on urination).

Estimated Cost: $$$

Renal Function Tests

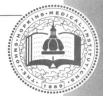

Description

• Analysis of blood and urine samples can be essential for the evaluation of kidney (renal) function. The following are some of the basic renal function tests.

• **Blood urea nitrogen (BUN)** provides a rough measurement of the glomerular filtration rate, the rate at which blood is filtered in the kidneys (see page 27 of the body atlas). Urea is formed in the liver as an end product of protein metabolism and is carried to the kidneys for excretion. Nearly all kidney diseases cause inadequate excretion of urea, elevating BUN levels in the blood. (Other causes of high BUN levels include gastrointestinal bleeding and steroid treatment.)

• **Creatinine** is a breakdown product of creatine, an important component of muscle. The production of creatinine depends on muscle mass, which varies very little. Creatinine is excreted exclusively by the kidneys, and its level in the blood is proportional to the glomerular filtration rate. The serum creatinine level (serum is the clear liquid that remains after whole blood has clotted) provides a more sensitive test of kidney function than BUN because kidney impairment is almost the only cause of elevated creatinine.

• **Creatinine clearance rate** determines how efficiently the kidneys are clearing creatinine from the blood and serves as an estimate of kidney function. For this test, urine and serum levels of creatinine are measured, as well as the volume of urine excreted over a 24-hour period. The creatinine clearance rate is then calculated and expressed as the volume of blood, in milliliters, that can be cleared of creatinine in 1 minute. A low creatinine clearance value indicates abnormal kidney function.

Purpose of the Test

• To evaluate kidney function and aid in the diagnosis of kidney disease.

• To monitor the progression of renal insufficiency.

• The BUN-to-creatinine ratio may aid in the evaluation of a person's state of hydration.

Who Performs It

• A doctor, a nurse, or a lab technician draws the blood sample.

Special Concerns

• A diet rich in meats can cause transient elevations of serum creatinine and creatinine clearance.

• A high-protein diet or dehydration elevates BUN levels.

• Exercise may increase creatinine clearance.

• Some medications may affect BUN levels, serum creatinine, and creatinine clearance.

Before the Test

• Be sure to inform your doctor of all medica-

Results

▼

➡ Your blood and urine samples are sent to a laboratory for analysis. A physician will review the results of the tests for any evidence of kidney disease or other abnormalities. (For more on laboratory testing, see Chapter 1.)

➡ Blood and urine tests are usually the first step in assessing potential kidney disorders. Abnormal results often necessitate additional imaging tests, such as a renal ultrasound (see page 76) or nuclear scan (see page 313), to evaluate kidney structure and function.

➡ If an abnormality is found and the doctor can make a definitive diagnosis, appropriate treatment will begin.

Renal Function Tests

tions, herbs, or supplements you are taking. You may be advised to discontinue certain of these agents before the test.

• Do not eat an excessive amount of meat before the creatinine clearance test, and avoid strenuous physical exercise during the urine collection period for this test.

What You Experience

• A sample of your blood is drawn from a vein, usually in your arm, and sent to a laboratory for analysis. (For more on this procedure, called venipuncture, see page 32.)

• To perform the creatinine clearance test, timed urine specimens are collected in a special container over a 24-hour period (this process is described on page 34).

Risks and Complications

• None.

After the Test

• You may leave the testing facility.

• Resume your normal diet and any medications withheld before the test, according to your doctor's instructions.

• Blood may collect and clot under the skin (hematoma) at the puncture site; this is harmless and will resolve on its own. For a large hematoma that causes swelling and discomfort, apply ice initially; after 24 hours, use warm, moist compresses to help dissolve the clotted blood.

Estimated Cost: $

Renal Nuclear Scan
(Kidney Scan)

Description

• After intravenous injection of a small amount of radioactive material, a special camera records the radiotracer as it circulates through the kidneys and ureters (illustrated on page 26). Data obtained by the camera can provide an image of kidney structure, and can also be recorded by a computer and analyzed to assess kidney function and blood flow. Different types of renal scans, using various radiotracers, are performed depending on what information is needed; often several types are done in succession. (For more on nuclear scans, see Chapter 2.)

Purpose of the Test

• To evaluate kidney function in a more accurate manner than blood tests alone.
• To detect kidney abnormalities, such as obstruction or reflux of urine back into the kidney.
• To identify whether high blood pressure is caused by impaired blood flow to the kidney (renovascular hypertension).
• To detect organ rejection in a transplanted kidney.

Who Performs It

• A physician or a nuclear medicine technician.

Special Concerns

• This test is a safe alternative for people who cannot undergo intravenous pyelography (see page 225) due to iodine allergy or poor kidney function.
• Renal scanning should be done at least 24 hours after intravenous pyelography.
• The test should not be done in pregnant or breastfeeding women.

Before the Test

• If you take an antihypertensive medication, ask your doctor if it should be withheld before the test.

• Good hydration is important for this test. The doctor will ask you to drink 2 or 3 glasses of water before it begins.
• You will be instructed to empty your bladder and remove all metal jewelry.

What You Experience

• The examiner injects a radiotracer into a vein, usually in your arm. This material will circulate through your bloodstream to the kidneys. (Other than the minor discomfort of this injection, the procedure is painless.)
• You may experience brief, mild nausea and flushing after the radiotracer enters your bloodstream.
• You will be asked to sit or lie down on a table, depending on the type of scan to be done. You must remain still throughout the procedure, which may cause some numbness or stiffness. (Ask the doctor if a pillow or pads can be placed on the table for your comfort.)
• A large scanning camera is passed over the kidney area at various intervals, recording the gamma rays emitted by the radiotracer. There may be a break of several hours before certain scans are taken.

Results

▼

➡ A physician will examine the recorded images and other test data for any evidence of kidney disease or other abnormalities.
➡ If a definitive diagnosis can be made, appropriate treatment will be initiated.
➡ Abnormal results may also necessitate additional tests, such as intravenous pyelography, renal arteriography (see page 95), or an abdominal CT scan (see page 76).

Renal Nuclear Scan

• If several types of scans are being performed in succession, you may need additional injections of radiotracers. In addition, some tests require scanning the kidney after the injection of an antihypertensive drug (typically captopril [Capoten]).

• Depending on what information is needed, kidney scanning may take from 1 to 4 hours.

• If your kidney function is being assessed, urine collections may be performed at specified times during and/or after the scan.

Risks and Complications

• The trace amounts of radioactive material used in this test are not associated with any significant risks or complications.

• In rare cases, infection may develop at the injection site. Inform your doctor of any redness or swelling.

After the Test

• Empty your bladder immediately after the procedure is finished. Most of the radioactive material is excreted in the urine within 6 to 24 hours. Drinking plenty of fluids facilitates this process.

• Most patients may go home the same day of the test and resume their normal activities. Some may require overnight hospitalization.

• Blood may collect and clot under the skin (hematoma) at the injection site; this is harmless and will resolve on its own. For a large hematoma that causes swelling and discomfort, apply ice initially; after 24 hours, use warm, moist compresses to help dissolve the clotted blood.

Estimated Cost: $$$

Retrograde Pyelography
(Retrograde Ureteropyelography)

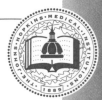

Description
• This test combines the use of a long, flexible viewing tube called a cystoscope with contrast x-rays to visualize the kidneys and ureters (illustrated on page 26). The cystoscope is inserted through the urethra into the bladder; fiberoptic cables permit direct visual inspection of these structures. A catheter is then threaded through the scope so that a contrast dye can be infused directly into the ureters to delineate them on x-ray films. Retrograde pyelography is most often performed when intravenous pyelography (see page 225) produces inconclusive results, or when it cannot be performed because of impaired kidney function or another reason. (For more on contrast x-rays, see Chapter 2.)

Purpose of the Test
• To evaluate the structure and integrity of the kidneys and ureters.
• To identify the cause of obstructions in the kidneys or ureters, such as tumors, narrowing, scarring, blood clots, or stones.

Who Performs It
• A urologist or a radiology technician.

Special Concerns
• Pregnant women should not undergo this test because exposure to ionizing radiation may harm the fetus.
• Retrograde pyelography is the preferred test to examine the urinary tract in people who are allergic to iodine or shellfish, and therefore may be hypersensitive to iodine-based contrast dyes. Allergic reactions rarely occur with this test, because none of the dye is absorbed into the bloodstream.
• This test must be performed carefully to prevent further damage to the ureter in individuals who have a slowing or stoppage of normal urine flow (urinary stasis) caused by ureteral obstruction.

• The presence of feces, gas, or residual barium from recent contrast x-rays of the gastrointestinal system can obscure visualization of the urinary tract.

Before the Test
• Be sure to tell your doctor if you have a known shellfish or iodine allergy or have ever had an adverse reaction to x-ray contrast dyes.
• If you are receiving a local anesthetic, you should have a liquid breakfast on the morning of the test.
• If general anesthesia is required, do not eat or drink after midnight on the day before the test.
• An intravenous (IV) catheter may be inserted into a vein in your arm to provide fluids and/or to administer a general anesthetic during the procedure.

What You Experience
• You will lie on your back on an examination table with your knees bent and feet resting in stirrups.
• After local or general anesthesia has been

Results
▼

➡ The doctor will examine the x-ray films for evidence of any abnormalities, such as a ureteral obstruction.

➡ If a definitive diagnosis can be made, your doctor will recommend an appropriate course of treatment.

➡ In some cases, additional diagnostic tests, such as a renal CT scan (see page 76), renal nuclear scan (see page 313), or ureteroscopy (see page 375), may be needed to further evaluate abnormal results.

administered, the doctor carefully inserts the cystoscope through your urethra and into the bladder, and performs a visual examination.

• Next, a thin tube, or catheter, is threaded through the cystoscope into the ureter. (Sometimes both ureters are catheterized.)

• The contrast dye is injected through the catheter. If you are conscious, you may feel some discomfort during catheter insertion and when the dye is instilled.

• X-ray films are obtained. You must remain still to avoid blurring the pictures.

• As the catheter is slowly withdrawn, more contrast dye is instilled and additional x-rays are taken to visualize the complete length of the ureter.

• A delayed x-ray film is usually taken about 5 minutes after the last injection to check for retention of contrast dye, which indicates a ureteral obstruction.

• If an obstruction is present, a catheter may be left in place in the ureter so that it can drain.

• The procedure usually takes about 1 hour.

Risks and Complications

• Possible complications include urinary tract infection, temporary blockage of the ureter due to swelling, and, rarely, inadvertent perforation of the bladder or ureter.

• Rarely, some people may experience an aller-gic reaction to the iodine-based contrast dye, which can cause symptoms such as nausea, sneezing, vomiting, hives, and occasionally a life-threatening response called anaphylactic shock. Emergency medications and equipment are kept readily available.

After the Test

• If no complications develop, you are usually free to leave the testing facility. Your doctor will instruct you to keep track of your urine output and report any urinary retention.

• Your urine may contain blood at first, causing a slight pink tinge; this should resolve after you have voided 3 times. If blood persists or you see bright red blood or blood clots, notify your physician.

• Urination is often painful or difficult for the first few times after the test. You may be instructed to take tub baths to help ease any discomfort, and painkillers will be prescribed, as needed.

• You are encouraged to increase your intake of fluids to help prevent urinary retention and accumulation of bacteria in your bladder.

• Inform your doctor immediately if you experience pain in the area of the kidneys, chills, or fever.

Estimated Cost: $$

Rheumatology Blood Tests

Description

• Analysis of a blood sample can provide important information about rheumatologic conditions, which are marked by inflammation in the joints, muscles, connective tissues, and other structures. The following blood tests are commonly performed to detect or evaluate rheumatologic disorders, including rheumatoid arthritis (RA), systemic lupus erythematosus (SLE), scleroderma, blood vessel inflammation (vasculitis), and gout.

• **Antibody tests** for autoimmune disorders are often necessary. Many rheumatologic conditions—including RA, SLE, and scleroderma—are caused by an abnormal autoimmune response where the body mistakenly releases immune cells to attack healthy tissues. For more on these tests, see page 89.

• **Complete blood count**—a general test that measures the amounts of various blood cells—can provide clues to the presence of inflammation, which tends to increase levels of white blood cells and platelets and decrease the amount of red blood cells. (This test is described in more detail on page 164.)

• **Blood chemistry screen** (see page 108) is another general test that can help to identify problems in the body's organs, especially the kidneys. Certain types of inflammatory arthritis, including RA, can affect kidney function, as can certain arthritis drugs.

• **Erythrocyte sedimentation rate (ESR)** refers to the rate at which red blood cells, or erythrocytes, settle at the bottom of a test tube to form a sediment. The ESR is increased in many rheumatologic disorders, particularly those associated with vasculitis.

• **Rheumatoid factor,** a type of antibody present in the blood of many individuals with RA, is thought to play a major role in the tissue destruction associated with this disease. About 80% of patients with RA test positive for rheumatoid factor, so this test is considered extremely useful for confirming a diagnosis of this type of arthritis.

• **Uric acid** is the final breakdown product of purines—the building blocks of RNA and DNA. The blood test for this substance is primarily used to detect gout, a form of arthritis that typically affects the joints of the feet and hands. Uric acid levels may also be elevated in some kidney disorders and other conditions that are associated with excessive tissue destruction.

Purpose of the Test

• To diagnose and monitor rheumatologic and autoimmune disorders.

Who Performs It

• A doctor, a nurse, or a lab technician draws the blood sample.

Special Concerns

• As many as 25% of healthy elderly people have slightly elevated rheumatoid factor lev-

---

Results

▼

➥ Your blood sample is sent to a laboratory for analysis. A physician will review the results for evidence of a rheumatologic disorder. (For more on laboratory testing, see Chapter 1.)

➥ If an abnormality is found and your doctor can make a definitive diagnosis, appropriate treatment will begin.

➥ In many cases, abnormal results on one or more of these blood tests may necessitate additional procedures, such as joint (see page 229) or muscle (see page 261) biopsy, to establish a diagnosis.

els, and the antibody may also be produced as a result of chronic inflammation unrelated to RA, certain infectious disorders, and certain other diseases.

• In addition to rheumatologic disorders, various other factors may affect ESR values, including age, menstruation and pregnancy, anemia, kidney disease, thyroid disease, certain infections, hormone disorders, cancer, and certain medications and vitamins.

• Uric acid levels may be elevated due to starvation, stress, alcohol abuse, and increased intake of high-purine foods (such as liver, kidney, sweetbreads, and anchovies). Certain medications and vitamins may also alter the test results.

Before the Test

• Report to your doctor any medications, vitamins, or supplements you are taking. You may be advised to discontinue certain of these agents before the test.

• You must fast for 8 hours before a blood test for uric acid.

What You Experience

• A sample of your blood is drawn from a vein, usually in your arm, and sent to a laboratory for analysis. (For more on this procedure, called venipuncture, see page 32.)

Risks and Complications

• None.

After the Test

• Immediately after blood is drawn, pressure is applied (with cotton or gauze) to the puncture site.

• Resume your normal diet and any medications withheld before the test.

• Blood may collect and clot under the skin (hematoma) at the puncture site; this is harmless and will resolve on its own. For a large hematoma that causes swelling and discomfort, apply ice initially; after 24 hours, use warm, moist compresses to help dissolve the clotted blood.

Estimated Cost: $

Schirmer Tearing Test

Description
• This test is used to assess the volume of the tear (lacrimal) glands in people with chronically dry eyes. A thin strip of filter paper is inserted inside each lower eyelid; the amount of moisture absorbed by the paper provides a measure of tear production in the eyes.

Purpose of the Test
• To measure tear secretion in people with suspected tearing deficiency.

Who Performs It
• An ophthalmologist, an optometrist, a nurse, or a lab technician.

Special Concerns
• Closing the eyes too tightly during the test will increase tearing, altering the results.
• The Schirmer test is quick and simple, but provides only a rough estimate of tear secretion. A positive result for tearing deficiency requires corroboration by a special microscopic examination of the eye (slit-lamp examination) that uses a colored dye, called the rose bengal stain, for confirmation.

Before the Test
• If you wear contact lenses, remove them before the test.
• Do not use eye drops for 1 hour before the procedure.

What You Experience
• You will sit in an examining chair.
• You will be instructed to look up, and the examiner will gently insert a thin strip of filter paper inside the lower lid of each eye. The strips are left in place for 5 minutes. Blinking normally or keeping your eyes lightly closed does not interfere with the test, but avoid squeezing or rubbing your eyes.
• The test strip is removed, and the amount of moisture absorbed by the strip is measured.
• In some cases, the test is repeated after anesthetic eye drops have been instilled in each eye.
• The procedure takes about 10 to 15 minutes.

Risks and Complications
• None.

After the Test
• If anesthetic eye drops were administered, do not rub your eyes for at least 30 minutes to avoid injuring the cornea.
• Do not reinsert your contact lenses for at least 2 hours after the test.
• You may resume your normal activities.

Estimated Cost: $

Results
▼

➡ The doctor will review the test results to determine whether tearing deficiency is present. Possible causes of insufficient tearing include Sjögren's syndrome (a chronic inflammatory disorder marked by dry eyes and mouth) and dry-eye syndrome, which may be a side effect of certain drugs or may be caused by allergies or other disorders.

➡ If the results are negative, no further testing is required.

➡ If the results are positive, your doctor may order a slit-lamp examination with rose bengal stain (see under Special Concerns) if it has not already been done. If Sjögren's syndrome is suspected, a lower lip biopsy (see page 242) may be done to confirm the diagnosis.

Scrotal Ultrasound
(Ultrasonography of the Testes)

Scrotal Ultrasound

Description
• A device called a transducer is passed over the scrotum, directing high-frequency sound waves (ultrasound) at the structures within, including the testicle, epididymis (the tube that transports sperm from the testicle), and blood vessels. The sound waves are reflected back to the transducer and electronically converted into real-time images displayed on a viewing monitor. These images are then saved on film or video and reviewed for abnormalities. (For more on how ultrasound works, see Chapter 2.)

Purpose of the Test
• To evaluate scrotal abnormalities, including masses; pain or trauma; testicular torsion (twisting of the spermatic cord that contains blood vessels that supply the testes); an absent or undescended testicle; inflammation; abnormal blood vessels; and fluid accumulation.
• To measure testicle size.
• To monitor men with previous testicular cancer or infection.
• Used for guidance during needle biopsy of a suspicious testicular mass.

Who Performs It
• A doctor or a technician who is trained in ultrasound.

Special Concerns
• None.

Before the Test
• You will be asked to disrobe and put on a hospital gown.

What You Experience
• You will lie on your back on an examining table.
• The doctor will perform a brief manual exam, gently palpating the scrotum on both sides.

• The penis is lifted, placed on the abdomen, and covered. A rolled up towel or the examiner's hand will be placed under the scrotum for support.
• A water-soluble gel is applied to your scrotal skin to enhance sound wave transmission.
• The examiner then moves the transducer back and forth over your scrotum to obtain different views. (This is usually painless, unless the scrotum is very tender.)
• Once clear images are obtained, they are recorded on film or video for later analysis.
• The test is repeated on the other side.
• The test takes 20 to 30 minutes.

Risks and Complications
• Ultrasound is painless, noninvasive, and involves no exposure to radiation. There are no associated risks.

After the Test
• The examiner removes the conductive gel from your skin.
• You may resume your normal activities.

Estimated Cost: $$

Results
▼
➥ A physician reviews the images and video for evidence of any abnormality.
➥ If a definitive diagnosis can be made, appropriate treatment will be initiated.
➥ If ultrasound fails to yield a definitive diagnosis, additional tests, such as a needle biopsy, may be needed to provide more specific information or to further evaluate abnormal findings.

Sex Hormone Tests

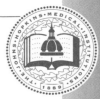

Description

• Measuring blood levels of the major sex hormones—estrogen and progesterone in women and testosterone in men—can aid in the evaluation of a variety of conditions, including fertility problems and certain cancers with sex-hormone-producing tumors. Because abnormal levels of sex hormones are sometimes associated with dysfunction elsewhere in the endocrine system—primarily the pituitary and adrenal glands (see page 18)—this test may be performed in conjunction with other hormone tests (see pages 83 and 293).

• **Estrogen**—predominantly in the form estradiol—is produced by the ovaries (see page 28) in response to signals from the pituitary gland, starting at puberty. The primary function of estradiol is to modulate the course of the menstrual cycle: Its secretion gradually increases over the first 2 weeks, reaches its peak during ovulation, and drops sharply right before the menstrual period. (Another form of estrogen, estriol, is the major estrogen produced during pregnancy.) After the menopause, estrogen levels drop to a consistently low level.

• **Progesterone,** another female hormone produced by the ovaries, causes the lining of the uterus (endometrium) to thicken and develop in preparation for a fertilized egg. Levels begin to rise rapidly after ovulation; if egg implantation fails to occur, progesterone (and estrogen) levels drop sharply and menstruation occurs about 2 days later. In pregnant women, the placenta releases large amounts of progesterone to maintain the pregnancy.

• **Testosterone** is the principal male sex hormone (androgen) secreted by the testes, starting at puberty. (In women, the adrenal glands and ovaries produce small amounts.) Levels begin to plateau at around age 40, and gradually decrease to one-fifth the peak level at age 80.

Results

➥ The blood sample is sent to a laboratory for analysis. Your doctor will consider the results in the context of your age, your symptoms and physical exam, and the results of other tests. (For more on laboratory testing, see Chapter 1.)

➥ Abnormally high estrogen levels can occur with estrogen-producing tumors or severe liver disease such as cirrhosis. Low levels may indicate ovarian failure, pituitary dysfunction, or menopause. In men, elevated estrogen levels may result from testicular tumors.

➥ Elevated progesterone levels are associated with ovulation, pregnancy, ovarian cysts, certain adrenal gland disorders, or progesterone-producing tumors. Low levels may indicate dysfunction of the ovaries or pituitary gland or problems with a pregnancy.

➥ Abnormally high testosterone levels are associated with benign and malignant adrenal gland tumors and hyperthyroidism (overactive thyroid gland). Low levels may result from pituitary gland dysfunction, testicular or prostate cancer, orchiectomy (removal of the testes), estrogen therapy, or cirrhosis of the liver. In women, elevated testosterone levels may be caused by ovarian or adrenal tumors or polycystic ovary syndrome.

➥ Depending on the suspected problem, additional tests are likely to be necessary in order to establish a diagnosis.

➥ If a definitive diagnosis can be made, appropriate treatment will be initiated.

Sex Hormone Tests

Sex Hormone Tests continued

Purpose of the Test

Estrogen:
• To evaluate menopausal status.
• To aid in the diagnosis of tumors that are known to secrete estrogen, such as certain ovarian tumors.
• To evaluate infertility or menstrual problems such as amenorrhea (loss of menstrual periods).
• To monitor fetal health in pregnant women.
• To aid in the evaluation of feminization (the development of female characteristics such as enlarged breasts) in men.

Progesterone:
• To aid in confirming ovulation and evaluate ovarian function in infertility studies.
• To monitor placental health during high-risk pregnancies.

Testosterone:
• To evaluate male infertility or sexual dysfunction.
• To help determine the cause of hypogonadism (decreased testosterone secretion).
• To aid in the evaluation of virilization (the development of male characteristics such as male-type baldness) in women.

Who Performs It
• A nurse or technician will draw the blood sample.

Special Concerns
• In men, testosterone levels vary slightly with the time of day—highest around 7 AM and lowest at 8 PM. The timing of blood sample collection must be carefully scheduled to coincide with or avoid times of peak secretion.
• Estrogen and progesterone tests may be repeated at specific times to coincide with different phases of the menstrual cycle.
• A recent nuclear scan (see page 46) may affect the results of estrogen and progesterone blood tests, since these hormones are often measured with a laboratory technique that utilizes a radioactive isotope (radioimmunoassay).
• A variety of medications—particularly hormone replacement therapies—can alter levels of estrogen, progesterone, and testosterone and interfere with the results.

Before the Test
• Inform your doctor about any medications, herbs, or supplements you are taking. You may be asked to discontinue certain agents before the test.
• Tell your doctor if you've recently undergone a nuclear scan.

What You Experience
• A sample of your blood is drawn from a vein, usually in your arm, and sent to a laboratory for analysis. (For more on this procedure, called venipuncture, see page 32.)

Risks and Complications
• None.

After the Test
• Immediately after blood is drawn, pressure is applied (with cotton or gauze) to the puncture site.
• You may resume any medications withheld before the test.
• Blood may collect and clot under the skin (hematoma) at the puncture site; this is harmless and will resolve on its own. For a large hematoma that causes swelling and discomfort, apply ice initially; after 24 hours, use warm, moist compresses to help dissolve the clotted blood.

Estimated Cost: $

Sigmoidoscopy
(Flexible Sigmoidoscopy, Proctoscopy, Anoscopy)

Description
• In this test, a flexible, lighted viewing tube (sigmoidoscope) is passed into the anus, rectum, and the lowest portion of the large intestine, or sigmoid colon (illustrated on page 25). Less often, a rigid scope is used, usually to examine just the anus or rectum. Fiberoptic cables permit the doctor to visually inspect the lining of these organs for any signs of disease or abnormality; in some cases, instruments are passed through the scope to obtain tissue biopsies or stool samples for microscopic examination. Sigmoidoscopy may also be done therapeutically, for example, to remove polyps.

Purpose of the Test
• To detect and evaluate inflammatory or infectious bowel disease, hemorrhoids, polyps, tumors, ulcers, and other bowel abnormalities in people with symptoms such as blood or mucus in the stool, recent changes in bowel habits, or abdominal pain.
• Performed routinely—for example, every 3 to 5 years—to screen for colorectal cancer or precancerous polyps in adults age 50 and older; may be done earlier and more often in those with a family history of the disease or a positive fecal occult blood test (see page 199). (For more on screening tests, see Chapter 3.)
• To remove hemorrhoids or polyps, or reduce twisting (volvulus) in the lower bowel.

Who Performs It
• A gastroenterologist or another physician.

Special Concerns
• Although sigmoidoscopy may provoke some anxiety, the procedure usually causes only mild to moderate discomfort.
• You should wait at least a week after having a barium test, such as a barium enema (see page 104), before undergoing sigmoidoscopy;

the presence of barium interferes with visual inspection of the colon.
• The procedure may not be possible in people with painful anorectal conditions, such as fissures or hemorrhoids, diverticulitis (inflammation in the sacs of the colon), or very active bleeding in the bowel or rectum.

Before the Test
• Consume only clear liquids (for example, water, bouillon, or gelatin) for 12 to 48 hours before the procedure, according to your doctor's instructions. You may have to fast on the morning of the procedure. In addition, some patients may also be prescribed an oral cathartic such as magnesium citrate.
• The morning of the procedure, you may need to self-administer a cleansing enema before

Results
▼

➡ During visual inspection of the bowel, the doctor will note any abnormalities such as bleeding, inflammation, abnormal growths, or ulcers.

➡ Various laboratory tests are often necessary to pinpoint a diagnosis. For example, stool samples may be cultured (see page 166) to identify the presence of infectious organisms. Biopsied tumors and excised polyps are examined under a microscope for signs of cancer or another abnormality. (For more on microscopic examination, see Chapter 1.)

➡ If precancerous polyps or a malignancy are detected, you should undergo a more extensive procedure, called colonoscopy, to examine the entire length of the colon (see page 159).

Sigmoidoscopy

leaving your home, or you may be given an enema at the testing facility. This preparation will provide the examiner with a better view during the test.

• If you are very anxious, you may receive a sedative injection, but this is not usually required.

• If you have an anal fissure or local inflammation, you may be given a local anesthetic jelly shortly before the procedure.

What You Experience

• You lie on your side on a table, with your knees drawn to your chest, and you are draped to minimize any embarrassment.

• The doctor begins by inserting a gloved, lubricated finger into your rectum to perform a manual examination.

• Next, the lubricated scope is gently inserted into your anus and through your rectum and the lower portion (up to 25 inches) of your colon. You may feel some abdominal cramping or the urge to defecate as the instrument is inserted and advanced. Breathe deeply and slowly through your mouth to relax your abdominal muscles and reduce this discomfort.

• The doctor may instill a small amount of air through the scope to dilate the intestinal passage for better viewing. This may cause you to feel bloated and to pass gas.

• As the scope is slowly withdrawn, the doctor carefully inspects the lining of your colon, rectum, and anus, looking for any abnormalities.

• If appropriate, a biopsy forceps or other instrument may be inserted through the scope to obtain tissue or stool specimens. Polyps may be entirely removed using an electrocautery device. (These procedures are painless, since the colon lining contains no pain fibers; however, if a biopsy of the anal canal is needed, a local anesthetic is given since this area is sensitive to pain.) Tissue and fluid samples will be sent to a laboratory for analysis.

• The procedure lasts 15 to 30 minutes.

Risks and Complications

• When performed by a skilled professional, flexible sigmoidoscopy is typically safe and well-tolerated.

• Possible complications include pain in the lower bowels, bleeding, infection, and, rarely, perforation of the rectum or colon (which requires surgical repair).

After the Test

• You may leave the facility promptly after the test is completed. (Patients who have been given a sedative may need to wait until the medication wears off, and arrange for someone to drive them home.)

• You may experience flatulence or gas pains after the procedure.

• If a biopsy was performed, you may have a small amount of rectal bleeding for several hours.

• Contact your doctor immediately if you develop fever, rectal bleeding, or abdominal pain and distention.

Estimated Cost: $$

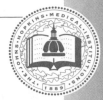

Skeletal CT Scan
(Computed Tomography Scan of the Bones)

Description

• In this test, a body scanner delivers x-rays to selected bones or joints—such as the shoulder, spine, hip, or pelvis—at many different angles. A computer compiles this information to construct highly detailed, cross-sectional images, which are then displayed on a TV monitor and recorded on x-ray film. In some cases, a contrast dye may be injected to enhance detail of the bones and the soft tissue inside and around the bones on the images. (For more on CT scanning, see Chapter 2.)

• A variation of this test, called myelography, involves injection of a contrast dye directly into the spinal canal to provide fine detail of the spine, spinal cord, and surrounding tissues. This procedure is described on page 263.

Purpose of the Test

• To identify abnormalities in the upper and lower spine, such as herniated discs and spinal stenosis (a narrowing of the spinal canal), that may be causing back pain and/or referred pain to the lower extremities.

• To detect and assess the extent of primary or metastatic bone tumors, and tumors in the soft tissue surrounding bones.

• To diagnose joint abnormalities, such as fractures through the joint surface and certain tumors, that are difficult to detect with other methods.

• To determine the location of an abscess.

• To evaluate skeletal changes in osteoporosis and other metabolic bone diseases.

Who Performs It

• A radiology technician.

Special Concerns

• Pregnant women should not undergo this test because exposure to ionizing radiation may harm the fetus.

• People with allergies to iodine or shellfish may experience an allergic reaction to iodine-based contrast dyes.

• Painkillers may be administered to people with significant bone or joint pain if remaining still during the exam is likely to cause discomfort.

• People who experience claustrophobia may find it difficult to undergo a CT scan, which takes place in a narrow, tunnel-like structure.

• This test may not be possible for severely overweight individuals (over 300 lbs).

Before the Test

• Inform your doctor if you have an allergy to iodine or shellfish. You may be given a combined antihistamine-steroid preparation to reduce the risk of an allergic reaction to the contrast dye.

• Tell your doctor if you suffer from claustrophobia. He or she may prescribe a sedative to help you tolerate the procedure.

• If a contrast dye is to be used or if sedation is anticipated, you will be instructed to fast for 4 hours before the test.

Results
▼

➥ A physician will examine the recorded images for evidence of abnormalities in the bones or joints being examined.

➥ If a definitive diagnosis can be made, appropriate treatment will be initiated, depending on the specific problem.

➥ In some cases, additional tests may be needed to establish a diagnosis and determine the extent of the problem. For example, magnetic resonance imaging (see page 327) may provide better detail of the soft tissues near the spine.

• You will be asked to remove your clothes, jewelry, and any metal objects and put on a hospital gown.

What You Experience
• You will lie on your back on a narrow table that is then advanced into the CT scanner.
• The scanner, which encircles you, rotates around you taking pictures at different intervals and from various angles. You will feel the table move during the test.
• You must remain as still as possible because any movement can distort the images on the scan.
• The examiner may advise you on how to control your breathing at several points during the procedure.
• A contrast dye may be administered through an intravenous (IV) needle or catheter inserted in a vein in your arm. You may feel a brief warm, flushing sensation after the injection; rarely, some people experience nausea and possibly vomiting.
• The test typically takes 30 to 60 minutes.

Risks and Complications
• CT scanning involves exposure to low levels of radiation.

• Some people may experience an allergic reaction to the iodine-based contrast dye, which can cause symptoms such as nausea, sneezing, vomiting, hives, and occasionally a life-threatening response called anaphylactic shock. Emergency medications and equipment are kept readily available.

After the Test
• You are free to resume your normal diet and activities.
• If a contrast dye was used, you are encouraged to drink clear fluids to avoid dehydration and help flush the material out of your system.
• Blood may collect and clot under the skin (hematoma) at the dye injection site; this is harmless and will resolve on its own. For a large hematoma that causes swelling and discomfort, apply ice initially; after 24 hours, use warm, moist compresses to help dissolve the clotted blood.
• Delayed allergic reactions to the contrast dye, such as hives, rash, or itching, may appear 2 to 6 hours after the procedure. If this occurs, your doctor will prescribe antihistamines or steroids to ease your discomfort.

Estimated Cost: $$$

Skeletal MRI
(Magnetic Resonance Imaging of the Bones)

Description

• Skeletal MRI uses a strong magnetic field combined with radiofrequency waves to create highly detailed, cross-sectional images of selected bones and surrounding tissues. These scans, which appear as two-dimensional slices through the bone, are then examined for abnormalities. For certain studies, an MRI contrast dye such as gadolinium may be injected to provide better definition of soft tissues and blood vessels and thus enhance the images. (For more information on how MRI works, see Chapter 2.)

Purpose of the Test

• To diagnose tumors of the bone or the soft tissue inside or around the bone, such as muscles and ligaments.

• To pinpoint any changes in the bone marrow cavity.

• To assess various disorders of the spine, spinal cord, spinal nerves, or intervertebral discs, and to evaluate the spine before surgery.

• To help diagnose meniscal tears in the knee, as well as injuries of the knee and shoulder ligaments.

Who Performs It

• A radiologist or a qualified technician.

Special Concerns

• MRI is more expensive and less widely available than x-rays (see page 331) or CT scans (see page 325), but is preferable in most cases where differentiation of the soft tissue in and around bones is necessary.

• People who experience claustrophobia may find it difficult to undergo an MRI, which takes place in a narrow, tunnel-like structure. In some cases, an open MRI—a larger unit that is open on several sides—may be used as an alternative.

• This test may not be possible for severely overweight individuals (over 300 lbs), although some open MRI scanners can now accommodate larger patients.

• Because the MRI generates a strong magnetic field, it cannot be performed on people who have certain types of internally placed metallic devices, including pacemakers, inner ear implants, or intracranial aneurysm clips.

• The test is not commonly done in pregnant women because the long-term effects of MRI on the fetus are unknown.

Before the Test

• Tell your doctor if you suffer from claustrophobia. He or she may prescribe a sedative that can help you tolerate the procedure.

• You will be advised to empty your bladder before the test.

• Remove any magnetic cards or metallic objects, including watches, hair clips, belts, credit cards, and jewelry. You may be asked to disrobe and put on a hospital gown.

What You Experience

• You will lie down on a narrow, padded bed

Results

▼

➥ The MRI scans are displayed on a video monitor and then recorded on film. The doctor will examine the images for signs of any skeletal abnormality.

➥ If a definitive diagnosis can be made, appropriate treatment will be initiated, depending on the specific problem.

➥ In some cases, additional tests, such as a bone biopsy (see page 113), may be required to establish a diagnosis or determine the extent of a problem.

Skeletal MRI

that slides into a large, enclosed cylinder containing the MRI magnets.

• You must remain very still throughout the procedure because any motion can distort the scan.

• In some cases, you will receive an injection of contrast dye such as gadolinium before or during the procedure.

• There is a microphone inside the imaging machine, and you may talk to the technician performing the scan at any time during the procedure.

• You will hear loud thumping sounds as the scanning is performed. To block out the noise, you can request earplugs or listen to music on earphones.

• The procedure usually takes from 60 to 90 minutes.

Risks and Complications

• MRI does not involve exposure to ionizing radiation and is not associated with any risks or complications.

After the Test

• Most patients can go home right after the scan and resume their usual activities.

• Sedated patients may be monitored for a short period until the effects of the sedative have worn off.

Estimated Cost: $$$

Skeletal Nuclear Scan
(Bone Scan)

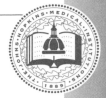

Description

• After intravenous injection of a small amount of radioactive material, a special camera records the distribution of radiotracer throughout the skeleton. This information is translated by a computer into two-dimensional images that are recorded on film. Nuclear scans can often identify skeletal abnormalities months before they would be detectable on x-rays. (For more on nuclear imaging, see Chapter 2.)

Purpose of the Test

• To identify primary bone tumors or metastatic cancer that has spread to the bone from other parts of the body, particularly when x-ray findings are normal but cancer is still suspected.

• To diagnose stress fractures that do not always appear on x-rays and to monitor fracture healing.

• To detect or evaluate bone infection, inflammation, arthritis, and other bone disorders.

• To pinpoint the site of an abnormality before a bone biopsy or surgery is performed.

• To aid in the evaluation of unexplained bone pain.

Who Performs It

• A nuclear medicine technician.

Special Concerns

• This test should not be performed in pregnant or breastfeeding women because of possible risks to the fetus or infant.

• It may not be possible to perform this scan in people with poor kidney function because their bones may not absorb sufficient amounts of the radiotracer.

• A skeletal injury that results from trauma may be missed if the scan is performed within the first 24 hours.

• Certain tumors, such as multiple myeloma (a tumor of the bone marrow), may not appear on a bone scan, and other tests will be needed to detect them.

Before the Test

• Remove any jewelry or metal objects before the test begins.

What You Experience

• The doctor injects a very small amount of a radiotracer into a vein, usually in your arm. (Other than the minor discomfort of this injection, the procedure is painless.) You may experience brief, mild nausea and flushing as the material enters your bloodstream.

• You will wait for 1 to 3 hours before the scan is performed. During this time, you will be encouraged to drink several glasses of water to help the kidneys filter out any radioactive

Results

▼

➥ A doctor examines the scans for any abnormalities and interprets these findings in conjunction with your medical and surgical history, x-ray findings, and laboratory test results. Healthy bone is characterized by uniform absorption of the radiotracer throughout the body, while areas of increased uptake appear as "hot spots" on the scans, indicating new bone growth associated with various abnormalities, including tumors, arthritis, fractures, infections, and degenerative bone and joint changes.

➥ If a definitive diagnosis can be made, appropriate treatment will be initiated.

➥ In some cases, additional tests, such as a bone biopsy (see page 113), may be needed to further evaluate abnormal results.

material that is not picked up by the bone.

• Immediately before the scanning, you should empty your bladder to eliminate any radiotracer that might obstruct the view of the underlying pelvic bones.

• You will be asked to lie down on an examining table. A large scanning camera is passed over your body, recording the gamma rays emitted by the radiotracer in the bones.

• You must remain still during the scan, which may cause some numbness or stiffness. (Ask the doctor if a pillow or pads can be placed on the table for your comfort.) At several points during the procedure, the examiner may instruct you to change your position.

• The scan itself usually takes about 30 to 60 minutes.

Risks and Complications

• The trace amount of radioactive material used in this test is not associated with any significant risks or complications.

• In extremely rare cases, patients may be hypersensitive to the radiotracer and may experience an adverse reaction.

After the Test

• You may resume your normal activities after the test.

• Drink extra fluids to help your body eliminate the radiotracer. Most of the radioactive material is excreted in the urine within 6 to 24 hours.

• Blood may collect and clot under the skin (hematoma) at the dye injection site; this is harmless and will resolve on its own. For a large hematoma that causes swelling and discomfort, apply ice initially; after 24 hours, use warm, moist compresses to help dissolve the clotted blood.

Estimated Cost: $$$

Skeletal X-ray
(Bone Radiography)

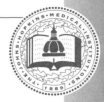

Description
• X-rays are passed through the bones or skeletal region being examined, producing images of these structures on a special type of film. When the test is used to examine the spinal column alone, it is termed a spinal x-ray. Examination of the entire skeleton is known as a skeletal survey. (For more on x-rays, see Chapter 2.)

Purpose of the Test
• To detect bone fractures and other abnormalities after a traumatic injury.
• To detect primary bone cancer or cancer that has metastasized (spread) to the bone.
• To detect infectious diseases of the bones, including the spinal vertebrae.
• To evaluate the intervertebral disc spaces in the lower spine.
• To assess abnormal curvature of the spine (scoliosis), degenerative disease of the spinal structures, and other spinal deformities.
• To diagnose different types of arthritis.

Who Performs It
• A radiology technician.

Special Concerns
• Pregnant women should not undergo this test because exposure to ionizing radiation may harm the fetus.

Before the Test
• Remove any jewelry or metal objects before the test. If necessary, you will be asked to disrobe and put on a hospital gown.
• If you are having a spinal x-ray and have long hair, clip your hair up beforehand so that it does not hang over your chest or shoulders.
• If you are having a skull x-ray, be sure to remove your glasses, contact lenses, hairpins, and dentures.
• In some cases, a protective lead shield may be placed over parts of the body not being scanned in order to minimize exposure to radiation.

What You Experience
• A technician will position you in front of an x-ray machine—either sitting, standing, or lying down on a table, depending on which bone(s) are being examined.
• You will be asked to remain perfectly still and hold your breath while the x-ray is being taken. Any movement can distort the image.
• You may be instructed to assume different positions as additional x-rays are obtained from different angles or of different bones, depending on the purpose of the test.
• The test usually takes 5 to 10 minutes. A full skeletal survey may take up to 1 hour.

Risks and Complications
• X-ray exams involve minimal exposure to radiation.

After the Test
• If the test is elective, you may return home and resume your normal activities.

Estimated Cost: $$

Results
▼

➡ A doctor will examine the x-ray films for evidence of any abnormalities.

➡ If a definitive diagnosis can be made, appropriate treatment will be initiated, depending on the specific problem.

➡ In many cases, additional tests, such as a skeletal MRI (see page 327), a CT scan (see page 325), or a bone scan (see page 329), may be required for further evaluation.

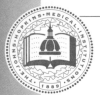

Skin Biopsy

Skin Biopsy

Description

• A small sample of skin tissue is removed, under local anesthesia, for examination under a microscope; the specimen is usually taken from an area that appears altered because of disease (lesion). Three different techniques may be used:

• **Shave biopsy** removes the outer layer of a lesion with a sharp scalpel.

• **Punch biopsy** uses a hollow, cylindrical instrument, called a punch, to remove a circular core of tissue from the center of a lesion.

• **Excisional biopsy** is the removal of the entire lesion with a surgical knife; this procedure may also function as a primary treatment.

Purpose of the Test

• To identify benign and malignant (cancerous) growths.

• To diagnose chronic bacterial and fungal skin infections.

• To diagnose inflammatory and autoimmune skin disorders, including psoriasis, systemic lupus erythematosus, and autoimmune blistering diseases.

• To serve as a form of therapy, by removing skin cancers, warts, moles, and other growths.

Who Performs It

• A dermatologist, a plastic surgeon, or another physician.

Special Concerns

• Results are more likely to be inconclusive if a small tissue sample is taken in an effort to reduce the scar size, or if the biopsy site was not selected properly.

Before the Test

• Inform your doctor of any drugs you are currently taking and whether you have any allergies to medication.

• If you are scheduled to have a large biopsy, such as an excisional biopsy, your doctor will advise you to discontinue any drugs (such as aspirin or ibuprofen) and herbal remedies that may promote bleeding, as well as alcohol, a few days before the procedure.

What You Experience

• After injecting a local anesthetic into the biopsy site to numb the area, the doctor removes the tissue sample.

• If a large tissue sample is obtained (which is most common in excisional biopsies and some punch biopsies), the area may be closed with stitches.

• In cases where a large lesion (such as a cancer) is removed, a skin graft may be needed.

• The biopsy usually takes about 5 to 10 minutes, but may take as long as 60 minutes if the procedure is complex.

Risks and Complications

• Skin biopsy leaves a scar, which can range

Results
▼

➡ The skin specimen is sent to a pathology laboratory and examined under a microscope for abnormal changes. (For more on microscopic examination, see Chapter 1.)

➡ If the biopsy reveals cancerous cells, treatment to completely remove the malignant lesion will be instituted (unless excisional biopsy was already performed to remove the entire lesion).

➡ If the biopsy findings indicate the presence of a specific autoimmune or inflammatory disorder, appropriate therapy will be started.

➡ If the biopsy findings are inconclusive, an additional biopsy may be needed.

from slight to obvious. Let your doctor know before surgery if you tend to form large scars, or keloids, in response to a skin injury; he or she will follow postoperative measures that may reduce scarring.

• Rarely, infection may occur after the biopsy, or nerve damage may develop if the biopsy is deep.

After the Test

• The doctor will check the biopsy site for bleeding, and may give you pain-relieving medication if needed.

• If no stitches were required, an antibiotic ointment is applied and a dressing placed over the site. The doctor will advise you to clean the area, reapply the ointment, and change the dressing at least once a day until healing occurs, usually in 5 to 28 days.

• If stitches were necessary, the doctor may leave the dressing in place or periodically change it until the stitches are removed, usually 3 to 14 days later. During this time, keep the biopsy site clean and dry. You may also have to avoid exercise or heavy lifting for several weeks.

Estimated Cost: $$

Skin Biopsy continued

Skin, Hair, or Nail Culture

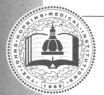

Description

• A sample of skin, hair, fingernails, or toenails is obtained using a scalpel or other instrument. The specimen is sent to a laboratory so that it can be grown in a suitable culture medium to identify potential infectious organisms. (For more on cultures, see page 166.)

Purpose of the Test

• To determine whether an abnormality of the skin, hair, or nails is caused by a bacterial, fungal, mycobacterial, or viral infection.

Who Performs It

• A doctor.

Special Concerns

• Previous therapy with antibacterial, antifungal, or antiviral drugs may lead to false-negative results.

• The herpes zoster virus (which causes chicken pox and shingles) is very fragile and almost never grows in a culture, in some cases leading to false-negative results.

• Certain bacteria or fungi that are cultured may not in fact be responsible for the infection, leading to false-positive results.

Before the Test

• No special preparation is required.

What You Experience

• If your skin is the site of the suspected infection, the doctor scrapes the outer layer of abnormal skin with a scalpel.

• When the scalp is affected, the doctor gently removes diseased hairs with a forceps and also scrapes your scalp with a scalpel.

• For nail infections, the examiner scrapes the inner surface of the nail below the tip or clips off the portion of the nail that appears abnormal.

• You may experience some minor discomfort while the sample is being collected.

• Sample collection usually takes only about 1 minute.

Risks and Complications

• None.

After the Test

• You may resume your normal activities.

Estimated Cost: $

Results

▼

➡ The skin, hair, or nail specimen is placed in culture media in the laboratory and is then observed for the growth of microorganisms. (For more on laboratory testing, see Chapter 1.)

➡ If organisms are observed growing in culture, they are identified and classified to provide a definitive diagnosis, and appropriate therapy is begun.

➡ If the test is negative but the problem persists, your doctor may test another tissue sample.

Skin Tests for Allergies

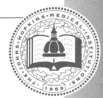

Description
• In these tests, a very small amount of a substance suspected of causing an allergy is applied through the skin to determine whether it will elicit an allergic reaction. Several different methods are used to prepare the skin before administering the allergen: A needle may be used to make one or more scratches in the skin (scratch test); to prick the skin and pick up the superficial layer of skin (prick test); or to make a small puncture in the skin (puncture test). Alternatively, the allergen solution may be injected between layers of the skin (intradermal test).

Purpose of the Test
• To identify allergies to specific substances—such as house dust mites, animal dander, pollens, latex, or certain drugs or foods.

Who Performs It
• A doctor, a nurse, or a lab technician.

Special Concerns
• Several factors may blunt an allergic skin test response, including dehydration and the use of certain drugs, such as antihistamines, tricyclic antidepressants, and phenothiazines. This may lead to false-negative results.
• Redness and swelling may result from skin irritation rather than allergy, leading to false-positive results. This is of special concern when testing with higher concentrations of allergens or drugs. (For more on false-positives and false-negatives, see page 35.)

Before the Test
• Report to your doctor any medications that you are currently taking. You may be asked to discontinue certain drugs for 3 to 7 days before the test. Long-acting antihistamines (for example, hydroxyzine or cetirizine) should be discontinued for 2 to 3 weeks.

What You Experience
• A normal-appearing patch of skin on your forearm or back is cleansed with alcohol.
• The examiner then applies a solution containing a particular allergen to your skin, using the scratch, prick, or puncture methods. If you are having an intradermal test, the examiner will inject a lower concentration of the allergen solution under your skin.
• Numerous allergen solutions may be tested in a single session, with the drops placed in parallel rows about an inch apart.
• After about 15 minutes, the test sites are examined for a positive reaction—indicated by the presence of a red, raised area called a wheal.
• The different test methods may be performed at separate times or sequentially in a single session. The tests may be repeated if the initial findings are negative but an allergy is strongly suspected.

Risks and Complications
• These tests are generally safe, although the

Results
▼

➥ The examiner inspects the test sites for redness and swelling. A strong skin response is regarded as evidence of an allergic sensitivity.

➥ If a specific allergy is diagnosed, your doctor may advise you to avoid the allergen, use anti-allergy medication, or have a series of allergy shots to increase your tolerance.

➥ If skin tests are negative or inconclusive, but an allergy is still a strong possibility, your doctor may recommend blood tests (see page 110) or provocation (challenge) tests (see page 276).

intradermal test carries a slightly higher risk of provoking a significant allergic reaction than the other methods.

• Very rarely, particularly sensitive individuals will experience a life-threatening condition called anaphylactic shock (characterized by symptoms such as respiratory distress, decreased blood pressure, and shock). Emergency medications and equipment are kept readily available.

After the Test

• The examiner will ask you to wait for up to 30 minutes to ensure you are not having a severe allergic reaction.

• Inform your doctor immediately if you experience wheezing, lightheadedness, severe itching, or shortness of breath during or after the testing.

• Skin at the testing site(s) may itch for several hours. If you are highly allergic, you may experience swelling, particularly after intradermal testing. Antihistamines and topical steroids are often given to minimize these symptoms.

• Keep the skin that was used for the test clean until it heals completely.

Estimated Cost: $ to $$

Sleep Studies
(Polysomnography)

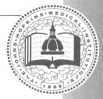

Description
• In this test, your heart rate, breathing, brain and muscle activity, and other body functions are monitored as you sleep. Typically, you are observed by means of electrocardiography (ECG; see page 174), electroencephalography (EEG; see page 175), electromyography (EMG; see page 177), and oximetry (see page 278).

Purpose of the Test
• To diagnose sleep disorders, including apnea (recurrent episodes of breathing cessation during sleep), in people who display typical symptoms such as excessive snoring, daytime sleepiness, and chronic fatigue, as well as those who have documented abnormal heart rhythms (arrhythmias) during sleep.

Who Performs It
• A nurse or a technician in a special sleep study center.

Special Concerns
• None.

Before the Test
• Avoid caffeine and alcohol for several days before the test.

What You Experience
• The test takes place during your normal sleeping hours in a specially designed sleep laboratory. The lab is constructed to block out external sounds and the temperature is easily controlled.
• Electrodes (small wires) are applied to your skin. They will monitor your heart rate and rhythm (ECG), brain waves (EEG), and muscle activity (EMG). This may require shaving areas of body hair in some men.
• You are attached to monitors that measure your air flow, breathing effort, and the amount of oxygen present in your blood. This equip-

ment is not uncomfortable, and should not disturb your sleeping pattern.
• The monitors and electrodes are removed when you wake.

Risks and Complications
• There are no risks or complications associated with this test.

After the Test
• Most patients can go home right after the study and resume their usual activities.

Estimated Cost: $$$

Results

▼

➡ Your doctor will examine and interpret the results. Based on this analysis, you may be diagnosed with a sleep disorder, such as obstructive sleep apnea (caused by complete obstruction of the upper airway that stops breathing for at least 10 seconds at a time during sleep) or central sleep apnea (characterized by the cessation of breathing not due to an obstructed airway).

➡ Depending on which type of sleep apnea is diagnosed, your doctor will make treatment recommendations.

Sleep Studies

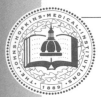
Small Bowel Biopsy
(Small Intestine Biopsy)

Small Bowel Biopsy

Description

• In this test, a tissue sample is extracted from the small intestine, or small bowel, and sent to a laboratory for analysis. To obtain the sample, you must swallow a capsule attached to a long, thin polyethylene tube; when it reaches the small intestine (illustrated on page 24), suction is applied to pull the tissue specimen into the capsule. This method permits biopsies from areas that are out of reach via esophagogastroduodenoscopy (see page 194) and allows for larger samples to be obtained.

Purpose of the Test

• To assist in the diagnosis of diseases of the intestinal lining, such as bacterial infections that cause diarrhea and malabsorption of nutrients.

Who Performs It

• A physician who is trained in endoscopic procedures.

Special Concerns

• Although small bowel biopsy may provoke some anxiety and cause slight discomfort, it is not painful and complications are rare.
• Small bowel biopsy may not be safe in people with certain bleeding disorders. Blood coagulation studies (see page 157) may be performed to ensure you are a proper candidate for the procedure.

Before the Test

• Do not eat or drink anything for at least 8 hours before the test.
• Inform your doctor if you regularly take anticoagulants or nonsteroidal anti-inflammatory drugs (such as aspirin, ibuprofen, or naproxen). These medications must be discontinued for some time before the test to reduce the risk of bleeding complications.

What You Experience

• You will begin the test sitting up on a table.
• A local anesthetic (such as lidocaine) is sprayed onto the back of your throat to suppress the gag reflex as the capsule and tube are inserted.
• The doctor inserts the lubricated capsule and tube into your throat and then asks you to flex your neck and swallow to aid in the advancement of the tube down through your esophagus.
• You will not be able to speak when the tube is inserted, but your breathing will not be affected.
• Next, you will lie on your right side as the doctor advances the capsule and tube into your stomach, through the pylorus (the opening of the stomach into the small intestine), and finally into the small intestine. Continuous x-ray imaging, or fluoroscopy (see page 205), is used to guide the progress and positioning of the device.
• When the capsule is in the proper position, you will be asked to roll onto your back so that the doctor can verify the capsule's placement using fluoroscopy.

Results

▼

➥ Biopsy specimens are sent to a pathology laboratory and examined under a microscope for changes that indicate a bacterial or parasitic infection or another abnormality. (For more on microscopic examination, see Chapter 1.)

➥ This test usually results in a definitive diagnosis. Your doctor will recommend an appropriate course of treatment, depending on the specific problem.

• To obtain the biopsy sample, a syringe is attached to the outer end of the tube and suction is applied. The suction draws a small piece of tissue into the capsule and then closes off the capsule, which cuts off the tissue from the intestinal lining.

• The tube is slowly withdrawn, and the tissue sample is sent to a laboratory for analysis.

• The procedure lasts 45 to 60 minutes.

Risks and Complications

• When performed by a skilled professional, small bowel biopsy is typically safe and well-tolerated.

• Rare but serious complications of this procedure include bleeding, blood infection, and perforation of the bowel (which requires surgical repair).

After the Test

• You may leave the testing facility promptly after the test is completed.

• Do not eat or drink anything until your gag reflex returns, usually in a few hours. (Touching the back of the throat with a tongue depressor tests for this reflex.)

• You may have black, tarry stools due to bleeding for a short period of time.

• Contact your doctor immediately if you develop a fever or abdominal pain.

Estimated Cost: $$$

Small Bowel Biopsy continued

Smell and Taste Testing

Smell and Taste Testing

Description
• The sense of smell is made possible by nerve cells located in the nose. When stimulated by particular odors, these specialized cells transmit certain messages to the brain, which interprets the information in order to distinguish particular aromas. The sense of taste works in a similar manner, as nerve cells in the taste buds of the mouth and throat react to particular foods or beverages. Both of these senses may be impaired by aging, illness, injury, and other factors. Smell and taste testing is performed to help determine the extent of any such sensory loss; this is done by measuring the lowest concentration of a test substance that you can detect and identify.

Purpose of the Test
• Smell testing is performed to detect smell disorders, including reduction in the ability to smell (hyposmia); total loss of smelling ability (anosmia); and smell distortion (dysosmia) such as perceiving a pleasant smell as being unpleasant.
• Taste testing is performed to detect taste disorders, including a reduction in the ability to taste (hypogeusia); total loss of tasting ability (ageusia); and persistent abnormal taste in the mouth (dysgeusia).

Who Performs It
• An otolaryngologist or another specially trained physician.

Special Concerns
• If you are having difficulty tasting food, you may actually have a smelling disorder. Most taste problems are actually caused by a loss of smelling ability, since the flavor of foods is highly dependent on their aroma.
• Smelling and tasting disorders rarely occur together in the same individual.

Before the Test
• No special preparation is necessary before these tests.

What You Experience
Smell testing:
• You will be asked to "scratch and sniff" a series of paper slips, and then to identify each odor from a list of possibilities.
• You may also be asked to compare certain of the smells, or to describe how the intensity of a smell grows when the concentration

Results
▼

➡ Your doctor will assess the test results and determine whether your sense of taste or smell is impaired. If so, your medical history usually provides a clear explanation for the problem. Possible causes include serious upper respiratory or sinus infections, nasal polyps, certain medications, tobacco smoking, dental problems, previous radiation therapy for cancer of the head or neck, and traumatic injury to the head. In addition, a number of systemic disorders, such as diabetes, hypertension, and degenerative nerve conditions such as Parkinson's disease, may also lead to loss of taste or smell.

➡ Some cases of impaired smell or taste are treatable, while others are not. When treatment is possible, it is directed at the underlying cause of the disorder.

➡ In rare cases, further testing, such as a CT scan (see page 212) or an MRI (see page 214) of the head, is needed to determine the cause for a taste or smell disorder.

of a particular substance is strengthened.
• This test takes about 30 minutes.

Taste testing:
• You will be asked to taste and then identify various substances, which cover the four basic taste sensations—sweet, sour, bitter, and salty.
• In some cases, you will sip a substance and spit it out, and then describe the taste.
• Alternatively, the test may involve applying different chemicals directly to specific areas of the tongue.
• You may also be asked to compare certain tastes, or to describe how the intensity of taste

grows when the concentration of a particular substance is strengthened.
• This test takes about 30 minutes.

Risks and Complications
• There are no risks or complications associated with this test.

After the Test
• You are free to leave the testing facility and resume your normal activities immediately after the test is completed.

Estimated Cost: $$

Smell and Taste Testing continued

Sonohysterogram

(Sonohysterography, Hysterosonography)

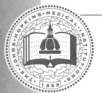

Sonohysterogram

Description

• In this relatively new test, sterile saline solution is slowly infused into a woman's uterus while the organ is being examined using transvaginal ultrasound (described on page 285). The saline slightly distends the uterine cavity and enhances the quality of the ultrasound images, providing more detailed views of the uterus and endometrium (the tissue lining the uterus). (For more on how ultrasound works, see Chapter 2.)

Purpose of the Test

• To evaluate abnormalities of the uterus and endometrium—for example, benign growths (such as polyps or fibroids), cancer, or endometrial thickening—that were first identified by pelvic or transvaginal ultrasound.
• To evaluate abnormal vaginal bleeding in peri- or postmenopausal women.
• To evaluate fertility problems in women.
• To monitor the uterus in certain women who take the drug tamoxifen (Nolvadex) for breast cancer (this drug has been associated with an increased risk of developing uterine cancer).
• To examine the condition of the uterus after uterine surgery.

Who Performs It

• A gynecologist or a radiologist.

Special Concerns

• This procedure should not be done in pregnant women and may not be possible in women with cervical stenosis (narrowing of the lower end of the uterus) or large fibroid growths of the uterus.
• Women with active pelvic inflammatory disease (PID, an infection of the uterus, fallopian tubes, and adjacent structures) should not undergo this test until the disease is brought under control.
• If the test is being performed to assess fertil-

ity problems, it should be done during the first 10 days of the menstrual cycle. To evaluate the uterus for the presence of polyps, the test should be done in the latter part of the menstrual cycle.

Before the Test

• Some women—including those with chronic PID or heart problems—may be prescribed an antibiotic medication to take on the day before the procedure, in order to reduce the risk of infection.
• Your doctor may advise you to take an over-the-counter nonsteroidal anti-inflammatory drug (NSAID), such as ibuprofen, about 1 hour before the test.
• You will be asked to undress from the waist down and put on a drape or hospital gown.
• Empty your bladder before the test.

What You Experience

• You will assume a position similar to the one used for a pelvic exam—lying on your back with your knees bent and feet placed in stirrups. Breathe slowly and deeply and try to relax

---

Results
▼

➡ A gynecologist or a radiologist reviews the recorded images and video for evidence of any abnormality.

➡ If a definitive diagnosis can be made, appropriate treatment will be initiated.

➡ If this test fails to yield a definitive diagnosis, other diagnostic tests, such as a hysteroscopy (see page 122) and endometrial biopsy (see page 185), may be needed to provide more specific information or to further evaluate abnormal findings.

---

your pelvic muscles throughout the procedure.

• A preliminary ultrasound exam is performed to ensure the test can continue safely. A sterile latex condom is placed over a special oblong transducer, and a small amount of lubricant gel is applied to the device. The transducer is gently inserted into the vagina and rested against the cervix. The examiner manipulates the device to obtain different views of the uterus on a viewing monitor.

• The transducer is withdrawn, and a lubricated speculum—a metal or plastic instrument that pushes apart the walls of the vagina to provide the examiner with a view of the cervix—is inserted into the vagina. This may feel cold and cause some pressure.

• The cervix is cleansed with an antiseptic (which will cause a brief, cold sensation), and a thin, flexible tube (catheter) is then passed through the vagina and into the uterus.

• A balloon at the tip of the catheter is inflated with saline to hold the device in place. Sterile saline is then infused through the catheter into the uterus. You may feel some mild to moderate cramping due to the saline infusion.

• After the speculum is removed, the ultrasound transducer is reinserted into the vagina and more images are obtained. These pictures are recorded on film or video for later analysis.

• The transducer and catheter are then gently withdrawn.

• The test takes about 15 minutes.

Risks and Complications

• There are no risks associated with ultrasound itself.

• The most common side effect is mild to moderate cramping. Rare but serious complications associated with the insertion of a catheter and infusion of saline include perforation of the uterus and infection.

After the Test

• You may return home and resume your normal activities.

• Mild bleeding (spotting) and cramping are common after this test. NSAIDs, such as ibuprofen, should ease any discomfort.

• Inform your doctor immediately if you develop abnormal bleeding, fever, or abdominal pain.

Estimated Cost: $$

Sonohysterogram continued

Stress Echocardiography

Stress Echocardiography

Description
• In this test, detailed images of the heart are obtained before, during, and after a cardiac stress test (see page 147) using a device called a transducer that is placed on the chest. (The transducer emits high-frequency sound waves, or ultrasound, and converts the sound waves echoed back from the heart into images.) Exercise on a stationary bike or treadmill is the most common form of stress testing. Stress echocardiography can detect heart muscle that is not contracting as strongly as expected, indicating possible blockages in the coronary arteries. (For more on how ultrasound works, see Chapter 2.)

Purpose of the Test
• To aid in the evaluation of possible coronary artery disease.
• To determine appropriate levels of exercise for people with angina (chest pain due to inadequate delivery of oxygen to the heart muscle) or other symptoms of heart disease.
• To evaluate heart function and exercise capacity after a heart attack, angioplasty, or bypass surgery.
• To evaluate the heart prior to major surgery.

Who Performs It
• A doctor assisted by a nurse or a technician.

Special Concerns
• People who cannot exercise adequately because of orthopedic, arthritic, or lung disorders may instead be given dobutamine, a drug that increases the heart rate.
• People who have unstable angina or severe aortic valvular heart disease may not be able to undergo this test.
• Standard transthoracic echocardiography (see page 367) may not produce accurate results in obese people or those who have thick chests, chronic obstructive pulmonary disease, or chest wall abnormalities. For such patients, transesophageal echocardiography (see page 365) or a cardiac nuclear scan (see page 144) may be a better option.

Before the Test
• Antianginal drugs (such as nitroglycerin, beta-blockers, and calcium channel blockers) can affect test results by increasing your exercise tolerance. Your doctor may ask you to discontinue these medications for 1 or 2 days before the test.
• Do not eat, drink, or smoke for 4 hours before the test.
• Wear comfortable shoes and loose, lightweight clothing.
• Immediately before the test, you will be asked to disrobe above the waist. (Women may wear a loose-fitting hospital gown that opens in the front.)

What You Experience
• After you lie down on an examination table, ECG leads (see page 174) are applied to your chest to monitor your heart rate and rhythm during the test.
• A water-soluble gel is applied to your chest

Results
▼
➥ A physician will examine the recorded images and video for evidence of any cardiac abnormality.
➥ If a definitive diagnosis can be made based on this test, treatment will be started with diet, exercise, or medication.
➥ In some cases, more invasive tests, such as cardiac catheterization (see page 140), may be needed to further evaluate abnormal results.

to permit better transmission of the sound waves. The examiner then moves the transducer across your chest to obtain images of your heart while at rest.

• For an exercise stress test, you begin by walking on a treadmill or pedaling a stationary bicycle. The pedaling tension on the cycle or the speed and grade of the incline on the treadmill are gradually increased until you reach a target heart rate set by your doctor.

• For a dobutamine stress test, an intravenous (IV) line is inserted into a vein in your arm. The doctor infuses the drug and gradually increases the dose to mimic the effects of intensifying exercise. Another drug called atropine is sometimes needed to further increase your heart rate to the desired level.

• The examiner obtains additional images of the heart at various stages of stress testing and at the end of the procedure.

• The test concludes when you achieve an adequate heart rate or develop significant symptoms, such as angina or fatigue.

• The test takes 20 to 90 minutes.

Risks and Complications

• Although generally safe, this procedure carries a small amount of risk. Rare complications include severe angina, heart attack, abnormal heart rhythms, a drop in blood pressure, and fainting.

• Dobutamine may cause flushing, palpitations, headache, and nausea, but these effects usually resolve quickly once the infusion is stopped.

• Atropine can cause dry mouth and dilatation of the pupils, which may persist for an hour or so after the test.

After the Test

• You will rest until your blood pressure, heart rate, and other vital signs return to normal. The ECG leads and conductive gel are then removed from your chest.

• If you received dobutamine, the IV line is removed from your arm and pressure is applied to the infusion site for several minutes. Blood may collect and clot under the skin (hematoma) at the infusion site; this is harmless and will resolve on its own. For a large hematoma that causes swelling and discomfort, apply ice initially; after 24 hours, use warm, moist compresses to help dissolve the clotted blood.

• If there are no complications, you may resume your normal activities.

Estimated Cost: $$$

Stress Echocardiography continued

T-tube and Operative Cholangiography

Description

• Cholangiography is the x-ray examination of the bile ducts (biliary tract) after administration of a contrast dye to delineate these channels on the images. (For more on contrast x-rays, see Chapter 2.) The procedure may be performed either during gallbladder removal surgery (operative cholangiography) or postoperatively (T-tube cholangiography).

• **Operative cholangiography** involves injecting the contrast dye directly into the common bile duct during open surgery. X-ray films are then used to guide the surgeon and to identify any stones or other obstructions for immediate removal.

• **T-tube cholangiography** is typically performed 5 to 10 days after gallbladder removal. Contrast dye is injected through a T-shaped rubber tube placed in the common bile duct during surgery, and x-rays are then taken to detect any residual stones or other abnormalities.

Purpose of the Test

• To detect stones and other abnormalities in the bile ducts, such as strictures (narrowings), abnormal growths, and fistulae (abnormal openings).

Who Performs It

• Operative cholangiography is performed by a surgeon, usually accompanied by a radiologist.
• T-tube cholangiography can be performed by an x-ray technician, a nurse, or a doctor.

Special Concerns

• Pregnant women should not undergo this test because exposure to ionizing radiation may harm the fetus.
• People with allergies to iodine or shellfish may experience an allergic reaction to the iodine-based contrast dye.
• Severe obesity or the presence of gas overlying the bile ducts may obscure the x-ray findings.

• Residual barium in the abdomen due to a recent contrast x-ray study of the digestive tract may interfere with visualization of the bile duct.

Before the Test

• Inform your doctor if you have an allergy to iodine or shellfish. You may be given a combined antihistamine-steroid preparation to reduce the risk of an allergic reaction to the contrast dye.
• Fasting is usually not required before T-tube cholangiography, but the standard preoperative restrictions on food and drink apply before operative cholangiography.
• You will be asked to disrobe and put on a hospital gown.

What You Experience
Operative cholangiography:

• During gallbladder removal surgery, a catheter or thin needle is inserted into a bile duct and contrast dye is infused directly into the biliary tract.
• X-ray films are obtained during the operation and immediately reviewed by the surgeon.

Results
▼

➡ The doctor examines the x-ray images for evidence of any bile duct abnormality.

➡ If bile duct stones or other abnormalities are detected with operative cholangiography, the surgeon can correct the problem before closing the incision.

➡ If residual stones are detected with T-tube cholangiography, they can be extracted through the tube tract. If no abnormalities are detected, the tube is removed.

➡ In some cases, additional tests may be needed to further evaluate abnormal results.

• If stones or other obstructions are detected on x-rays, they are removed by the surgeon before the incision is closed.

T-tube cholangiography:

• After gallbladder removal surgery, a T-tube is left in place to facilitate drainage. Cholangiography typically occurs 5 to 10 days later.

• You will lie on your back on an x-ray table. An antiseptic solution is used to cleanse the T-tube.

• The contrast dye is injected into the T-tube. You may feel a bloating sensation in the upper right abdomen as it is injected.

• X-rays and fluoroscopy (see page 205) are used to visualize the biliary tract. You are instructed to assume various positions as x-ray films are obtained.

• The procedure takes about 15 minutes.

Risks and Complications

• Both tests involve exposure to low levels of ionizing radiation.

• Some people may experience an allergic reaction to the iodine-based contrast dye, which can cause symptoms such as nausea, sneezing, vomiting, hives, and occasionally a life-threatening response called anaphylactic shock. Emergency medications and equipment are kept readily available.

• In extremely rare cases, blood infection (sepsis) may occur.

After the Test

• If the T-tube is left in place, a sterile, closed drainage system is attached to it.

• If the tube is removed, a nurse applies a sterile dressing and records any drainage. The dressing is changed as necessary.

• You may gradually resume your normal activities.

Estimated Cost: $$$$

T-tube and Operative Cholangiography continued

Tensilon Test

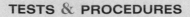

Description

• This test evaluates the response of muscles to the drug Tensilon (edrophonium chloride) in order to aid in the diagnosis of myasthenia gravis, a chronic disease in which the muscles weaken due to an impaired ability to respond to nerve signals. To stimulate a muscle, nerve cells release a chemical messenger—the neurotransmitter acetylcholine—which is later broken down by the enzyme acetylcholinesterase. In people with myasthenia gravis, there are a reduced number of receptors for acetylcholine and the chemical is degraded before it can fully activate a muscle. Tensilon blocks the action of acetylcholinesterase, and thus can prolong muscle stimulation and temporarily improve muscle strength. An increase in muscle strength after an injection of Tensilon strongly suggests a diagnosis of myasthenia gravis.

Purpose of the Test

• To assist in the diagnosis of myasthenia gravis.
• To help differentiate between a myasthenic crisis (a worsening of the disease that necessitates therapy with anticholinesterase drugs) and a cholinergic crisis (caused by an overdose of anticholinesterase drugs). Both conditions are marked by severe muscle weakness and breathing difficulty.

Who Performs It

• A physician.

Special Concerns

• A number of medications, including prednisone, anticholinergics, procainamide, quinidine, and muscle relaxants, can interfere with test results.
• Because Tensilon can produce certain adverse reactions, people with low blood pressure, slow heart rate, sleep apnea (temporary cessation of breathing during sleep), or mechanical obstruction of the intestine or urinary tract may not be candidates for this test.
• In some cases, the drug Prostigmin (neostigmine)—used for the treatment of myasthenia gravis—is also administered to confirm a positive diagnosis established by the Tensilon test.

Before the Test

• Report to your doctor any medications, herbs, and supplements that you are taking. You may be advised to discontinue certain of these agents before the test. In general, do not take any medication within 4 hours of the procedure.
• An intravenous (IV) needle or catheter is inserted into a vein in your arm immediately before the test begins.

What You Experience

To diagnose myasthenia gravis:

• A small dose of Tensilon is injected through the IV line. You may be asked to perform certain exercises, such as counting toward 100

Results

➥ The doctor will evaluate the results to determine if they support a diagnosis of myasthenia gravis; if you are experiencing a myasthenic or a cholinergic crisis; or if an adjustment in your anticholinesterase therapy is necessary.

➥ If a definitive diagnosis can be made, treatment will be started or the dose of your current medication will be modified.

➥ In some cases, additional tests, such as electromyography (see page 177), will be needed to confirm a diagnosis of myasthenia gravis.

until your voice diminishes or holding your arms above your shoulders until they drop. After your muscles have been fatigued, a larger dose of Tensilon is given.

• You will then be asked to perform some repetitive movements, such as opening and closing your eyes and crossing and uncrossing your legs, while the examiner looks for an increase in muscle strength. If the drug does not restore power to your muscles within 1 or 2 minutes, the dose is increased. The test may be repeated 3 to 4 times.

• The procedure takes about 15 to 30 minutes.

To differentiate between a myasthenic and a cholinergic crisis:

• A small amount of Tensilon is infused through the IV line, and the dose is gradually increased while the examiner observes you for signs of improved muscle strength (indicating a myasthenic crisis) or worsening muscle weakness (suggesting a cholinergic crisis).

• If the test confirms a myasthenic crisis, the drug neostigmine is given immediately. If you are having a cholinergic crisis, the drug atropine is administered.

• The procedure takes about 15 to 30 minutes.

To assess oral anticholinesterase therapy:

• Tensilon is infused through the IV line 1 hour after you take your last dose of anticholinesterase medication, and you are care-fully observed for muscle response and any adverse reactions.

• The procedure takes about 15 to 30 minutes.

Risks and Complications

• Tensilon may produce side effects such as nausea, abdominal discomfort, dizziness, blurred vision, and rapid, frequent blinking of the eyelids.

• Less often, the drug may cause potentially serious complications, including respiratory failure and heart rhythm abnormalities, in sensitive individuals. Appropriate resuscitation equipment is kept nearby to treat such adverse reactions.

After the Test

• The effects of Tensilon subside quickly and are completely gone after 30 to 60 minutes.

• You may resume your normal activities and any medications that were withheld before the test, according to your doctor's instructions.

• Blood may collect and clot under the skin (hematoma) at the IV infusion site; this is harmless and will resolve on its own. For a large hematoma that causes swelling and discomfort, apply ice initially; after 24 hours, use warm, moist compresses to help dissolve the clotted blood.

Estimated Cost: $$

Tensilon Test continued

Thoracentesis
(Pleural Fluid Analysis)

Thoracentesis

Description
• A needle is used to aspirate fluid from the pleural space, which lies between the lungs and the chest wall. The fluid sample is sent for laboratory analysis to identify the cause of pleural effusion (excess fluid in the pleural space). This procedure may also be performed therapeutically to relieve symptoms caused by accumulation of pleural fluid.

Purpose of the Test
• To determine the cause of pleural effusion and help select an appropriate treatment.
• To relieve symptoms, such as pain and breathing difficulty, which can result from accumulation of pleural fluid.

Who Performs It
• A physician.

Special Concerns
• Thoracentesis may be performed in a hospital or an outpatient setting.
• This procedure may not be safe in people with bleeding disorders.
• A chest x-ray (see page 156) or ultrasound scan (see Chapter 2) may be performed before the test in order to help the doctor locate the pleural fluid and guide needle placement. Alternatively, fluoroscopy (see page 205), may be done during the procedure.

Before the Test
• Report to your doctor any medications, herbs, or supplements you are taking. You may be advised to discontinue certain drugs before the test. In addition, tell your doctor if you are taking any antimicrobial drugs, such as antibiotics.

What You Experience
• You are asked to remove your shirt and put on a hospital gown. The doctor will advise you to remain still and avoid coughing or breathing deeply during the procedure to reduce the risk of needle damage to the lung or pleura.
• The doctor will position you in a way that facilitates access to the pleural space—usually sitting upright on a bed or chair with your arms raised and supported on a table, and sometimes lying partially on your side with your arms overhead.
• The skin at the site of injection is cleansed with an antiseptic, and a local anesthetic is administered to numb the area.
• The aspiration needle is inserted between two ribs through the chest wall into the pleural space. You will feel pressure during insertion, and may have a very brief sensation of sharp pain as the needle enters the pleural space. In general, only mild discomfort is experienced.
• Once the needle is inserted, a clamp may be

Results
▼

➡ The specimen containers may be sent to several different laboratories for examination. The gross appearance of the fluid will be considered, and it will be analyzed for bacteria, white and red blood cells, the presence of unusual cells, and other components. (For more on fluid analysis, see Chapter 1.)

➡ Your doctor may be able to diagnose the cause of the pleural effusion based on results from these laboratory tests, although this is not always possible. Potential causes include pneumonia, tuberculosis, pancreatitis (an inflamed pancreas), cancer, and congestive heart failure.

➡ Appropriate treatment will be initiated, depending on the problem.

attached to hold it in place. The fluid is withdrawn through the needle into a syringe, and specimen containers are sent immediately to a laboratory for analysis.

• The needle is withdrawn and a small bandage is applied.

• The procedure takes 15 to 60 minutes.

Risks and Complications

• Possible serious complications include pneumothorax (leakage of air outside the lungs and into the pleural cavity, resulting in a collapsed lung); bleeding; infection; inadvertent puncture of the lung or a blood vessel; or, if a large amount of fluid was withdrawn, pulmonary edema (accumulation of fluid in the lungs).

• The use of ultrasound or fluoroscopy to guide needle insertion may reduce the risk of complications.

After the Test

• Your vital signs will be monitored and you will be observed for any signs of complications for a period of time after the procedure.

• A chest x-ray will be done to ensure that a pneumothorax has not developed.

Estimated Cost: $$

Thoracentesis continued

Thoracoscopy
(Thoracoscopic Lung or Pleural Biopsy)

Thoracoscopy

Description
• In this surgical procedure, a thin, flexible viewing tube (called a thoracoscope) is inserted through a small incision in the chest. Fiberoptic cables permit the surgeon to visually inspect the lungs, mediastinum (the area between the lungs), and pleura (the membrane covering the lungs and lining the chest cavity). In addition, surgical instruments may be inserted through other small incisions in the chest, to perform both diagnostic and therapeutic procedures.

Purpose of the Test
• To visually inspect the lungs, pleura, or mediastinum for evidence of abnormalities.
• To obtain tissue biopsies or fluid samples from the lungs, pleura, or mediastinum in order to diagnose infections, cancer, and other diseases.
• Used therapeutically to remove excess fluid in the pleural cavity or pleural cysts, or to remove a portion of diseased lung tissue (wedge resection).

Who Performs It
• A chest surgeon or pulmonary specialist and a surgical team.

Special Concerns
• You may undergo various preoperative tests, such as pulmonary function tests (see page 306), chest x-ray (see page 156), and electrocardiography (see page 174), to ensure that you are an appropriate candidate for this procedure.
• Thoracoscopy may not be safe for people who have had previous lung surgery, who have severe bleeding disorders, or who cannot breathe with just one lung (since one lung must be partially or completely deflated during the procedure).
• This procedure is associated with fewer risks, less postoperative pain, and faster recovery than open chest surgery (thoracotomy); however, if bleeding or other complications occur, or the procedure cannot be completed satisfactorily, an open thoracotomy may be required.

Before the Test
• Tell your doctor if you regularly take anticoagulants, nonsteroidal anti-inflammatory drugs (such as aspirin, ibuprofen, or naproxen), or any other medications. You may be instructed to discontinue certain drugs before the test. Also mention any herbs or supplements that you take.

Results
▼

➥ Depending on the suspected problem, tissue and fluid specimens may be sent to different laboratories for inspection. For example, biopsied tissue may be inspected under a microscope for signs of unusual cells, or may be cultured (see page 166) for infectious organisms. (For more on laboratory testing, see Chapter 1.)

➥ If a malignant lung tumor is suspected, biopsy specimens may be examined during the procedure via frozen section (see page 39). If lung cancer is detected, additional surgical procedures may be performed immediately to remove all or part of the affected lung.

➥ If a definitive diagnosis can be made, appropriate treatment will be initiated.

➥ If the doctor cannot make a diagnosis, additional tests, such as a bronchoscopy (see page 134) or open lung biopsy (see page 245), may be needed.

• Do not eat or drink anything for 12 hours before the test.
• Immediately before the test, an intravenous (IV) needle or catheter is inserted into a vein in your arm, and you are placed under general anesthesia.

What You Experience

• A thin tube is inserted through your mouth and into your lungs. The lung on the operative side is partially or completely deflated to create space between the lung and chest wall and provide the surgeon with a clear view of the area.
• The surgeon makes several small incisions in your chest, and inserts drainage tubes to remove blood during the procedure. The scope is passed into the space between the lung and chest wall; fiberoptic cables transmit images of the area onto a TV screen in the operating room. The scope may be moved to different locations as needed.
• Following inspection of the lung and pleura, the doctor may insert surgical instruments through small incisions to remove tissue or fluid for diagnostic examination or as a therapeutic measure.
• The scope and other instruments are removed, the collapsed lung is re-expanded, and all the incisions but one are closed with stitches or adhesive tape. A thin tube is placed in the remaining incision and left there for 1 to 2 days, in order to drain air and fluid from the chest.
• The procedure takes 2 to 4 hours.

Risks and Complications

• Thoracoscopy requires general anesthesia, and thus carries the associated risks.
• Rare complications include excessive bleeding, infection, perforation of the diaphragm, and pneumothorax (leakage of air outside the lungs and into the pleural cavity, resulting in a collapsed lung).

After the Test

• You will remain in the hospital up to several days until you recover from the effects of surgery and anesthesia. During this time, your vital signs will be monitored, and you will be observed for any signs of complications.
• You may be given pain-relieving medication to allay the discomfort associated with surgery.
• A chest x-ray (see page 156) will be performed to ensure complete reinflation of the lung.

Estimated Cost: $$$

Thoracoscopy continued

Thyroid Biopsy

Thyroid Biopsy

Description

• In this test, a tissue sample is removed from the thyroid gland—which is located in the neck (see page 18)—for microscopic examination. Several techniques may be used, including **fine needle aspiration biopsy,** which uses a long, thin needle to withdraw (aspirate) a specimen, and **open biopsy,** which accesses the thyroid surgically through a small incision.

Purpose of the Test

• To determine whether a thyroid growth is benign or malignant (cancerous).

Who Performs It

• Needle biopsy is conducted by a physician.
• Open biopsy is performed by a surgeon and surgical team.

Special Concerns

• Open biopsy may require general anesthesia, but is sometimes done with a local anesthetic injection. Performed less frequently than needle biopsy, it is generally done in cases where a larger piece of tissue is needed to confirm a diagnosis, or when complete removal of the thyroid is likely to be necessary.
• Thyroid biopsy should be done with caution in people with bleeding disorders.

Before the Test

• Tell your doctor if you regularly take anticoagulants or nonsteroidal anti-inflammatory drugs (such as aspirin, ibuprofen, or naproxen). You will be instructed to discontinue them for some time before the test. Also mention any other medications, herbs, or supplements that you take.
• Do not eat or drink anything for 12 hours before an open biopsy. No fasting is necessary before a needle biopsy.
• For general anesthesia, an intravenous (IV) needle or catheter is inserted into a vein in your arm and the medication is administered. In some cases, a thin tube attached to a breathing machine will be inserted through your mouth and into your windpipe to ensure you breathe properly during the procedure.

What You Experience

Fine needle aspiration biopsy:
• You will lie on your back on an examining table with a pillow placed under your shoulder blades.
• The skin at the needle insertion site is cleansed with an antiseptic, and a local anesthetic is injected to numb the area. This injection may cause mild discomfort. Do not swallow as the anesthetic is being administered.
• The doctor inserts a thin needle through the skin into the thyroid, and withdraws a thin column of cells. You may feel pressure as the needle is inserted.

Results

▼

➡ Tissue samples are sent to a pathology laboratory and examined under a microscope for abnormal cells. (For more on microscopic examination, see Chapter 1.) Possible findings include Hashimoto's disease (inflammation caused by immune cells that mistakenly attack thyroid tissue), benign tumor, and cancer.

➡ This test usually provides a definitive diagnosis. Your doctor will recommend appropriate medical or surgical treatment.

➡ In rare cases, the cells obtained by a fine needle biopsy are insufficient to make a diagnosis. The procedure may need to be repeated, or an open biopsy may be required.

• Additional samples may be obtained.
• Pressure is placed on the needle insertion site until bleeding has stopped, and a small bandage is applied.
• The procedure takes about 30 minutes.

Open biopsy:

• You are positioned on your back on an operating table.
• If the procedure does not require general anesthesia, the skin on your neck will be cleansed with an antiseptic, and a local anesthetic is injected to numb the area. This injection may cause mild discomfort.
• An incision is made in your neck.
• A piece of tissue from a thyroid mass is removed with surgical instruments. The specimen may be sent for immediate microscopic inspection via frozen section (see page 39); if malignant cells are detected, surgery is performed at once to excise the entire gland.
• The incision is stitched closed.
• The length of this procedure may vary widely, depending on whether general or local anesthesia is used.

Risks and Complications

• The most common complications after needle biopsy are swelling or discoloration due to collection of blood under the skin (hematoma) at the needle insertion site (which may cause discomfort, but is harmless) and temporary difficulty swallowing.
• Serious complications, such as inadvertent puncture of other structures in the neck or infection, are rare.

• Open thyroid biopsy using a general anesthetic carries all the risks associated with general anesthesia.

After the Test

• No recovery time is usually needed after a fine needle biopsy. After an open biopsy, you will remain in a recovery room for several hours. During this time, your vital signs will be monitored and you will be observed for any signs of complications.
• You may feel more comfortable in a semi-sitting position with your head partially raised and supported. To avoid straining the biopsy site, you should place both hands behind your neck for support as you sit up.
• You may be given pain-relieving medication such as acetaminophen to allay any discomfort around the biopsy site.
• You may return home. If you received general anesthesia, arrange for someone else to drive you.
• Keep the biopsy site clean and dry. You may shower and wet your neck the day after the procedure.
• For swelling and discomfort resulting from a hematoma after a fine needle biopsy, apply ice initially; after 24 hours, use warm, moist compresses to help dissolve the clotted blood.
• Inform your doctor immediately if you develop persistent bleeding, excessive swelling, or unusual pain at the biopsy site; difficulty breathing; or signs of infection (such as fever, headache, dizziness, or malaise).

Estimated Cost: $$ to $$$$

Thyroid Biopsy continued

Thyroid Hormone Tests
(Thyroid Panel)

Thyroid Hormone Tests

Description

• The thyroid—a butterfly-shaped endocrine gland located at the front of the neck (illustrated on page 18)—is essential for growth and development in children and is the primary regulator of body metabolism. The functions of the thyroid—which include maintaining the correct metabolic rate for cells to function and helping to control the body's use of food for energy—are primarily carried out by two major hormones, T3 and T4. Blood tests to measure thyroid hormones are most useful for evaluating disorders of thyroid function, including overactivity (hyperthyroidism) and underactivity (hypothyroidism).

• **Thyroxine (T4)** controls body metabolism, helps to oversee physical and mental development, and plays a part in resistance to infection and vitamin requirements. It is secreted by the thyroid in response to the release of thyroid-stimulating hormone by the pituitary gland (see below).

• **Triiodothyronine (T3)**—a more potent molecule than T4—is essential for maintaining the rate of chemical reactions, or metabolic rate, in all cells in the body. Most T3 is produced by tissues throughout the body (primarily the liver) through the removal of an iodine atom from T4; the rest is secreted directly by the thyroid. Although T3 is present in smaller quantities and is metabolically active for a shorter time than T4, its impact on body metabolism is of greater magnitude.

• **Thyroxine-binding globulin (TBG)** is the major thyroid hormone protein carrier. Most of the T4 and T3 in the blood is bound to proteins, primarily TBG; the remaining fraction, which circulates freely and thus is known as free T4 and T3, makes up the active portion of these hormones. When TBG levels are elevated—as in pregnancy or in those taking estrogen replacement therapy or oral contraceptives—less free (and active) T3 and T4 is available. To compensate, the thyroid responds by releasing more T3 and T4. By measuring TBG, it is possible to determine whether abnormal T4 and T3 levels are the result of this normal response or whether there is true thyroid dysfunction.

• **The T3 uptake test** provides an indirect measurement of T4 levels, as well as the amount of available protein (primarily TBG) that can bind to T3 and T4. In this test, radioactive T3 (RT3) is added your blood sample in the laboratory; by measuring how much RT3 can attach to thyroid hormone-binding proteins, the amount of T4 that is already bound to the proteins can be indirectly quantified. The results of this test are only useful when considered together with other thyroid hormone tests.

Results

▼

➡ Your blood sample is sent to a laboratory for analysis. The doctor will review the results for evidence of a thyroid disorder. (For more on laboratory testing, see Chapter 1.)

➡ Elevated T3 and T4 levels indicate hyperthyroidism, while low levels of these hormones suggest hypothyroidism. Abnormal TSH levels suggest that thyroid dysfunction results from problems originating in the pituitary gland or hypothalamus.

➡ If an abnormality is found and the doctor can make a definitive diagnosis, appropriate treatment will begin.

➡ In some cases, abnormal results on one or more of the thyroid hormone tests will necessitate additional tests—such as a thyroid nuclear scan (see page 358)—to establish a diagnosis.

• **Thyroid-stimulating hormone (TSH)**, also known as thyrotropin, is a hormone secreted by the pituitary gland in the brain in response to hormonal signals from the hypothalamus (another part of the brain). The function of TSH is to stimulate the release of both T4 and T3 by the thyroid gland. Problems with TSH secretion lead to abnormal T4 and T3 levels, and thus result in thyroid dysfunction.

Purpose of the Test

T4, T3, and TSH:

• To evaluate thyroid function.

• To help diagnose hyperthyroidism (particularly in people with typical symptoms such as rapid heartbeat, weight loss, and dizziness) and hypothyroidism (which causes symptoms such as fatigue, sensitivity to cold, and weight gain).

• To monitor the effectiveness of drug therapy for thyroid dysfunction.

• TSH helps to distinguish between primary (originating in the thyroid) and secondary (originating in the pituitary or hypothalamus) hypothyroidism.

TBG and T3 uptake:

• To evaluate thyroid function and aid in the assessment of patients with abnormal T3 and T4 levels.

Who Performs It

• A nurse or a technician will draw the blood sample.

Special Concerns

• A variety of medications and hormone supplements may interfere with the results of these tests. In addition, pregnancy causes increased levels of TBG, T4, and total (but not free) T3.

• Because TSH levels vary throughout the day—generally peaking at around midnight—this test is scheduled for a particular time of day, usually in the morning.

• A recent nuclear scanning test (see page 46) may affect the results of certain thyroid hormone tests, since these chemicals may be measured with a laboratory technique that utilizes a radioactive isotope (radioimmunoassay).

Before the Test

• Report to your doctor any medications, herbs, or supplements you are taking. You may be advised to discontinue certain of these agents before the test.

• Tell your doctor if you've had any recent procedures, such as a nuclear scan, that introduced radioactive material into your bloodstream.

What You Experience

• A sample of your blood is drawn from a vein, usually in your arm, and sent to a laboratory for analysis (see page 32).

• For a TSH test, the blood sample is typically drawn in the morning.

Risks and Complications

• None.

After the Test

• Immediately after blood is drawn, pressure is applied (with cotton or gauze) to the puncture site.

• Resume your normal activities and any medications withheld before the test.

• Blood may collect and clot under the skin (hematoma) at the puncture site; this is harmless and will resolve on its own. For a large hematoma that causes swelling and discomfort, apply ice initially; after 24 hours, use warm, moist compresses to help dissolve the clotted blood.

Estimated Cost: $

Thyroid Hormone Tests continued

Thyroid Nuclear Scan

Thyroid Nuclear Scan

Description

• In this test, a small amount of radioactive material is introduced into your body, and a special type of camera records the absorption of the radiotracer by the thyroid gland. (Usually, a form of radioactive iodine is given by mouth.) The camera data are translated by a computer into two-dimensional images that are displayed on a viewing monitor and recorded on film. This test is most often done to examine a thyroid growth, or nodule, that was detected on another imaging test or by palpating the gland. (For more on nuclear imaging, see Chapter 2.)

Purpose of the Test

• To evaluate the size, structure, position, and function of the thyroid gland, usually in conjunction with other thyroid tests.
• To detect thyroid growths, or nodules, and aid in determining whether they are benign or malignant.

Who Performs It

• A physician, a nurse, or a nuclear medicine technician.

Special Concerns

• People with allergies to iodine or shellfish may experience a severe allergic reaction to radioactive iodine; another radiotracer will be used.
• Women who are pregnant or nursing should not undergo this test because exposure to the radiotracer may harm the fetus or infant.
• A diet deficient in iodine can cause increased uptake of radioactive iodine; on the other hand, ingestion of iodine-containing foods such as iodized salt or shellfish can interfere with its uptake. Recent exposure to x-ray contrast dyes (see page 41) may also affect test results because these agents may contain large quantities of iodine.

• The presence of kidney disease, severe diarrhea, or vomiting, as well as various medications (including thyroid drugs, cough medicines, multivitamins, some oral contraceptives, phenothiazines, and corticosteroids) may affect test results.

Before the Test

• Inform your doctor if you have an allergy to iodine or shellfish, and whether you have undergone any contrast x-ray procedures or nuclear scans in the previous 60 days.
• Report to your doctor any medications, herbs, or supplements you are taking. You may be advised to discontinue certain of these agents for a specified period before the test.
• You will be instructed to avoid ingesting iodized salt, iodinated salt substitutes, and seafood for 1 week before the test.
• If this test requires you to take radioactive

Results

▼

➡ A physician will examine the scans for evidence of abnormalities. Nodules exhibiting increased iodine uptake are deemed "hot spots" (indicating a possible benign tumor), while nodules that take up little or no iodine, or "cold spots," may be cysts, cancer, or another abnormality. Diffuse increased uptake may indicate hyperthyroidism (overactive thyroid).

➡ If a definitive diagnosis can be made, appropriate therapy will be started.

➡ In most cases, a diagnosis must be confirmed with blood tests for thyroid hormones (see page 356), ultrasound (see page 360), or a biopsy (see page 354).

iodine orally, you will be asked to fast for 12 hours beforehand.

• On the day of the test, wear a comfortable, loose-fitting shirt.

• Immediately before the scan, you will be asked to remove your dentures and any jewelry that could interfere with visualization of the thyroid.

What You Experience

• You will ingest an oral radiotracer either in a beverage or in pill form, and you will be asked to return for the scanning procedure 4 to 24 hours later.

• You will lie on your back on an examination table with your neck pushed forward, or hyperextended. (A pillow is placed under your neck to make this position more comfortable.)

• A scanning camera is placed over your neck to record the gamma rays emitted by the radiotracer in the thyroid. The device projects images of the gland on a viewing screen, and these pictures are recorded on x-ray film. Several views will be obtained from different angles.

• The scanning procedure itself takes about 20 or 30 minutes.

Risks and Complications

• The trace amount of radioactive material used in this test is not associated with any significant risks or complications.

After the Test

• Resume your normal diet and any medications withheld before the test, according to your doctor's instructions.

Estimated Cost: $$

Thyroid Nuclear Scan continued

Thyroid Ultrasound
(Thyroid Ultrasonography)

Description
• A device called a transducer is passed over your neck, directing high-frequency sound waves (ultrasound) at the thyroid gland. The sound waves are reflected back to the transducer and electronically converted into images displayed on a viewing monitor. The images are then saved on film or video and reviewed for abnormalities. This test is most often done when a thyroid growth, or nodule, is detected on another imaging test or by palpating the gland. (For more on how ultrasound works, see Chapter 2.)

Purpose of the Test
• To determine whether a thyroid nodule is a fluid-filled cyst or a solid tumor; cysts are usually benign, while tumors may be malignant (cancerous).
• To monitor the size and condition of a thyroid nodule during treatment.
• To monitor thyroid cancer patients for cancer recurrence or cancer spread to the lymph nodes.

Who Performs It
• A doctor or a technician who is trained in ultrasonography.

Special Concerns
• None.

Before the Test
• No special preparation is necessary.

What You Experience
• You will lie on your back on an examination table.
• A pillow is placed under your shoulder blades to push the neck forward.
• A water-soluble gel is applied to the skin on your neck to enhance sound wave transmission.
• The examiner then moves the transducer back and forth over your neck to obtain different views of the thyroid.
• Once clear images are obtained, they are recorded on film or video for later analysis.
• The test takes about 15 to 30 minutes.

Risks and Complications
• Ultrasound is painless, noninvasive, and involves no exposure to radiation. There are no associated risks.

After the Test
• The examiner removes the conductive gel from your skin.
• You are free to resume your normal diet and activities.

Estimated Cost: $$

Results
▼

➡ A radiologist reviews the recorded images and video for evidence of abnormalities.

➡ If a thyroid nodule is found to be a fluid-filled cyst, it can be aspirated (drained) with a needle.

➡ If the mass is mixed or solid, a tumor may be present. A fine needle aspiration biopsy (see page 354) is usually required to establish a definitive diagnosis.

Tilt Table Test

Description

• This test examines people who have had repeated episodes of fainting. You are placed on a table that starts in a horizontal position and is then tilted upward at different angles. By monitoring your heart rate, blood pressure, and symptoms, a doctor can determine whether vasopressor syncope is responsible for your fainting. In this condition, the nerves controlling blood pressure and heart rate respond abnormally to changes in position by producing a sudden drop in blood pressure.

Purpose of the Test

• To determine whether vasopressor syncope is responsible for fainting episodes.

Who Performs It

• A doctor assisted by a technician.

Special Concerns

• Antihypertensive drugs or diuretics may interfere with interpretation of test results.
• People who are dehydrated or who have low blood volume may show changes in blood pressure and heart rate similar to those caused by vasopressor syncope.

Before the Test

• You will be asked to avoid food and fluids for a specified period to prevent nausea during the test.
• Tell your doctor if you take any antihypertensive or diuretic drugs, and if you experience nausea or diarrhea in the 24 hours before the test.

What You Experience

• An intravenous (IV) line is inserted into a vein in your arm so that you can be given fluids and medications during the test. ECG leads (see page 174) and a blood pressure cuff are used to monitor your heart rate and blood pressure.
• You are strapped in place on the tilt table with loosely fitting Velcro belts.
• As you lie flat for about 15 minutes, blood pressure and pulse measurements are obtained. The examiner then tilts the table in stages to an almost upright position. You remain in this position for 30 to 45 minutes, and then are returned to a flat position.
• If you do not experience symptoms, the examiner may administer an adrenaline-like medication and then repeat the tilt.
• The examiner will ask you about the presence of any symptoms, such as lightheadedness or dizziness, and observe you for fainting episodes.

Risks and Complications

• Because you are held by safety straps and your blood pressure and heart rate are monitored continuously, fainting does not pose any serious risk. Most people who do faint wake up as they are lowered to the horizontal position.

After the Test

• The test can be quite tiring. Arrange for someone to drive you home afterward.

Estimated Cost: $$

Results

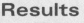

➡ The doctor will review the data to determine whether vasopressor syncope is causing your recurrent fainting episodes. If the doctor can make this diagnosis, medication may be prescribed to treat this condition.

➡ If another diagnosis, such as an abnormal heart rhythm (arrhythmia) is suspected, additional tests, such as Holter monitoring (see page 221) or electrophysiology studies (see page 182), may be needed.

Tilt Table Test

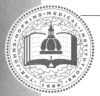
Tonometry

Tonometry

Description
• This test estimates the fluid pressure within the eye, or intraocular pressure (IOP), with a special instrument, called a tonometer, that exerts gentle pressure on the cornea (the transparent disc in front of the iris and pupil of the eye). Tonometry is included as part of a full eye examination. Several techniques may be used.
• **Applanation (Goldmann) tonometry**—considered the most accurate method—measures the amount of force necessary to flatten a specific area of the cornea. The higher the IOP, the greater the force required to flatten the cornea.
• **Schiotz (or indentation) tonometry** uses a preset amount of weight to gently press a plunger into the cornea, making a slight indentation. The amount of corneal indentation, which is proportional to IOP, is measured.
• **Noncontact (or air-puff) tonometry** determines IOP by blowing a small puff of air toward the eye and recording the air rebounding from the corneal surface. It is not as accurate as the other tonometry methods.
• **Pneumotonometry** uses a special device that is applied to the side of the eye. The amount of pressure required to flatten the tip indicates pressure inside the eye.

Purpose of the Test
• To measure intraocular pressure.
• To aid in the diagnosis of glaucomas, vision-threatening disorders marked by an elevation in IOP that can gradually (or suddenly) destroy the optic nerve.
• To detect low IOP, which can be caused by injury, inflammation, detachment of the retina, or poor blood supply to the eye.

Who Performs It
• An ophthalmologist, an optometrist, or a specially trained nurse or technician.

Special Concerns
• If you have an irregularly-shaped or deformed cornea, a special tonometer must be used.

Before the Test
• If you wear contact lenses, remove them before the test.
• Loosen or remove any restricting clothing around the neck, such as a neck tie.

What You Experience
Applanation tonometry:
• The examiner will administer topical anesthetic eye drops, as well as eye drops containing a special dye (called fluorescein).
• You will sit in a chair in front of a slit-lamp microscope, an instrument that permits the examiner to view both the front and inside of the eye. Your head will be positioned comfortably against a chin rest and padded forehead bar.

Results
▼
➡ IOP is measured in millimeters of mercury (mm Hg). Normally, IOP falls between 10 and 20 mm Hg. Higher levels may indicate glaucoma or ocular hypertension (elevated IOP that has not yet caused optic nerve damage).
➡ If IOP is normal, no further testing is needed.
➡ If IOP is elevated, an ophthalmologist must perform other tests to confirm a diagnosis of glaucoma, including visual inspection of the optic nerve with a magnifying device called an ophthalmoscope and visual field testing, or perimetry (see page 389).
➡ If IOP is low, further testing will be needed to determine the cause of the low pressure.

• You will be asked to direct your eyes at the bottom of the examiner's ear.

• The tonometer, which is mounted on the slit lamp, is moved in front of the eye so that the tip touches the cornea. The examiner adjusts the amount of force applied until the device flattens the central cornea by a standard amount. This reading is an indication of IOP.

• The test is repeated on the other eye.

• The procedure takes 1 to 2 minutes.

Schiotz tonometry:

• The examiner will administer topical anesthetic eye drops.

• You will lie on your back on an examination table, and will be instructed to look upward.

• The examiner will gently retract the skin around the eye to help hold the eyelids open.

• The Schiotz tonometer is a hand-held device consisting of a weight, a calibrated scale, a plunger, and a concave (curved) footplate that rests snugly on the cornea. The examiner will carefully lower the device into place, and a preset amount of weight is used to press the plunger gently into the cornea and make a slight indentation.

• Corneal resistance, which is proportional to IOP, deflects the plunger upward.

• The test is repeated on the other eye.

• The procedure takes 1 to 2 minutes.

Noncontact tonometry:

• The noncontact tonometer, as its name implies, does not come into contact with the eye so a topical anesthetic is unnecessary.

• A small puff of air is blown against the cornea. A pressure sensor in the tonometer records the amount of air rebounding off the corneal surface.

• The test is repeated on the other eye.

• The procedure takes 1 to 2 minutes.

Pneumotonometry:

• You are asked to look straight ahead.

• A special tonometer directs a stream of air into the sensing tip. The amount of air pressure required to flatten the tip indicates IOP.

• The instrument prints a tracing on a piece of graph paper.

Risks and Complications

• All of these methods are painless and pose virtually no risk to the cornea. Any minor corneal scratches by the tonometer usually heal within 24 hours.

After the Test

• If anesthetic eye drops were applied, do not rub your eyes for at least 30 minutes or until the numb sensation wears off to avoid injuring your cornea.

• If you wear contact lenses, do not reinsert them for at least 2 hours after the test.

• You may resume your normal activities.

Estimated Cost: $

Tonometry continued

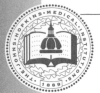

Transcranial Doppler Ultrasound
(Transcranial Duplex Ultrasound)

Transcranial Doppler Ultrasound *(sidebar)*

Description
• This test uses a technique called Doppler ultrasound to evaluate blood circulation in the brain. A device called a transducer is passed lightly across different areas of your head, directing high-frequency sound waves (ultrasound) at particular cerebral arteries. The sound waves are reflected back at frequencies that correspond to the velocity of blood flow, and are converted into audible sounds and graphic recordings.
• **Duplex scanning** combines Doppler ultrasound with real-time ultrasound imaging of the arteries. Images are displayed on a viewing monitor and may also be recorded on film or video for later examination. (For more on Doppler and duplex ultrasound, see Chapter 2.)

Purpose of the Test
• To evaluate blood flow in the brain.
• To identify abnormalities, such as narrowing (vasospasm), blockages, or arteriovenous malformation (a congenital blood vessel defect), in arteries within the brain.
• To monitor progression of cerebral vasospasm.

Who Performs It
• A radiologist, a neurologist, or a trained technician.

Special Concerns
• None.

Before the Test
• No special preparation is necessary.

What You Experience
• You will either lie on a bed or table or sit in a reclining chair.
• A small amount of water-soluble gel is applied to the skin on certain portions of your face and head to enhance the transmission of sound waves.

• The examiner then moves the transducer back and forth over your head—typically, the forehead, eye socket region, and base of the skull—to obtain different views of the artery or arteries being studied.
• Once clear images are obtained, they are recorded on film or video for later analysis.
• The test usually takes less than 1 hour.

Risks and Complications
• Ultrasound is painless, noninvasive, and involves no exposure to radiation. There are no associated risks.

After the Test
• The examiner removes the conductive gel from your skin.
• You may resume your normal activities.

Estimated Cost: $$

Results
▼

➡ A radiologist reviews the recorded images and other test data for evidence of any abnormality. High blood flow velocity suggests that blood flow is too turbulent or that the blood vessel is too narrow. This finding may indicate a blockage, vasospasm, or an arteriovenous malformation.

➡ If a definitive diagnosis can be made, appropriate treatment will be initiated.

➡ In many cases—particularly before surgical treatment—additional tests, such as arteriography of the cerebral blood vessels (see page 95), are required to further evaluate abnormal findings and to provide more specific information.

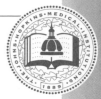

Transesophageal Echocardiography
(TEE)

Description
• Transesophageal echocardiography (TEE) combines the use of a thin, flexible, lighted viewing tube (endoscope) with ultrasound imaging to visualize the heart and nearby structures. The endoscope, which is passed into the mouth and down the esophagus, is used to position a tiny device called a transducer behind the heart. The transducer directs high-frequency sound waves (ultrasound) at the heart; the sound waves that are echoed back from the heart are then electronically converted into real-time images displayed on a viewing monitor. These images may be recorded on film or video and reviewed for abnormalities. (For more on how ultrasound works, see Chapter 2.)

Purpose of the Test
• To identify vascular disease in the chest cavity, such as aneurysm, dissection, or atherosclerosis in the aorta (which is a risk factor for stroke).
• To visualize and evaluate heart conditions, including congenital heart disease; endocarditis (inflammation of the lining membrane of the heart); blood clots; cardiac tumors; and disease of the heart valves or problems with prosthetic valves.

Who Performs It
• A doctor.

Special Concerns
• Because TEE uses high-frequency sound waves and avoids interference from chest wall structures, it can provide higher quality images of the heart than conventional transthoracic echocardiography (see page 367).
• People with esophageal abnormalities, such as obstruction (strictures), enlarged blood vessels (varices), or scleroderma; bleeding disorders; previous radiation therapy to the chest; or severe neck arthritis are not candidates for TEE.

Before the Test
• Avoid eating or drinking anything for 6 hours before the test.
• Remove any dentures or oral prostheses immediately before the test.

What You Experience
• You will lie down on your left side.
• You are connected to monitors that keep track of your blood pressure and heart rate during the procedure.
• A sedative medication is injected into a vein in your arm.
• A topical anesthetic is sprayed on the back of your throat to suppress the gag reflex (however, you may still gag when the endoscope is inserted).
• A plastic mouthpiece is then inserted to hold your mouth open and to prevent you from biting down on the endoscope.
• The doctor inserts the endoscope containing the transducer into your mouth and asks you to swallow it. You may have to swallow

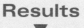

Results
➡ The doctor will examine the recorded images and video for any sign of a cardiac or aortic abnormality.
➡ If a definitive diagnosis can be made based on these images, appropriate treatment will be initiated.
➡ In some cases, more invasive tests, such as cardiac catheterization (see page 140), may be needed to further evaluate abnormal results.

several times to move it downward to the correct position.

• The transducer may be moved several times during the test to obtain different views of the heart.

• The test takes about 60 minutes in total.

Risks and Complications

• Ultrasound involves no exposure to radiation.

• You may have a sore throat for a few days after the test.

• There is a small risk of bleeding in the esophagus; if this occurs during the test, it will be discontinued. In rare cases, perforation of the esophagus may occur.

After the Test

• You will lie down, and your vital signs will be monitored until the sedative wears off.

• TEE does not necessitate an overnight hospital stay. However, someone should drive you home after the procedure.

• Do not eat or drink until your gag reflex returns, usually in a few hours. (Touching the back of the throat with a tongue depressor tests for this reflex.)

• Avoid drinking alcohol for a day or two after the test, since it can increase the sedative effect.

Estimated Cost: $$$

Transesophageal Echocardiography continued

Transthoracic Echocardiography

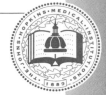

Description

• A device called a transducer is passed over the chest, directing high-frequency sound waves (ultrasound) at the heart. The sound waves are reflected back to the transducer and electronically converted into images displayed on a viewing monitor. The images can also be saved on film or video and then examined for abnormalities. This test often includes three different techniques: **M-mode,** which provides a one-dimensional, vertical view of the heart; **two-dimensional,** which produces a cross-sectional view of cardiac structures; and **color flow Doppler imaging,** which gives a picture of blood flow. (For more on ultrasound, see Chapter 2.)

Purpose of the Test

• To detect and evaluate heart conditions, including heart valve abnormalities, congenital heart defects, cardiomyopathy, atrial tumors, and pericardial effusions (excessive fluid around the heart).
• To measure the size of the heart's chambers.
• To assess cardiac function and heart wall motion after a heart attack.

Who Performs It

• A doctor, a nurse, or a technician trained in ultrasound.

Special Concerns

• This test may not produce accurate results in people who are obese or who have thick chests, chronic obstructive pulmonary disease, or chest wall abnormalities. Transesophageal echocardiography (see page 365) may be a better option for such patients.

Before the Test

• Immediately before the test, remove your clothing and jewelry above the waist.

What You Experience

• After you lie on an examination table, a water-soluble gel is applied to your chest to allow better transmission of the sound waves.
• The examiner places the transducer on your chest and applies some pressure while guiding it over specific areas of your chest.
• You may be repositioned during the procedure and asked to breathe in a certain way.
• The procedure is painless and usually takes about 45 minutes.

Risks and Complications

• Ultrasound is painless, noninvasive, and involves no exposure to radiation. There are no associated risks.

After the Test

• The examiner removes the gel from your chest, after which you may leave and resume your normal activities.

Estimated Cost: $$

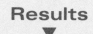

Results

▼

➥ The doctor will examine the recorded images and other test data for any evidence of a cardiac abnormality.
➥ If a definitive diagnosis can be made, appropriate treatment will be started.
➥ In some cases, more invasive tests, such as cardiac catheterization (see page 140), may be needed to further evaluate abnormal results.

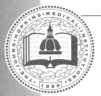

Tuberculin Test
(PPD Skin Test, Mantoux Test)

Tuberculin Test

Description
• In this test, the tuberculin antigen is injected in the skin of your forearm. If you have been exposed to tuberculosis (TB)—an infectious disease caused by a microorganism called *Mycobacterium tuberculosis*—your body's immune response will cause an inflammatory reaction at the injection site. However, the tuberculin test cannot distinguish between active and dormant tuberculosis infection, and the results are not definitive. In adults, this test is most often performed in people who have had a chest x-ray (see page 156) that suggests possible tuberculosis, or in those with a suspected recent exposure.

Purpose of the Test
• To detect previous infection with the bacterium *M. tuberculosis* and to determine the need for further testing.
• To distinguish tuberculosis from other infections that affect the lungs.

Who Performs It
• A nurse or a doctor.

Special Concerns
• Multipuncture tuberculin tests, such as the tine test, are most often used for screening purposes in apparently healthy individuals. However, a positive reaction with these less accurate tests generally requires tuberculin injection for confirmation.
• This test is not generally done after a diagnosis of tuberculosis has been made, or in individuals known to have had a positive skin test reaction in the past.
• People whose immune system is compromised due to old age, poor nutrition, or chronic illness; those who were recently vaccinated for measles, rubella, mumps, or another infectious disease; and those receiving treatment with steroid medications may not react to this test despite exposure to tuberculosis; this is known as a false-negative result (see page 35).
• False-negative results are also possible if tuberculosis exposure occurred less than 10 weeks before the test.

Before the Test
• Your doctor or another health care provider will interview you regarding your medical history before the test. You should mention previous active tuberculosis and the results of prior skin tests.

What You Experience
• You sit with your arm extended on a table or some other flat surface.

Results

➥ A positive reaction to the tuberculin test will appear as a red, raised area at the injection site. Redness alone without the raised area, however, does not constitute a positive test.

➥ If you do have a positive skin reaction, the cause is not always tuberculosis—it may result, for example, from infection with another, related bacterium. For this reason, additional tests, such as a sputum culture (see page 166) and chest x-rays, will be necessary to confirm the diagnosis.

➥ If the reaction is borderline, the skin test may be repeated.

➥ If the skin reaction is negative, but you have other signs suggesting possible tuberculosis, additional tests may be performed.

• The person performing the test will clean your upper forearm with alcohol, let it dry, and administer the tuberculin injection. The injection may cause brief discomfort.

• The site is often circled with indelible ink for easy identification.

• You must return to the testing site in 2 to 3 days, since skin reactions to the tuberculin antigen typically develop within this period. You may experience some itching during the interim, but do not scratch the area.

Risks and Complications

• Rarely, this test may cause an acute allergic reaction.

• In people with an active tuberculosis infection or those who have previously been vaccinated against the disease, reaction to the skin test may be severe, causing skin breakdown or ulceration.

After the Test

• You may leave the testing facility immediately after the injection has been administered.

• A follow-up appointment will be scheduled for 2 to 3 days after the injection.

• Call your doctor if a severe skin reaction occurs.

Estimated Cost: $

Tuberculin Test continued

Tumor Markers

Description

• The term tumor marker refers to any substance that can be detected in higher than normal amounts in the blood, urine, or tissues of some patients with certain types of cancer. Tumor markers alone, however, are not sufficient to diagnose cancer for several reasons: Their levels can be raised in benign conditions; they are not elevated in every person with cancer (particularly in early-stage disease); and many markers are not specific for a particular cancer (i.e., their levels can be raised in more than one type of cancer). At present, most tumor markers are not used to diagnose cancer, but rather to monitor progression of the disease, evaluate the response to treatment, and check for tumor recurrence.

Purpose of the Test

• To help determine the extent of malignant disease.
• To monitor the effectiveness of anticancer therapy and detect recurrent disease before symptoms appear.
• The tumor marker prostate specific antigen (PSA) is now commonly used as a screening test to help diagnose prostate cancer. (See Chapter 3 for more information on the PSA test and screening tests in general.)

Who Performs It

• A doctor, a nurse, or a lab technician will draw the blood sample.

Special Concerns

• False-positive results are common with many tumor marker tests. For example, CA-125, a marker for ovarian cancer, is also elevated in nonmalignant disorders such as cirrhosis, pancreatitis, endometriosis, and pelvic inflammatory disease.
• False-negative results are also common. For instance, CA 19-9 is a marker for pancreatic or hepatobiliary cancer (affecting the liver and bile ducts), but its level is not elevated in about 30% of patients with pancreatic cancer or 35% of those with hepatobiliary cancer. (For more on false-positives and false-negatives, see page 35.)
• Many tumor markers are not specific for a particular cancer. CEA, for example, is a marker for colorectal, pancreatic, gastric, lung, breast, and ovarian cancers.
• Borderline test results may pose a problem. For example, it is not clear whether all men with borderline PSA values—which may indicate prostate cancer or benign prostate conditions—should undergo a biopsy. In such cases, newer variations of the PSA test, such as the percent free PSA test, PSA velocity, and PSA density, may help clarify whether a biopsy is necessary.
• Certain medications may alter the results of the various tests.

Results

➡ Your blood sample is sent to a laboratory for analysis. A variety of techniques may be used to isolate different tumor markers and quantify their levels. For example, a technique called serum protein electrophoresis—which uses an electrical field to differentiate blood proteins according to their size, shape, and electrical charge—is used to detect elevated immunoglobulin levels. (For more on laboratory testing, see Chapter 1.)

➡ A tumor marker assay is often used as an initial step in the diagnosis of cancer or cancer recurrence. Abnormal results necessitate additional tests, such as imaging studies and biopsy, to establish a diagnosis and determine the extent of the problem.

• Pregnancy, normal menstruation, cigarette smoking, and various benign disorders may alter the levels of some tumor markers.

Before the Test

• Report to your doctor any medications, herbs, or supplements you are taking. You may be advised to discontinue certain of these agents before the test.

What You Experience

• A sample of your blood is drawn from a vein, usually in your arm, and sent to a laboratory for analysis. (For more on this procedure, called venipuncture, see page 32.)

Risks and Complications

• None.

After the Test

• Immediately after blood is drawn, pressure is applied (with cotton or gauze) to the puncture site.

• You are free to leave the testing facility.

• Resume taking any medications that were withheld before the test, according to your doctor's instructions.

• Blood may collect and clot under the skin (hematoma) at the puncture site; this is harmless and will resolve on its own. For a large hematoma that causes swelling and discomfort, apply ice initially; after 24 hours, use warm, moist compresses to help dissolve the clotted blood.

Estimated Cost: $

Tumor Markers continued

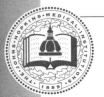

Tzanck Smear

Description
• In this test, which is used to determine whether skin lesions are caused by a herpes virus, a blister is scraped and its contents are smeared on a slide. The slide is then stained and viewed under a microscope.

Purpose of the Test
• To diagnose infections caused by herpes viruses, including herpes simplex (which causes fever blisters, cold sores, and genital sores) and varicella-zoster virus (responsible for chickenpox and shingles).

Who Performs It
• A doctor.

Special Concerns
• A positive result only indicates the presence of herpes simplex (which causes fever blisters) or herpes zoster (which causes chickenpox and shingles), but does not distinguish between the two.

Before the Test
• No special preparation is necessary.

What You Experience
• The doctor scrapes a sore and spreads the contents on a slide. You will experience minor discomfort while the sample is being collected.

Risks and Complications
• None.

After the Test
• You may resume your normal activities.

Estimated Cost: $

Results
▼

➡ The specimen slide is colored with a special dye and examined under a microscope, either at the doctor's office or at a pathology laboratory. The examiner looks for abnormally large cells (called giant cells) that are characteristic of herpes virus infections. (For more on microscopic examination, see Chapter 1.)

➡ If the characteristic giant cells are observed upon microscopic examination, your doctor will institute appropriate antiviral therapy.

➡ If results are negative, a viral culture (see page 166) may be ordered in an effort to detect the herpes virus, or your doctor may conclude that you do not have a herpes infection.

Tzanck Smear

Upper GI and Small Bowel Series

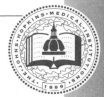

Description

• In this test, you ingest a liquid mixture containing barium sulfate, a contrast dye that delineates your upper gastrointestinal (GI) tract on x-rays and reveals any abnormalities. (See the illustration on page 24.) Examination of the esophagus, the stomach, and the upper part of the small intestine (duodenum) is known as an upper GI series. In some cases, the flow of barium is followed through the entire 20-foot length of the small intestine; this is called a small bowel series. This test is often performed in conjunction with a barium swallow (see page 106) and enteroclysis (see page 190). (For more on contrast x-rays, see Chapter 2.)

Purpose of the Test

• To examine the upper GI tract in people with symptoms such as difficulty swallowing, regurgitation, burning or gnawing stomach pain, diarrhea, weight loss, vomiting of blood, and black, tarry stool.
• To detect abnormalities of the upper GI tract, such as strictures (narrowings), ulcers, tumors, inflammatory conditions, esophageal diverticula (abnormal pouches), and hiatal hernia (a condition in which a portion of the stomach protrudes upward through the diaphragm).

Who Performs It

• A radiologist.

Special Concerns

• Patients with an intestinal obstruction should not undergo this procedure.
• When perforation of the upper GI tract is suspected, barium is not used because leakage of the dye could worsen any existing infection. A water-soluble contrast agent, diatrizoate (Gastrografin), is usually substituted.
• Pregnant women should not undergo this test because exposure to ionizing radiation may harm the fetus.

• Patients with a poor swallowing reflex may inadvertently aspirate barium into their lungs. Your swallowing reflex may be assessed before the test.
• Patients with unstable vital signs must be closely monitored during this test.

Before the Test

• Be sure to inform your doctor of all medications you are taking. You may need to discontinue certain medications for up to 24 hours before the test.
• Do not eat or smoke after midnight on the day before the test.
• Remove any metallic objects, such as jewelry, watches, dentures, or hairpins, before the test begins.

What You Experience

• In a radiology room, you are strapped securely to a tilting x-ray table.
• You are asked to drink a thick, milkshake-like liquid containing the barium sulfate. The barium has a chalky taste, but is usually flavored to increase its palatability.
• The x-ray table is tilted into various positions to ensure that the dye sufficiently coats the GI

Results

▼

➡ The doctor will examine the recorded x-ray images for signs of any abnormality, including strictures, tumors, or ulcers.

➡ If a definitive diagnosis can be made, appropriate treatment will be initiated.

➡ In some cases, additional tests, such as a biopsy or endoscopic retrograde cholangiopancreatography (see page 187), may be needed to further evaluate abnormal results.

tract. Your abdomen may also be palpated to ensure your stomach is adequately coated.

• The radiologist observes the flow of the barium through your esophagus, stomach, and, if necessary, duodenum via fluoroscopy (see page 205), which transmits continuous, moving x-ray images onto a viewing screen.

• Spot x-ray films are taken of any significant abnormalities. As each x-ray is taken, you will be instructed to hold your breath and remain very still.

• In some cases, you may be asked to swallow a carbonated powder, which creates carbon dioxide in your stomach and enhances visualization of the stomach lining, during the test.

• The test is painless, but you may occasionally experience a feeling of bloating or nausea.

• The procedure takes about 30 to 60 minutes.

Risks and Complications

• Although radiation exposure is minimal, you receive a higher dose of radiation than during standard x-ray procedures.

• The barium may accumulate and block the intestines if it is not excreted within a few days.

After the Test

• Drink plenty of fluids to help eliminate the barium. Your doctor may also give you a mild laxative to purge your body of the contrast agent.

• Your stool will be chalky and light-colored initially, but should return to normal color after 1 to 3 days.

• Inform your doctor if you experience abdominal fullness or pain after the procedure.

• If diatrizoate was used rather than barium, you may experience transient diarrhea.

• You may resume your normal diet, medications, and activities.

Estimated Cost: $$

Ureteroscopy

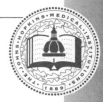

Description

• In this test, a flexible viewing tube (called a ureteroscope) is passed through the urethra and bladder and up the ureter—the tube that connects the bladder to the kidney (illustrated on page 26). Fiberoptic cables permit direct visualization of the ureter and kidney. In addition, various instruments may be passed through the scope to take tissue samples for laboratory examination or to perform therapeutic procedures, such as removal of stones in the ureter or kidney.

Purpose of the Test

• To inspect the ureter and kidney for the presence of small tumors and to remove tissue samples to confirm or rule out a diagnosis of cancer.

• Used therapeutically to remove stones in the ureter or kidney or scar tissue that is blocking the flow of urine from the kidney.

Who Performs It

• A urinary tract specialist (urologist) or another physician.

Special Concerns

• Ureteroscopy is usually performed in a hospital or outpatient facility under general or spinal anesthesia.

• This procedure should be postponed if you currently have a urinary tract infection.

Before the Test

• Drink plenty of fluids on the night before the test, but do not eat or drink anything after midnight.

• At the testing facility, you will be asked to disrobe and put on a hospital gown.

• An intravenous (IV) needle or catheter may be inserted into a vein in your arm immediately before the procedure begins, and any needed medications, such as a sedative or general anesthesia, will be administered.

• If spinal anesthesia is used, the anesthetic medication will be injected into your lower spinal column to numb the lower half of your body. You will remain conscious throughout the procedure.

• If general anesthesia is being used, a thin tube attached to a breathing machine will be inserted through your mouth and into your windpipe to help you breathe.

What You Experience

• You will lie on your back with your knees bent, legs spread apart, and feet resting in stirrups.

• The ureteroscope is gently inserted into the urethra and passed through the bladder into the ureter. It may be guided as far as the kidney, if necessary.

• The doctor visually inspects the area for abnormalities.

• If appropriate, instruments may be passed through the scope to obtain a tissue biopsy for laboratory analysis or to perform therapeutic procedures (such as removal of a stone with a

Results

▼

➥ The doctor will note any abnormalities during the visual inspection of your urinary tract. If a stone is detected in your ureter or kidney, it will be removed during the procedure.

➥ If tissue samples were taken, the specimens will be sent to a pathology laboratory and examined under a microscope for the presence of unusual cells. (For more on laboratory tests, see Chapter 1.)

➥ This test usually results in a definitive diagnosis. Your doctor will recommend an appropriate course of medical or surgical treatment, depending on the specific problem.

small basket at the end of a wire or laser obliteration of the stone into smaller particles that can then pass out of your body in urine).

• A small flexible tube called a stent may be left in the ureter for 1 to 4 weeks after the procedure to help keep the channel open and allow urine to easily drain into the bladder.

• Once the procedure is complete, the ureteroscope is slowly withdrawn.

• The procedure usually takes about 30 to 45 minutes but may take longer if large or multiple stones need to be removed from the upper ureter or kidney.

Risks and Complications

• If general anesthesia is necessary, the procedure carries the associated risks.

• Rare complications include infection, inadvertent perforation of the bladder or ureter, and formation of a stricture (narrowing) or scar tissue weeks or months after a significant perforation.

After the Test

• You will remain in a recovery room until the effects of the anesthetic subside. During this time, your vital signs will be monitored, and you will be observed for any signs of complications.

• Arrange for someone to drive you home after the procedure.

• Drink plenty of fluids (but no alcohol) to prevent accumulation of bacteria in the bladder and to reduce the slight burning sensation that may occur during urination (which may persist for 1 or 2 days).

• You may be given an antibiotic to reduce the risk of infection.

• If you have a stent, you may experience a sense of increased urgency to urinate. Your doctor may prescribe medication to minimize this problem.

• It is common to have a pink tinge to your urine for about 24 hours (or the entire time that a stent remains in place). However, if bright red blood or blood clots are present, notify your doctor.

• Call your doctor immediately if you experience pain in your back, stomach, or side, urinary difficulties, chills, or fever.

• If you have a ureteral stent, your doctor will remove it in 1 to 4 weeks using a simple procedure that does not require anesthesia.

Estimated Cost: $$$ to $$$$

Urinalysis

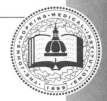

Description

• For urinalysis, an array of chemical and microscopic tests are used to examine a urine specimen. The results can aid in the diagnosis of kidney disorders, urinary tract infections, and metabolic diseases that result in the excretion of abnormal breakdown products in the urine. The following tests are commonly included:

• **Appearance, color, and odor** can provide clues to various disorders. For example, cloudy urine may be caused by the presence of pus, red blood cells, or bacteria. High levels of bilirubin (the main pigment in bile) may color the urine dark yellow, indicating possible liver disease.

• **Specific gravity** is a measure of how dilute or concentrated the urine is; abnormal levels can occur with kidney disease, dehydration, and other conditions.

Chemical analysis:

• **pH level** indicates the relative acidity or alkalinity of the urine. For example, a highly alkaline urine pH may be associated with certain bacteria that cause urinary tract infections.

• **Protein** is not normally found in the urine in large quantities. The presence of protein in the urine usually signifies that there is a structural abnormality, and may indicate a range of problems including kidney dysfunction.

• **Glucose,** when present in excessive amounts in the urine, usually indicates diabetes mellitus.

• **Ketones,** which are breakdown products of fat metabolism, may be found in the urine during starvation, after alcohol intoxication, and in people with poorly controlled diabetes.

• **Bilirubin,** a byproduct of the hemoglobin in red blood cells, indicates possible liver disease when found in the urine.

• **Nitrites** suggest a urinary tract infection, because many bacteria produce an enzyme that converts urinary nitrates to nitrites.

Microscopic examination:

• **Crystals** may appear in normal urine or in samples that have not been examined immediately, or may indicate a kidney stone or another problem. The type of crystal varies with the disease and the pH of the urine.

• **Casts**—plugs that form when a protein made in the renal tubules (see page 27) combines with cells or cellular debris—may sometimes be seen in the urine. Different types of casts (such as hyaline, granular, fatty, waxy, epithelial, red cell, and white cell casts) are linked with particular disorders.

• **White blood cells** in the urine suggest urinary tract inflammation, particularly in the kidney or bladder.

Results

▼

➥ The urine sample is frequently analyzed in your doctor's office with special chemical strips that react with substances in the urine and change color. The examiner then interprets the resulting color changes. A more detailed analysis, including microscopic examination, may also be done in-office or at a pathology laboratory. (For more on laboratory testing, see Chapter 1.)

➥ Your doctor will review the findings for evidence of kidney disease, urinary tract infection, and diabetes or another metabolic abnormality.

➥ Urinalysis is often a first step in assessing potential kidney or metabolic disorders. In many cases, additional tests may be needed to obtain a definitive diagnosis.

➥ If an abnormality is found and the doctor can make a definitive diagnosis, appropriate treatment will begin, depending on the problem.

Urinalysis

• **Red blood cells** in the urine signal bleeding within the genitourinary tract. Diseases affecting the bladder, ureters, or urethra are the most common causes.

Purpose of the Test
• To check for signs of kidney or urinary tract disease.
• To aid in the detection of metabolic or systemic diseases not related to kidney disorders.

Who Performs It
• You will usually be asked to collect the urine sample yourself.

Special Concerns
• Dietary factors, some medications, and strenuous exercise may interfere with interpretation of results.
• Recent injection with an x-ray contrast dye may alter the specific gravity, cause false-positive protein levels, and lead to crystals in the urine.

• Vaginal secretions in the urine can affect protein levels and cause false-positive results for white blood cells.

Before the Test
• Avoid strenuous exercise before the test.
• Inform your doctor about any medications you are currently taking. If a specific drug could alter the results, you may be advised to stop taking it before the test.

What You Experience
• A standard urine sample is collected in a sterile container (see page 34).

Risks and Complications
• None.

After the Test
• Resume taking any medications withheld before the test.

Estimated Cost: $

Urodynamic Testing

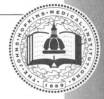

Description

• Urodynamic testing is used to evaluate lower urinary tract function in people who are experiencing problems with urination, such as incontinence, and to pinpoint the cause of the problem. Any of the following studies may be included, singly or in combination.

• **Uroflowmetry** is a simple, noninvasive test that utilizes an electronic recorder to measure the speed of urine flow (more precisely, the volume expelled from the bladder per second). If the rate is very slow, obstruction may be present along the urinary tract.

• **Cystometry** (or a cystometrogram) involves instilling fluid through a catheter into the bladder and evaluating the bladder's muscle and nerve function. Various parameters are measured, including the pressure within the bladder, the sensation of urgency that you feel when your bladder is filled, and muscle contractions by the bladder wall.

• **Urethral pressure profile,** sometimes done as part of cystometry, uses a special probe to measure the pressures along the urethra, the canal through which urine flows from the bladder out of the body, and to locate any obstruction.

• **Pressure-flow studies** measure bladder pressure and urine flow rate during urination by placing a recording device into the bladder and, in many cases, another into the rectum. A high pressure with a low urine flow indicates obstruction; low pressure with a low flow indicates a problem with the bladder itself, such as nerve or muscle dysfunction.

• **Electromyographic studies** are used to evaluate the function of the external urinary sphincter and pelvic floor muscles, which help to control the outflow of urine from the bladder. Several sensors, or electrodes, are used to measure the electrical activity of these muscles at rest, during contraction, and during urination. These tests are usually done simultaneously with cystometry and pressure-flow studies.

• **Video urodynamic studies** combine the use of real-time x-rays, or fluoroscopy (see page 205), with cystometry and pressure-flow studies. Instead of a fluid such as saline, the bladder is filled with a liquid contrast dye that appears opaque on x-rays and delineates the bladder and urethra on the images. This procedure is reserved for complex cases or when the more standard tests have not yielded satisfactory results.

Purpose of the Test

• To evaluate lower urinary tract function and determine the type and nature of urinary dysfunction in people with incontinence and other urinary problems.

Who Performs It

• A doctor, a nurse, or a lab technician.

Special Concerns

• Certain medications may alter the results of several urodynamic tests.
• Cystometry, urethral pressure profile, pressure-flow studies, and video urodynamic studies should not be done in people with an active urinary tract infection.

Results

➥ A physician will review the data from the various urodynamic studies to determine what type of urinary dysfunction is present.

➥ If a definitive diagnosis can be made, appropriate therapy will be started.

➥ Additional tests, such as cystography (see page 168) and cystoscopy (see page 170), may be needed to further evaluate any abnormal findings and establish a diagnosis.

• Movement during electromyographic studies may distort the recordings.

• Pregnant women should not undergo video urodynamic studies because exposure to ionizing radiation may harm the fetus.

Before the Test

• Report to your doctor any medications, herbs, or supplements you are taking. You may be advised to discontinue certain of these agents before the test.

• Before uroflowmetry, do not urinate for several hours and increase your intake of fluids so that you have a full bladder when the test begins.

• Before video urodynamic studies, be sure to tell your doctor if you are possibly pregnant or have a known shellfish or iodine allergy or have ever had an adverse reaction to x-ray contrast dyes.

What You Experience

Uroflowmetry:

• You will be escorted to a private room with a special uroflowmetry commode that measures the flow rate as you urinate.

• You are left alone. After pushing the start button and waiting for 5 seconds, you should begin to urinate. When you are finished, count to 5 and press the button again.

• To maximize the accuracy of results, remain still as you urinate and avoid straining.

• The test takes about 10 minutes.

Cystometry:

• Just before the procedure, you will be asked to urinate.

• You will lie down on an examining table.

• A thin, soft tube, or catheter, is carefully passed through your urethra and into the bladder, and any residual urine is measured and recorded.

• After the fluid is drained from your bladder, the catheter is connected to a device called a cystometer, which monitors bladder pressure.

• Next, saline solution or water (or in some cases carbon dioxide gas) is slowly introduced into the bladder at a controlled rate, usually while you are in a seated position. During this process, bladder pressures are recorded.

• The doctor will ask you to indicate when you first feel the urge to urinate and then when you feel urgency, indicating your bladder is full.

• You may be asked to cough or strain to determine the presence of any leakage.

• The fluid is then drained and the catheter removed if no additional tests are required.

• The test usually takes about 45 minutes.

Urethral pressure profile:

• A catheter is gently inserted through your urethra and into your bladder, and attached to a machine that monitors pressure.

• Fluids or gas are instilled through the catheter. As the catheter is withdrawn slowly, pressures along the urethral walls are measured.

• A syringe pump maintains a constant infusion of the fluids or gas.

• The catheter is removed.

• The test usually takes less than 15 minutes.

Pressure-flow studies:

• You will lie down on an examining table, with your knees bent and feet resting in stirrups.

• A catheter equipped with a special pressure sensor is gently inserted through the urethra into the bladder. A similar device may be inserted into the rectum.

• Fluid is instilled through the catheter to fill the bladder. You should report when you first feel the urge to urinate, and when the sensation becomes urgent.

• When you feel a strong urge to urinate, you will be instructed to urinate around the catheter.

• The catheter(s) are withdrawn.

• The test takes about 10 minutes.

Electromyographic studies:

• You will lie down on an examining table.

• A special paste is applied, and several electrodes are taped in place on the skin; they are typically placed in the area around the urethra in women and around the anus in men. An additional electrode that serves as a ground is usually taped to your thigh.

• Less often, the external sphincter may be evaluated using needle electrodes inserted through the skin (this causes only mild discomfort) or an anal plug electrode.

• A catheter is gently inserted through your urethra and into your bladder.

• Electrical activity is recorded while you are relaxed and your bladder is empty.

• For additional measurements, you may be asked to cough; the examiner may gently tug on the catheter; and you may be asked to contract and relax the sphincter muscles so that voluntary activity can be assessed.

• Next, your bladder is filled with room-temperature water, the catheter is removed, and you will be asked to urinate.

• The electrodes are then removed, and the affected area is cleaned and dried.

• The test usually takes 30 to 60 minutes.

Video urodynamic studies:

• The test is usually performed while you are seated or standing.

• Cystometry is conducted as described above, with the only difference being that a radiographic contrast agent serves as the filling medium and fluoroscopy is used to produce an image of the lower urinary tract.

• The pressure and volume measurements recorded in cystometry are displayed simultaneously with fluoroscopic images of the lower urinary tract on a TV monitor. The data can also be stored on videotape for later review.

• To reduce radiation exposure, the total amount of fluoroscopic screening time is less than 20 seconds.

• The procedure takes about 20 to 40 minutes.

Risks and Complications
Uroflowmetry:
• There are no risks associated with this test.

Cystometry, urethral pressure profile, pressure-flow studies, electromyographic studies:
• Temporary mild irritation of the urethra is common. Other possible risks include infection.

Video urodynamic studies:

• Temporary, mild irritation of the urethra is common after this test. Other possible risks include infection.

• The test involves minimal radiation exposure.

• Rarely, some people may experience an allergic reaction to the iodine-based contrast dye, which can cause symptoms such as nausea, sneezing, vomiting, hives, and occasionally a life-threatening response called anaphylactic shock. Emergency medications and equipment are kept readily available.

After the Test
All tests:
• Resume your normal diet and any medications that were withheld before the test, according to your doctor's instructions.

Uroflowmetry:
• You may return home immediately.

Cystometry, urethral pressure profile, pressure-flow studies, electromyographic studies, video urodynamic studies:
• To relieve any post-test discomfort, your doctor may recommend a therapeutic bath in which you sit with your hips and buttocks immersed in warm, sometimes medicated water (sitz bath).

• Drink plenty of fluids to relieve any burning on urination that may occur after the test.

• In some cases, prophylactic antibiotics may be prescribed to prevent infection. Tell your doctor if you experience any symptoms of infection, such as fever and chills.

• If needle electrodes were used for electromyographic studies, blood may collect and clot under the skin (hematoma) at the needle insertion sites; this is harmless and will resolve on its own. For a large hematoma that causes swelling and discomfort, apply ice initially; after 24 hours, use warm, moist compresses to help dissolve the clotted blood.

Estimated Cost: $$ to $$$

Urodynamic Testing continued

Venography

Description

• In this test, a contrast dye is injected through a thin, flexible tube (catheter) into a particular vein or group of veins and a series of x-rays is obtained. Filled with the dye, the veins are differentiated from other bodily structures on the x-ray images. Venography is most commonly used to evaluate veins in the kidneys, lower extremities, and adrenal glands, as well as the portal vein in the liver. (For more on contrast x-rays, see Chapter 2.)

Purpose of the Test

Lower extremity venography:
• To identify and locate blood clots in the deep veins of the legs (deep vein thrombosis).
• To distinguish between a blood clot and an obstruction caused by a large pelvic tumor encroaching on the venous system.
• To assess congenital venous malformations.
• To evaluate the competence of valves in the leg veins (which can aid in identifying the causes of leg swelling).

Renal venography:
• To detect and evaluate blood clots, tumors, or abnormalities in the renal veins of the kidney.
• To collect blood samples from the renal vein to evaluate renovascular hypertension (increased blood pressure due to narrowing of the artery that leads to the kidney).

Adrenal venography:
• To obtain blood samples from the adrenal gland veins to aid in the detection of diseases such as Cushing's syndrome (marked by increased secretion of the hormone cortisol) and pheochromocytoma (a tumor marked by increased secretion of the hormones epinephrine or norepinephrine).

Portal venography:
• To diagnose and assess portal hypertension (high pressure in the portal vein, which empties into the liver).
• To detect and locate a suspected blood clot in the portal or splenic vein.
• To assess the progression of cirrhosis of the liver.
• To assess the patency of shunts that were constructed to treat portal hypertension (portal-systemic shunts).

Who Performs It

• A radiologist or another physician.

Special Concerns

• Pregnant women should not undergo this test because exposure to ionizing radiation may harm the fetus.
• People with allergies to iodine or shellfish may experience an allergic reaction to iodine-based contrast dyes.
• In people with kidney disorders or chronic dehydration, the contrast dye can worsen kidney function and may cause renal failure. To determine whether the dye can be administered safely, your doctor may perform a blood test to assess your kidney function (see page 311) before the test.
• This procedure may not be safe for people who have bleeding disorders. Coagulation studies (see page 157) may be performed

Results

▼

➡ A physician will examine the recorded images and other test data for evidence of venous abnormalities.

➡ This test usually establishes a definitive diagnosis. Based on the findings, your doctor will recommend an appropriate course of medical or surgical treatment.

prior to the test to ensure that your blood will clot normally.

• The presence of feces, gas, or residual barium in the abdomen from recent contrast x-rays may make it difficult to obtain clear pictures of abdominal veins.

Before the Test

• You may be asked to observe certain dietary restrictions for variable periods before the test, depending on the specific procedure.

• Report to your doctor any medications, herbs, or supplements you are taking. You may be advised to discontinue certain of these agents before the test.

• Inform your doctor if you have a known shellfish or iodine allergy or have ever had an adverse reaction to x-ray contrast dyes. You may be given preventive medication to reduce the risk of an allergic reaction, or a noniodinated dye may be used.

• An intravenous (IV) line is inserted into a vein in your arm so that any necessary medications can be administered during the procedure.

• Empty your bladder before the procedure.

• You will be given a sedative to help you relax during the examination.

What You Experience
Lower extremity venography (ascending):

• You are positioned lying down on a tilting x-ray table. The table is inclined so that your feet are elevated.

• The skin on the top of your foot is cleansed with an antiseptic, and a local anesthetic is injected. A tourniquet may be tied around the ankle to make the foot veins fill with blood.

• A catheter is inserted into a selected foot vein, and contrast dye is infused into the vein.

• The movement of the dye up the leg is followed using continuous x-ray imaging, or fluoroscopy (see page 205). Spot x-ray films are also obtained as the dye circulates through different regions of the leg.

• The catheter is withdrawn, and a bandage is applied to the insertion site.

• The procedure may take 30 to 45 minutes.

Lower extremity venography (descending):

• You are positioned lying down on a tilting x-ray table.

• The skin over a vein in your arm or neck is cleansed with an antiseptic solution, and a local anesthetic is injected.

• A catheter is inserted into the selected vein. Under the guidance of fluoroscopic imaging, it is carefully guided to a selected pelvic or leg vein.

• Contrast dye is injected through the catheter and the table is inclined so that your feet are lowered.

• The movement of the dye down the leg is followed using continuous x-ray imaging, or fluoroscopy. Spot x-ray films are also obtained to document any "leaking" valves in the veins of the legs.

• The catheter is withdrawn, and a bandage is applied to the insertion site.

• The procedure may take 30 to 45 minutes.

Renal and adrenal venography:

• You will lie on your back on an x-ray table.

• The skin over the catheter insertion site—usually the femoral vein in the groin—is cleansed with an antiseptic solution and (if necessary) shaved. A local anesthetic is injected to numb the area.

• A catheter is inserted into the femoral vein. Under the guidance of fluoroscopic imaging, it is carefully guided to either the renal or adrenal veins in the abdomen.

• A contrast dye is injected through the catheter. This may cause a transient burning or flushing sensation.

• As the contrast agent flows through the selected veins, a series of x-ray films is obtained.

• If applicable, blood samples are then obtained and sent to a laboratory for analysis.

• The catheter is withdrawn, and a bandage is applied to the insertion site.

• The procedure takes about 1 hour.

Portal venography:

• You will lie on your back on an x-ray table.

• The skin over the catheter insertion site—usually the femoral artery in the groin—is

Venography continued

cleansed with an antiseptic solution and (if necessary) shaved. A local anesthetic is injected to numb the area.

• A catheter is inserted into the femoral artery. Under the guidance of fluoroscopic imaging, it is carefully guided to a selected abdominal artery.

• A contrast dye is injected through the catheter. This may cause a transient burning or flushing sensation.

• Fluoroscopy is used to follow the flow of the dye from the selected artery into draining veins and then into the portal vein near the liver.

• The catheter is withdrawn, and a bandage is applied to the insertion site.

• The procedure takes about 1 hour.

Risks and Complications

• Possible risks include blood clot formation, bleeding, blood vessel damage, or infection at the site of catheter insertion.

• Some people may experience an allergic reaction to the iodine-based contrast dye, which can cause symptoms such as nausea, sneezing, vomiting, hives, and occasionally a life-threatening response called anaphylactic shock. Emergency medications and equipment are kept readily available.

• Renal failure may occur as a result of exposure to the contrast dye, especially in elderly patients with chronic dehydration or mild renal impairment.

• Cellulitis, or inflammation of connective tissue, and pain may occur if the contrast dye infiltrates into the tissues under the skin.

After the Test

• Your vital signs will be monitored until they are stable. Depending on the procedure, you may be advised to rest in bed for a certain period of time.

• Cold compresses can help to relieve any swelling or discomfort at the puncture site.

• You are encouraged to drink clear fluids to avoid dehydration and to help flush the contrast dye out of your system.

• You may resume your normal diet and any medications discontinued before the test, according to your doctor's instructions.

• If bleeding or any other complications develop, call your doctor or emergency medical service immediately.

Estimated Cost: $$ to $$$

Venous Doppler Studies

(Venous Duplex Ultrasound)

Description

• Venous Doppler studies use a technique called Doppler ultrasound to evaluate blood circulation in the veins of the arms or legs. A device called a transducer is passed lightly across different areas of your limbs, directing high-frequency sound waves (ultrasound) at superficial and deep veins. The sound waves are reflected back at frequencies that correspond to the velocity of blood flow, and are converted into audible sounds and graphic recordings.

• **Duplex scanning** combines Doppler ultrasound with real-time ultrasound imaging of the veins. Images are displayed on a viewing monitor and may also be recorded on film or video for later examination. (For more on Doppler and duplex ultrasound, see Chapter 2.)

Purpose of the Test

• To evaluate venous blood flow in the arms and legs in people with symptoms such as leg pain and swelling, swollen arms and legs, or varicose veins in the arms or legs.

• To aid in the diagnosis of venous abnormalities such as a suspected blood clot in a deep vein of the leg (deep vein thrombosis); narrowing or closure (occlusion) of a vein; or impaired blood flow (venous insufficiency).

Who Performs It

• A qualified vascular laboratory technician.

Special Concerns

• This test is often unable to detect blood clots in a calf vein. Venous plethysmography (see page 296) and venography (see page 382) are more accurate for this purpose.

Before the Test

• You will be asked to remove any clothes covering the area to be examined and put on a hospital gown.

What You Experience

• You will lie on either a bed or a table.

• A small amount of water-soluble gel is applied to the skin on the areas being examined to enhance sound wave transmission.

• The examiner then moves the transducer back and forth over the selected limb to record blood flow and obtain different views of the vein or veins being studied. You will be instructed to breathe normally as this is done.

• Once clear images are obtained, they are recorded on film or video for later analysis.

• Additional images will be obtained after the examiner applies brief pressure to compress and release certain veins, and as you perform certain breathing exercises to vary blood flow through the veins.

• The test usually takes 20 to 30 minutes.

Risks and Complications

• Ultrasound is painless, noninvasive, and involves no exposure to radiation. There are no associated risks.

After the Test

• The examiner removes the conductive gel from your skin.

• You may resume your normal activities.

Estimated Cost: $$

Results
▼

➥ A physician reviews the images and other test data for evidence of any abnormality.

➥ If a definitive diagnosis can be made, appropriate treatment will be initiated.

➥ In some cases, additional tests, such as venography, are required to further evaluate abnormal findings.

Venous Doppler Studies

Video Stroboscopy

Video Stroboscopy *(side tab)*

Description

• This test combines videotaping with a technique called stroboscopy to evaluate the function of the vocal cords, or larynx, in people with voice disorders. During speech, the vocal folds in the larynx vibrate too rapidly to permit examination with a normal light source. Stroboscopy overcomes this obstacle by using a strobe light to illuminate the larynx: The strobe emits light pulses at a rate slightly slower than the vibration frequency of the vocal folds, causing the folds to appear to move in slow motion. An examiner may then observe the movement and function of your larynx as you make particular sounds. This is done with either a flexible viewing tube (endoscope) passed through the nose or a rigid endoscope passed through the mouth. The scope contains an optical system and a tiny camera to record the exam on videotape for later review.

Purpose of the Test

• To identify the cause of hoarseness or voice dysfunction.
• To detect or evaluate vocal cord lesions and other abnormalities such as scar tissue, inflammation, or muscle tension disorders.

Who Performs It

• An ear, nose, and throat physician (otolaryngologist) or a speech pathologist.

Special Concerns

• None.

Before the Test

• No special preparation is necessary.

What You Experience

• You will be asked to sit upright, leaning a little bit forward from your hips.
• A topical anesthetic may be sprayed on your throat and, if necessary, in your nose to make the procedure more comfortable and suppress the gag reflex. (You may still cough or gag if the endoscope touches the back of your throat or tongue.)
• The examiner guides a flexible scope through one nostril into the throat, or holds your tongue gently with a piece of gauze and passes a rigid scope into your mouth.
• You will be instructed to perform particular vocal tasks, such as pronouncing vowels or singing, while the examiner uses the stroboscope to visualize your vocal cords. This examination is recorded on videotape.
• The procedure takes about 15 minutes.

Risks and Complications

• The procedure has no associated risks.

After the Test

• You may resume your normal activities.

Estimated Cost: $$$

Results

▼

➡ After the procedure, the doctor will review the videotape with you, explain the findings, and discuss potential treatment options.

Vision Tests

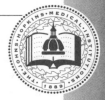

Description

• The following basic vision tests help to assess how well your eyes are functioning and to detect potential vision disorders. They are ordinarily included as part of a full eye examination. Techniques vary depending on whether you are a new or returning patient to the eye practitioner.

• **Visual acuity tests** help to evaluate your ability to distinguish the form and detail of an object or printed figure. This is usually done with Snellen charts, which are composed of standardized rows of different-sized letters. You are asked to read the letters on a chart from a distance of 20 feet. The smaller the letters you can identify, the better your visual acuity. The score 20/20 means you have normal vision at 20 feet.

• **The pinhole test** helps to determine whether reduced visual acuity is due to a refractive error (an inability of the cornea and lens of the eye to bend light rays into proper focus on the retina) or to an organic vision disorder. You look through a pinhole (in the center of a disk) at the Snellen chart. If visual impairment is due to a refractive error, your vision will improve when looking through the pinhole, which eliminates irregular light rays.

• **The Amsler grid**—a grid with a black dot at its center printed on a piece of paper—is an extremely sensitive test to detect blind spots, distortion, and other problems in central vision. You are asked to focus your eyes on the dot and note any blurring, distortion, or missing lines on the grid. This test helps to detect problems affecting the macula—the most sensitive area of the retina responsible for central vision and seeing fine detail.

• **Color vision tests** use plates made up of dot patterns in the primary colors superimposed on backgrounds of randomly mixed colors to assess the ability to recognize color differences. People with normal color vision are able to identify the number shown by the dot pattern. If color vision is defective, you will be unable to distinguish between the dot pattern and the background. Impaired color vision results from dysfunction of specialized cells, called cones, in the retina and disorders of the optic nerve.

Purpose of the Test

• Performed as part of a regular eye examination for glasses and routine screening for vision disorders such as cataracts, glaucoma, or eye changes associated with diabetes.

• To assess the eyes of people who report vision problems.

• To evaluate people with neurologic (nerve) disorders or other systemic conditions that may affect the eyes.

Who Performs It

• An ophthalmologist, an optometrist, a nurse, or an ophthalmic technician.

Special Concerns

• None.

Results

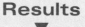

➡ An ophthalmologist or optometrist reviews the test data for evidence of any visual defect, and considers these findings along with your eye exam and any symptoms you report.

➡ In cases of simple vision dysfunction, such as myopia (nearsightedness), these tests will be sufficient to prescribe glasses or contact lenses.

➡ If a more serious vision disorder is suspected, an in-depth eye examination and more specialized tests will be necessary to establish a diagnosis.

Before the Test

• If you normally wear eyeglasses or contact lenses, wear them to the exam.

What You Experience

Visual acuity tests:

• You will sit in a chair 20 feet from an illuminated eye chart (letters may also be projected on a reflecting screen or displayed on a TV monitor).

• You are first tested while wearing your most recently prescribed glasses or contact lenses. You will be asked to read all the letters or numbers in each progressively smaller line until you cannot discern the figures. Each eye is tested separately (while the other eye is covered).

• If visual acuity is less than 20/20, the examiner will try different lenses to learn if a change of your glasses or contact lens prescription will improve visual acuity (a process known as "refraction"). The pinhole test (see below) is often used at the beginning of refraction as a quick test.

Pinhole test:

• For this test, you will usually wear your glasses or contact lenses.

• You will be asked to cover one eye. With the other eye, you will look at the eye chart through a pinhole in the center of a disk.

• Read aloud the smallest line of letters you can see on the chart.

• The procedure is repeated for the other eye.

Amsler grid:

• You will wear your regular, bifocal, or reading glasses or contact lenses for this test.

• You will be instructed to cover one eye, and the Amsler grid is held in front of the uncovered eye.

• You are asked to look directly at the black dot at the center of the grid.

• Report any irregularities that you see on the grid, such as wavy or blurred lines, blank spots, gray areas, or other distortions in the grid pattern. You may be asked to outline (with a pencil) any areas on the grid that appear distorted.

• The procedure is repeated for the other eye.

Color vision test:

• You will wear your glasses or contact lenses for this test.

• Each eye is tested separately.

• You will be given a test book containing color plates, and asked to read aloud the number or numbers shown in each color plate.

• The number of accurate responses is recorded.

Risks and Complications

• None.

After the Test

• You may resume your normal activities.

Estimated Cost: $

Visual Field Testing
(Perimetry)

Description
• Visual field testing defines the severity and shape of defects in both central and peripheral vision. Various techniques may be used, ranging from simple tests to more complicated ones that require special instruments.

• **Confrontation (or kinetic perimetry)** brings a test object from a nonseeing area (such as behind the head) into the field of vision. You will be asked to focus your eyes on a central point—such as the examiner's nose, the center of a dark screen (known as a "tangent screen"), or the center of a 2-foot bowl-shaped instrument called a perimeter—and to tell the examiner when you first see the object enter your visual field. Depending on the technique, different test objects are used (for example, the examiner's fingers, a pencil, or different-sized spots projected on the perimeter).

• **Static perimetry** uses a different type of bowl-shaped perimeter in which computer-driven programs cause spots of light to appear at multiple points. You are asked to press a button when you see a light.

• **Color testing** assesses your ability to recognize the color of test objects, red being especially important for identifying neurologic (nerve) disorders. The techniques of kinetic perimetry are employed, but with colored objects or lights.

Purpose of the Test
• To detect patterns of vision loss that indicate specific disorders, including diseases of the retina and optic nerve, glaucoma, brain tumors, and stroke.

• To monitor the course of visual field loss over time and the effectiveness of treatment for disorders such as glaucoma, optic neuritis (inflammation of the optic nerve), and brain tumors.

Who Performs It
• An ophthalmologist or a trained technician.

Special Concerns
• The simpler visual field tests (such as confrontation testing using the examiner's fingers as test objects) are used for people with decreased mental function due to a stroke, head injury, brain tumor, or infection. More complicated techniques (such as static perimetry) require a high level of alertness and sustained attention.

Before the Test
• No special preparation is needed.

What You Experience
• One eye is first covered with a patch.
• You are instructed to indicate when you see a test object in your visual field. The exact procedure varies depending on which technique is performed.
• The test is repeated in the other eye.
• The procedure takes about 30 minutes.

Risks and Complications
• None.

After the Test
• You may resume your normal activities.

Estimated Cost: $·

Results
▼

➡ An ophthalmologist reviews the data for evidence of a visual field defect. Certain diseases produce characteristic patterns of visual loss.

➡ The doctor considers these findings along with your symptoms, your eye exam, and the results of other tests to decide on the need for further testing, such as a brain CT scan (see page 121) or MRI (see page 119), or treatment.

Visual Field Testing

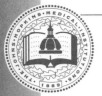

Wet Prep
(Wet Mount, Vaginitis Test)

Wet Prep

Description
• A sample of vaginal discharge is obtained with a cotton swab or wooden spatula and spread on glass slides, which are examined under a microscope. This test is typically done to identify suspected vaginal infections (vaginitis) in women who are experiencing symptoms such as vaginal itching, pain, odor, or abnormal discharge.

Purpose of the Test
• To identify viral, fungal, and parasitic infections of the vagina.

Who Performs It
• A gynecologist or a nurse practitioner.

Special Concerns
• None.

Before the Test
• Do not douche for 24 hours before the test.
• You will be asked to disrobe from the waist down and put on a drape or hospital gown.

What You Experience
• You will lie on an examining table, with your knees bent and feet resting in stirrups.
• A small metal or plastic instrument, called a speculum, is inserted into your vagina to hold the vaginal walls slightly open. (This may cause slight discomfort, but is not painful.) Relax and breathe deeply through your mouth to ease insertion.
• The examiner inserts a sterile, moist cotton swab or wooden spatula into the vagina to collect a sample of vaginal secretions; the sample is spread on glass slides, which are examined under a microscope.
• The speculum is withdrawn.
• The test usually takes about 2 to 3 minutes.

Risks and Complications
• There are no risks or complications.

After the Test
• You may dress and return to your normal activities.

Estimated Cost: $

Results

▼

➡ A physician will examine the slides under a microscope for the presence of unusual cells. (For more on microscopic examination, see Chapter 1.) Possible causes of vaginitis include yeast infection (caused by a fungus called *Candida albicans*), a parasitic infection called trichomoniasis, and bacterial infection.

➡ If a definitive diagnosis can be made, appropriate treatment will be initiated. In some cases, such as the parasitic infection trichomoniasis, your sexual partner should be treated as well.

Whitaker Test

Description

• In this test, a contrast dye is injected directly into one of your kidneys, and a series of x-ray films is taken as the material flows through the kidney and ureter (illustrated on page 26). The dye delineates these structures on the x-ray images and reveals any abnormalities. Pressures are also measured in the kidneys and bladder. Correlation of the pressure measurements with the x-ray findings can provide information about the flow of urine through the kidney and the presence of any obstructions. (For more on contrast x-rays, see Chapter 2.)

Purpose of the Test

• To identify and evaluate kidney obstructions, such as narrowing or stones.
• To help determine whether surgery is needed to remove a kidney obstruction.

Who Performs It

• A physician.

Special Concerns

• People who have an allergy to shellfish or iodine may experience an allergic reaction to the contrast dye.
• Pregnant women should not undergo this test because exposure to ionizing radiation may harm the fetus.
• This test may not be safe for people who have a bleeding disorder or a severe infection.
• The presence of feces, gas, or residual barium in the abdomen from recent contrast x-rays may hinder accurate needle placement and interfere with visualization of the upper urinary tract.

Before the Test

• Tell your doctor if you regularly take anticoagulant drugs. You may be instructed to discontinue them for some time before the test.

• Be sure to tell your doctor if you have a known shellfish or iodine allergy or have ever had an adverse reaction to x-ray contrast dyes.
• Do not eat or drink anything for at least 4 hours before the test.
• You will be asked to disrobe and put on a hospital gown.
• You may be given a mild sedative.
• You may be asked to empty your bladder just before the procedure.

What You Experience

• You will lie on your back on an examination table.
• A thin tube, or catheter, equipped with a special pressure sensor is gently inserted through the urethra into the bladder.
• The doctor takes a plain x-ray film of the urinary tract to locate the position of the kidney and ureter.
• A contrast dye is administered through an intravenous (IV) catheter inserted into a vein in your arm. (Upon injection of the dye, you may experience a brief flushing sensation and a metallic taste in your mouth.)
• When x-rays show that the contrast dye has entered the kidney, the skin over the kidney is cleansed with an antiseptic solution and draped. A local anesthetic is then injected to numb the area.
• You will be asked to hold your breath as the

Results
▼

➡ The doctor will examine the x-rays and pressure measurements to determine whether a kidney obstruction is present.
➡ A definitive diagnosis can usually be made after this test. Appropriate treatment will be initiated, depending on the specific problem.

doctor inserts a hollow needle into your kidney, using fluoroscopy or ultrasound imaging (see Chapter 2) as a guide. A pressure sensor is connected to this needle.

• Contrast dye is infused through the needle into your kidney, and serial x-ray films are obtained to visualize the kidney and ureter. You should remain still as each x-ray is taken.

• Pressures within the kidney and bladder are measured.

• The needle and catheter are then removed, and a small bandage is applied over the needle insertion site.

• The test takes about 60 to 90 minutes.

Risks and Complications
• X-rays involve minimal exposure to radiation.
• Possible complications include bleeding at the site of needle insertion.
• Some people may experience an allergic reaction to the iodine-based contrast dye, which can cause symptoms such as nausea, sneezing, vomiting, hives, and occasionally a life-threatening response called anaphylactic shock. Emergency medications and equipment are kept readily available.

After the Test
• A pressure dressing is applied to the site of needle insertion.

• You will rest in a recovery room for 15 to 30 minutes. Your vital signs will be monitored, and pain medication will be provided if necessary.

• If no complications develop, you are usually free to leave the testing facility. You will be advised to remain on your back for 12 hours after the test.

• You will be instructed to keep track of your urine output and report any urinary retention (inability to urinate due to swelling). At first, the urine may contain blood, causing a slight pink tinge; this should resolve after voiding a few times. If blood persists or you see bright red blood or blood clots, notify your physician.

• You may resume your normal diet and any medications withheld before the test.

• Delayed allergic reactions to the contrast dye, such as hives, rash, or itching, may appear 2 to 6 hours after the procedure. If this occurs, your doctor will prescribe antihistamines or steroids to ease your discomfort.

• You may be given prophylactic antibiotic drugs for several days to prevent infection.

• Report to your doctor any signs of infection, such as chills, fever, rapid breathing, or a feeling of faintness.

Estimated Cost: $$ to $$$

INDEX

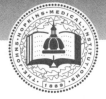

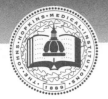

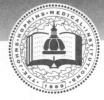

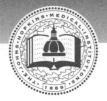

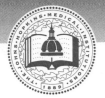

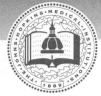

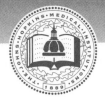